While great care has been taken to check drug dosages in this book, errors may have been overlooked. Furthermore, dosage schedules are continually revised, indications updated, and new side-effects documented. The reader is strongly urged to consult the current information provided by the licensing authority or the drug manufacturer before administering any unfamiliar drugs mentioned in this book.

Biological Treatments in Psychiatry

15—

Biological Treatments in Psychiatry

MALCOLM LADER

Professor of Clinical Psychopharmacology, University of London

and

REGINALD HERRINGTON

Senior Lecturer in Psychological Medicine, University of Glasgow

Oxford New York Tokyo

OXFORD UNIVERSITY PRESS

1990

Oxford University Press, Walton Street, Oxford OX2 6DP
Oxford New York Toronto
Delhi Bombay Calcutta Madras Karachi
Petaling Jaya Singapore Hong Kong Tokyo
Nairobi Dar es Salaam Cape Town
Melbourne Auckland

and associated companies in
Berlin Ibadan

Oxford is a trade mark of Oxford University Press

Published in the United States
by Oxford University Press, New York

British Library Cataloguing in Publication Data
Lader, M. H. (Malcolm Harold)
Biological treatments in psychiatry.
1. Man. Mental disorders. Drug therapy
I. Title II. Herrington, Reginald
616.8918
ISBN 0–19–261644–7
ISBN 0–19–261939–X pbk

Library of Congress Cataloging in Publication Data
Lader, Malcolm Harold.
Biological treatments in psychiatry/Malcolm Lader, Reginald Herrington.
(Oxford medical publications)
Includes bibliographical references.
1. Mental illness–Chemotherapy. 2. Psychopharmacology.
3. Electroconvulsive therapy. 4. Brain–Surgery. I. Herrington, Reginald N. II. Title.
III. Series. [DNLM: 1. Behavior–drug effects. 2. Electroconvulsive Therapy.
3. Mental disorders–drug therapy. 4. Psychotropic Drugs–therapeutic use.
5. Psychosurgery. WM 402 L15b]
RC483.L24 1990 616.89'1–dc20 90–6747
ISBN 0–19–261644–7 ISBN 0–19–261939–X (pbk.)

Set by B.P. Integraphics, Bath, Avon

Printed in Great Britain by
Courier International Ltd,
Tiptree, Colchester, Essex

Preface

It is a daunting task to attempt to provide the practising psychiatrist with information about physical therapies in his specialty and with guidelines about how to use them. However, this area of therapeutics has grown apace in the last 30 years with respect to both the number and complexity of the therapies, mainly drugs, available. The former largely represents the intense activity of the pharmaceutical industry in devising and marketing new therapies. The latter reflects the great strides in our knowledge of the workings of the brain in terms of its physiology and biochemistry.

Nevertheless, great gaps confront us in our understanding of the mechanisms of action of most of our current physical therapies and even more so in our comprehension of the pathogenesis of the whole range of psychiatric disorders. Even the indisputably organic conditions such as Huntington's chorea are only now being elucidated. The inevitable upshot of our ignorance is that our treatments must be evaluated empirically rather than rationally and this limitation was very much before us as we wrote this book.

We have tried to keep a balance between the uncritical claims of those enthusiasts who see physical treatments as the answer to most psychiatric problems and the therapeutic nihilism of the sceptics who see no solutions anywhere. We have sought throughout to apply well-accepted therapeutic principles from other more developed branches of pharmacology and medicine without setting up the rigid double-blind controlled trial as the only arbiter. To that end, we have devoted some chapters to clinical problems, clinical trials, and social aspects of prescribing in order to set therapeutic topics in context and to outline systematic ways of tackling practical problems.

Although aware of the serendipitous discovery and empirical use of almost all physical treatments in psychiatry, we believe that developments in neuropharmacology will eventually lead to much better treatments. Chapters are accordingly devoted to basic neuropharmacology, to behavioural studies, and to a resumé of biological aspects of psychiatry. Pharmacokinetic principles, a complex but none the less essential discipline for the proper use of drugs, are outlined.

The bulk of the book comprises chapters devoted to the many types of psychotropic drugs, classified according to main indication. We have dealt with anticonvulsants and mentioned a wide range of therapies as well as the classical antidepressants, antipsychotics, lithium, and sedative/hypnotics. Two chapters are devoted to special areas—the young and the elderly. Non-drug treatments include ECT and psychosurgery.

The book is written primarily for the psychiatrist-in-training but we hope the qualified psychiatrist will also find it useful. Others who may find it helpful include clinical psychologists, general practitioners, general physicians and other specialists, particularly neurologists. Although our approach mainly reflects that in the UK, we have culled the world literature for major studies and hope that overseas readers will find it relevant to their needs.

We would like to thank all those with whom we have discussed various points, especially our colleagues and our students from whom we have learnt so much. We are grateful to the various secretaries who over the years have typed successive drafts. We also thank the various staff of Oxford University Press, for their exceptional patience and unfailing help and courtesy. Finally, we should like to acknowledge our debt to our families who have lived with this book for so long and uncomplainingly gave us the time to bring it to completion.

London and Glasgow M.L.
September 1989 R.H.

Contents

1. Introduction

Psychopharmacology is both an old and a new subject. Old, because mankind has resorted to mind-altering drugs for the whole of recorded history and probably for thousands of years before that. New, because the study of mind-altering drugs using modern scientific methods essentially dates from around 1950, culminating in the discovery of the modern drugs used in psychiatry. Only the technological revolution separates neolithic man finding out that fermented wild grapes intoxicated him from the synthesizer of and experimenter with LSD, Hoffmann. The unknown Stone Age man who first discovered the analgesic and psychotropic effect of the opium poppy ranks with the chemists, pharmacologists, and clinicians who developed chlorpromazine, imipramine, lithium, and the benzodiazepines and discovered their therapeutic effects.

The introduction of drugs to treat psychiatric conditions was facilitated by the prior discovery and popularization of physical treatments. To understand the impact made by these new approaches it is necessary to review the historical antecedents. After the inhumane treatment of the insane in the seventeenth and eighteenth centuries, the Age of Enlightenment influenced men like Pinel and Tuke to strike off the manacles of their prisoner-patients. The wave of liberal concern for society's unfortunates in the second quarter of the nineteenth century, together with the increasing affluence of Victorian society, led to the construction of numerous lunatic asylums. These buildings, mostly designed to a recognizably common plan, are still visible outside our major towns and cities. Wherever possible they were sited on a hill, not as commonly supposed to isolate the patients from the community, but because such a situation was believed to protect against the epidemics, especially of tuberculosis, that ravaged all institutions in the nineteenth Century.

This isolation, however, took its professional toll not only of the patients, but also of the doctors and nurses, who had little contact with the outside world. Associations of lunatic asylum doctors were set up to lessen this professional neglect, but these doctors ruled as autocrats in their own little fiefs. The institutions dealt with insane people, committal being necessary for admission in most instances. Lesser degrees of mental illnesses, particularly the neuroses, were dealt with by family doctors or by neurologists. The institutions were unable to attract many able doctors, and the patients, nurses, and doctors all stagnated. Even so, some patients did recover and were discharged, but for most admission to the local asylum was a life sentence.

The establishment of medicine as a science-based technology which started in the late nineteenth century did not extend much to psychiatry, although the vitamin deficiency diseases such as pellagra became understood. The introduction of malarial therapy in the 1920s was the first physical treatment to show that mental illness, or at least some forms of it, was susceptible to the same sort of approach that was slowly proving successful in other branches of medicine. Although general paralysis of the insane is now a rarity, it was quite common in mental hospitals during the first quarter of this century.

The 1930s saw the introduction of three forms of physical therapy, two of which are extant. The casualty has been insulin coma therapy which became widely used for a while in the treatment of schizophrenia. Major resources were allocated to setting up special intensive therapy units which claimed good or even excellent results. Eventually, when a few sceptics got round to controlled evaluations it became apparent that any therapeutic effects were non-specific: they reflected skill in selecting patients of good prognosis and the general mood of optimism engendered by active treatment units in the midst of institutions otherwise providing little than custodial care. But the hope and optimism engendered by even insulin coma therapy added to the feeling that things were moving favourably in the area of mental illness.

Sometimes this optimism became not only infectious, but uncritically excessive. Prefrontal leucotomy, introduced slowly and cautiously, found its aficionados who simplified it and used it widely in patients with schizophrenia, anxiety and depression. So crude was the technique and so widespread its use that psychosurgery became discredited. Unfortunately, other forms of physical treatment including drug therapy, became tarred with the same brush and provided weapons with which antipsychiatry groups belaboured the psychiatric profession. Electroconvulsive therapy, the third of these therapies, proved very useful in severely depressed patients, but again, its too widespread and uncritical use has discredited it to the point where some countries or states within countries trammel its use even in severely depressed patients.

Another change in professional and public opinion was the realization that large institutions were not ideal places for the custody, let alone the therapy of the mentally ill. Indeed, evidence accrued that these institutions generated problems of their own, patients becoming 'institutionalized' with secondary handicaps and deficits. Efforts were made to rehabilitate the chronically ill patients who crowded the back wards of mental hospitals. Their numbers had swelled, not because of any increase in the incidence or change in nature of mental illness, but because improvements in hygiene and therapy were prolonging the lives of the inmates. Pious sentiments were expressed that the goal of therapy was rehabilitation back into the community and that the policy would be so successful that the mental hospitals could be emptied and closed down. That they still exist, albeit with reduced numbers of patients, is evidence of the uncritical futility of this approach. Furthermore, many of those discharged into the community are functioning poorly and are becoming 're-institutionalized' in the bedrooms of seaside boarding houses or are sleeping rough in the big cities.

Nevertheless, the move to transfer patients into the care of the community, compounded with the great promise of the new drugs introduced in the 1950s, led some to hail the imminence of the psychiatric millennium. With hindsight this was premature, but at the time great enthusiasm was generated by the new drugs and their use was vigorous. More sober appraisals suggested that the new drugs were only partially successful, and it is obvious that much remains to be known about the optimal practical use of these drugs.

Even larger lacunae exist in our understanding of the mechanism of action of these drugs. Because of their therapeutic effects, it is held firmly that elucidation of the modes of action would throw much light on the biological mechanisms presumed to be associated with mental illness. This hope is still being espoused, and as more is learned about basic neuropharmacological and neurochemical mechanisms, the older theories concerning drug action are being revised and updated.

One point cannot be stressed enough and relates to the scientific basis of these drugs' actions. The major discoveries were, by and large, made by lucky accident. The pharmacology followed. Thus, both psychopharmacology and our understanding of the scientific basis of physical treatments in psychiatry has developed empirically, not by rational deduction from scientific principles. The drugs were established as useful and even indispensable therapeutic advances, before enough was known about basic neuronal mechanisms to begin guessing at the mechanisms of action. Potentially new compounds are still screened on a battery of tests devised *post hoc* as providing characteristic profiles for the major groups of psychotropic drugs. Recently, the addition of receptor binding techniques to the behavioural pharmacological methods has simplified screening procedures, but in no way rationalized them. Drugs are still being discovered, either by the laborious process of synthesizing new organic chemicals and screening them routinely, or entirely by accident. No new therapies have been introduced successfully based on rational development from our knowledge of biochemistry.

2. Principles of Treatment

Psychiatric diagnosis

The management of any problem logically depends on the analysis of its nature and causes and on its likely development if left to itself. In clinical practice, diagnosis and prognosis precede treatment and 'of these diagnosis is by far the most important, for upon it the success of the other two depends' (Ryle 1948). Diagnosis contains two processes: first, the development of a system of classification of diseases or disorders, and secondly, the assignment of an individual patient to the appropriate category. Diagnosis or classification has a number of functions, notably to aid the communication amongst clinicians and scientists and to provide a key to existing knowledge about a particular disorder including knowledge of its course and response to treatment (that is, prognosis). To be useful a diagnostic system should provide the basis for describing important similarities and differences between patients. Diagnostic entities should be fairly homogeneous (although patients with the same diagnoses need have only some of a range of symptoms and signs) and it ought to be possible to allocate a diagnosis to most patients (clearly a diagnostic scheme accommodating only half the patients would be of limited use). In short, a diagnostic system aids the recognition of a disorder in an individual patient and allows knowledge gained from the management of previous patients with a similar disorder to be applied to him.

This is clearly the case in many areas of internal medicine where knowledge of abnormal processes allows their precise characterization and the close control of treatment (for example, pernicious anaemia or bacterial pneumonitis), but where knowledge is much less certain, as in the more minor illnesses in general practice, the importance and value of diagnosis is much reduced (Howie 1972). In the case of nervous disorders the situation is much more complex and uncertain, there is disagreement about what sort of information should be entered into the diagnostic process, and there is even a view that making a diagnosis inferring a primary malfunction within the person is inappropriate.

Nervous disorders come to notice through a wide range of complaints: physical symptoms, emotional changes, cognitive impairments, unusual beliefs, perceptual abnormalities, changes in behaviour and personality, antisocial behaviour, criminal acts, discord in family life and other social situations. A patient may be unaware of his problem and deny it when his attention is drawn to it by others or it may be subtly interwoven within a social nexus which itself has to be understood and analysed. In general medicine, symptoms are of interest mainly because their pattern and development allow the identification of underlying causes or disease process for which other evidence can often be obtained by examination of the patient or by laboratory investigations. This is true for some psychiatric conditions, particularly the organic psychoses, but what of other conditions where there are no physical abnormalities and laboratory or psychological tests seldom yield useful, critical information? It is still possible to view them with a 'disease' or 'medical' model, expecting that the analysis of the pattern of symptoms and their change over time will reveal a limited number of disorders for which some subtle neurological derangement can be hypothesized. However, it may be argued that such consistencies do not inevitably indicate a biological defect or pathological process but simply reflect the limited repertoire of human reactions to stress which, if its source is not obvious in the immediate environment, can be located in the imperfect development of personality or subtle malfunctions in social networks, particularly the family. The locus of the important pathology is therefore alleged to be in various places, from inside the person (and hence a variety of 'medical models' (Macklin 1973)) to society at large. Attempts have therefore been made to explain psychiatric disorder from a number of standpoints: the biological sciences—especially biochemistry, psychoanalysis, learning theory, social psychology, and sociology, each of which may be in vogue at a particular time or place, with a particular profession dealing with the mentally ill or with opinion makers and publicists. The practising psychiatrist is not usually ideologically rigid or committed and is often willing to use a model which allows him to deal with a particular illness in a particular setting although he may not always be explicitly aware that he is doing so (Lazare 1973). It is, for example, easy to view the psychoses, both organic and functional, from a medical perspective, the neuroses from psychoanalysis or learning theory, whilst social models best account for alcoholism, drug addiction, shoplifting, or chronic disability. Intelligently pursued, such eclecticism can bestow on the clinician an adaptability which allows him to survive the exigencies of the clinic and changes of fashion but if pursued without occasional reflection and review can obscure issues and only blunt therapeutic effectiveness.

The existence of several 'schools' of psychiatry and different models of mental illness and other abnormal behaviour has important sociopolitical and ethical consequences which influence the perception of abnormality and the need for treatment and also the types of management considered permissible. Psychosurgery, electroconvulsive therapy, drug treatments, and the use of instrumental or aversive conditioning methods have all been criticized on these grounds. The consistency of clinical appraisal and treatment has also suffered from the same causes, a matter of intense study and dispute during the past 20 years. Writing at a time when modern psychotropic drugs were just making their appearance, Stengel (1959) observed: 'a serious obstacle to progress in psychiatry is difficulty of communication. Everybody who has followed the literature and listened to discussions concerning mental illness soon discovers that psychiatrists, even those apparently sharing the same basic orientation, often do not speak the same language. They either use different names for the same concepts or the same term for different concepts, usually without being aware of it. It is sometimes argued that this is inevitable in the present state of psychiatric knowledge, but it is doubtful whether this is a valid excuse. The lack of a common classification of mental disorders has defeated attempts at comparing psychiatric observations and the results of treatments undertaken in various countries or even in various centres in the same country. Possibly, if greater attention had been paid to these difficulties, there might be a greater measure of agreement about the values of specific treatments than exists today.' Many studies during the ensuing years have explored and measured these deficiencies and it is instructive to consider some of them briefly before discussing the current situation.

The difficulty clinicians have in reaching the same precise diagnosis has been demonstrated in numerous studies (Kendell 1975). Agreement is understandably quite high in deciding between broad categories, such as psychosis versus neurosis, but it falls considerably when attempts are made to allot a patient to a more precise category within the broader divisions and this is especially so for the neuroses and personality disorders. Some of the disagreement can be removed if interviews are conducted in a particular way and if diagnostic criteria are agreed beforehand, but other factors such as social context or the influence of fellow professionals, which must exist in everyday practice, undoubtedly operate. The influence of such factors is demonstrated by an experiment in which three groups of psychiatrists were shown a video tape of an actor who had been trained to respond to questioning in a way considered typical of a normal individual. The tape was introduced in a different way to each audience and such biasing was shown to shift the range of diagnoses offered, stretching from normal personality to character disorder, various neuroses, and schizophrenia! (Temerlin 1968). Theoretical orientation of a psychiatrist, which undoubtedly contributes to such diagnostic confusion, also influences management plans as shown in a study (Mayou 1977) where questionnaire replies from 43 experienced psychiatrists showed considerable variation in the ways they would manage agoraphobia. Variation in the symptoms of the single illness as it evolves or from episode to episode may also be a source of variation in diagnosis. Diagnoses come into fashion, have their heyday and disappear (for example, neurasthenia) and even if a particular diagnosis endures its frequency of use may vary considerably, perhaps influenced by the availability of a particular treatment as seen in the shifts in the incidence of schizophrenia and manic depressive psychosis in the USA, probably associated with the introduction of lithium salts (Baldessarini 1970).

Clearly, this is not a very satisfactory state of affairs. There have been varied reactions to it. Some see these inadequacies as strong evidence that medical models are quite inappropriate. Some conclude that classifying nervous disorders into species of disease is incorrect, that there are no 'ideal' forms against which each patient is to be compared and that differences between people, including patients, arise from continuous variations (rather like height or intelligence) in a series of dimensions. Still others are impressed by the individuality of people, the unique genetic make up, life experiences, stresses, and so forth, so that classification into types of reaction or illness does considerable violence to the truth: there are no psychiatric disorders, only psychiatric patients (Menninger *et al.* 1958). Others, wishing to preserve a disease model respond either by splitting diagnostic categories, convinced that further refinement will improve consistency or, conceding that only the broad categories have any stability, lump conditions together to the ultimate limits of 'general neurotic syndrome' and 'unitary psychosis' (Crow 1986; Tyrer 1985).

During the past decade or so there has been a movement seeking to reinstate and strengthen the disease model of psychiatric illness, taking an empirical approach to the problems presented to psychiatrists, shorn of theory so far as is possible. This pragmatic approach sees little point in starting by settling the broad issues, such as what is meant by mental health or mental illness, any more than internal medicine has been greatly concerned with the definition of health and illness (Black 1968). It takes confidence from the fact that many classic descriptions of disease have stood the test of time, that diagnostic error and disagreement are not uncommon in general medicine (Koran 1975; Goldman *et al.* 1983), and it prefers to set limited objectives in the expectation that areas of firm knowledge will coalesce to form a more general understanding of psychiatric disorder. It takes a 'toughminded' approach to psychiatric thinking: 'just because it is difficult to make valid observations and accurate measurements, just because objectivity is so elusive, just because unintended error is so easy, it is necessary to be even more careful than would be necessary in a more developed field. Knowing that it is easy to form erroneous opinions when dealing with psychologic phenomena, knowing that it is more difficult to eliminate or reduce observer bias in studies of psychologic processes, we should demand more rather than less in the way of repeatedly demonstrated, systematic, controlled evidence' (Guze 1970). Much has already been achieved. Careful definition of symptoms and signs, structured interviewing procedures, agreement on which symptoms have precedence in the presence of others, and the instrumental definition of syndromes have greatly improved the agreement between observers, although such improved reliability does not necessarily imply improved validity (one is simply in greater agreement about something, but it may ultimately prove to be agreement about the wrong thing).

Accepting that the aetiology of psychiatric disorders, apart from the organic psychoses, is mostly unknown, recent efforts at categorical classification have centred on symptoms and, to some extent their development through time, whilst recognizing from the history of internal medicine that classification of symptoms can be misleading. A major effort in this direction is the *Diagnostic and Statistical Manual of Mental Disorders* of the American Psychiatric Association (3rd edn), 1980 (DSM-III), which defines disorders on the basis of operational criteria embodying descriptive psychopathology. However, it also recognizes that premorbid personality and recent stress probably play an important role in shaping the fine detail and the timing of an illness and, in order not to confound these with symptoms as many previous classifications have done, it adopts a multiaxial system where personality, associated physical illness, psychosocial stress, and current social functioning are independently rated. It therefore allows a very comprehensive assessment of the individual patient, thereby recognising that categorical diagnoses discard a lot of information about the individual person and thus deferring to the views of the psychobiological school of Meyer and Menninger. (DSM-III has not so far found itself about to incorporate insights of psychoanalysis by, for example, incorporating some assessment of ego defence mechanisms.) With this information, carefully collected on each individual, it is then possible to explore relationships with aetiological factors such as genetics, the course of the disorder and treatment response. Needless to say, DSM-III is not perfect, and it has been criticized (e.g. Vaillant 1984; Faust and Miner 1986) but it has many strengths, particularly the fact that it incorporates the views and experience of large numbers of psychiatrists and it is subject to continuing review and will change as evidence accrues.

One of the purposes of classification is to aid communication (Blashfield and Draguns 1976) and an account of present treatment techniques would be easier if those developing the subject accepted a universally agreed diagnostic (or other) system. As it is, much of the knowledge gained during the past 30 years or so has accrued from different perspectives, many studies failing to mention any diagnostic system which was employed, and even if this information were available the interpretation of the mountain of information recorded would be almost impossible. Nevertheless, a clinical concensus, although a rather impressionistic one, has arisen and, in the United Kingdom at least, this has developed through clinicians who have the 'neo-Kraepelinian' orientation of British texts, particularly Mayer-Gross *et al*. (1954). The views of an increasingly influential American school of similar orientation are clearly stated in the textbook by Goodwin and Guze (1974). This is the broad orientation of the authors of this text. We assert that psychiatric practice should be based on rigorous empirical study, that nervous illnesses do exist and are not simply social constructions, that they are due to many disorders the classification of which is a major scientific task which will lead to a knowledge of aetiology and effective treatment. At the present time, treatment must be guided by such fragmentary knowledge as we have. The awareness of ignorance is an important element of wise therapeutics.

The classification of psychotropic drugs

A vast number of chemical agents affect brain activity, behaviour, and mental life, both normal and abnormal, and in order to examine their use in therapeutics it is necessary to have a classification of psychotropic drugs. This has proved as difficult as the classification of psychiatric disorder (Shepherd 1980). An early attempt to do this was made by Lewin (1931) who described five categories which stood fairly independently of each other: euphoriants; phantastica or hallucinogens; inebriantia; hypnotica and excitantia which cause a general enhancement of mental capacities without disturbing consciousness. Such a classification was rather over-elaborate for clinical purposes at the time and most pharmacological and clinical texts for the ensuing twenty years were satisfied with two categories: depressants and stimulants. In the 1950s a series of drugs was introduced into psychiatric practice (mostly from other branches of medicine where their psychological effects had been incidently noticed) which had novel and more subtle mental and neurological effects: alteration of mood, suppression of hallucinations and delusions, the reduction of anxiety without sedation, and the production of unhelpful but striking neurological effects such as dystonia and parkinsonism. Clinicians witnessing these effects invented a plethora of new terms to describe them: anxiolytics, tranquillizers, antidepressants, mood normalizers, neuroleptics, antipsychotics, psychic energizers. It was clearly difficult to divine the essence of these effects. The terms proved difficult to define, were never universally favoured, and were soon attacked by pharmacologists (Weatherall 1962). Efforts to identify important or essential pharmacological actions which underlie these novel clinical changes have proved difficult because the drugs are pharmacologically 'dirty' and have innumerable effects within the brain and other tissues. It may be that their success in combating mental illness lies in a particular combination of pharmacological actions, but extensive study of pharmacological profiles involving increasingly sophisticated biological techniques and mathematical analysis, whilst it has had some success in selecting compounds for development of psychotropic agents (see Chapter 7), has not provided insights into the nature of the central action of these substances upon which a clinically useful classification can be based. Search amongst 'target symptoms', hypothesized neurophysiological mechanisms, batteries of behavioural or psychological tests, has proved no more fruitful. The structural chemist, pharmacologist, behavioural scientist, and psychiatrist have therefore to view these compounds from their own standpoint and the psychiatrist has to fall back on clinicopathological criteria alone.

From a clinical viewpoint there are some obvious differences. Some drugs have a symptomatic action. For example, propranolol blocks certain autonomic effects of anxiety, hypnotics promote sleep, antilibido agents reduce sexual drive. Other drugs affect groups of symptoms which tend to wax and wane together (i.e. syndromes) and these affect anxiety, mood disturbance, and hallucinations and delusions. None of these has a 'curative' action (which at present is only achieved by drugs interrupting known organic processes such as hypothyroidism) although the long-term course of chronic disorders such as schizophrenia is altered by drug treatment. Considering those drugs which have syndromal effects, and which constitute the core of clinical psychopharmacology, only a broad classification is possible: anxiolytics (sedatives, minor tranquillizers), antidepressants, mood stabilizers and antipsychotics (neuroleptics, major tranquillisers). Within each class some subclassification is possible: on the basis of pharmacokinetic differences (e.g. benzodiazepines), on the existence of incidental but useful properties such as sedation or stimulation (e.g. antidepressants, antipsychotics) or because of differences in chemical nature and pharmacology believed to indicate efficacy against a particular subcategory of illness such as depression (e.g. tricyclic antidepressants versus monoamine-oxidase inhibitors). Some drug effects probably occur only in illness. Clearly, an antipsychotic effect cannot be manifest in the absence of psychosis, but these drugs do not seem to alter thinking or perception. Likewise, antidepressant action does not affect normal mood or normal sadness. On the other hand, the sedative effects of benzodiazepines would occur in most people without anxiety, and the symptomatic effects of propranolol occur in the absence of illness and may be used by normal people outside clinical practice to improve violin playing or skill at playing snooker.

These therefore remain very broad categories and the practical difficulty is matching the individual patient to a particular drug. Whilst most cases of undoubted depressive illness respond to an antidepressant drug such as amitriptyline and most cases of acute psychosis to a neuroleptic such as chlorpromazine, the degree of response is highly variable and it is not uncommon to meet two patients with the same symptoms who do not respond to the same treatment. There are many possible reasons for this: pharmacokinetic differences, differences in biological sensitivity, and perhaps different pathophysiology may produce a similar pattern of symptoms in different people. Clearly, there are many sources of variation which lie between symptom patterns and the response of an individual to a particular drug and it is necessary to know more about aetiology and pathological mechanisms to make sense of known drug effects. This can be illustrated by considering the treatment of congestive cardiac failure where the cause of failure is not revealed. Relief of failure by diuretics, nitrates, nifedipine, prazosin, captopril, opiates, oxygen inhalation, reduced dietary sodium, and venesection (undoubtedly a physical method of treatment!), would be puzzling, especially if little was known about the relevant pharmacology. Certainly, simple correspondence between symptoms and pharmacological profiles would not be expected. Of course, some of the symptoms of failure, such as breathlessness or oedema, occur in other diseases, and the drugs used to treat failure may be used in other conditions such as oedema of other cause and arterial disease in various sites. Knowledge of the effects of cardiac failure and each drug on the pulmonary and systemic circulations, on venous and arterial pressures, the role of the renin-angiotensive system in promoting sodium and water retention and the influence of central nervous factors, including anxiety, promotes understanding of the role of each of these drugs and procedures in the management of cardiac failure. Moreover, biochemical, endocrine, and autonomic changes can be precisely measured when the changes effected by treatment, including harmful adaptive changes, can be monitored. The psychiatrist has to do his work without such insights and with few aids and there is still a good deal of art in his practice rather than science. However, one can see that because a particular drug may be beneficial in several conditions or because a single condition can be eased by several drugs it does not follow that clinical psychopharmacology is not a science or that the medical model is inappropriate. If a drug has beneficial effects on many disorders this may indicate that it influences different abnormalities or common mechanisms in complex systems. Lithium salts have such wide effects (Wood and Goodwin 1987) that it is not too surprising that they have found use in acute mania, depression, some schizophrenic disorders and aggressive states and that they affect mood and cognition in normal individuals (Judd *et al.* 1971). The improvement in depressive disorders by a range of treatments, electroplexy, sleep deprivation, antidepressants of diverse chemical nature and pharmacology, neuroleptics, lithium salts, even benzodiazepines, may indicate that conditions which have a similar presentation have quite different underlying pathophysiology or that the various agents block different aspects of the depressive process. Likewise the reduction of schizophrenic hallucinations with benzodiazepines, drugs which are generally considered to have no antipsychotic activity (Kramer 1967; Kahn et al. 1988) may result not from any fundamental effect on the psychotic process but with reduction of anxiety which exacerbates or provokes it. It is clear that a successful classification must await improved understanding of disease mechanisms and the relevant pharmacology.

Assessment of the patient

Psychiatric nosology and clinical psychopharmacology are undoubtedly rather inexact sciences and are the basis of only rather general guidelines in the treatment of the individual patient. Yet psychotropics are among the commonest groups of drugs prescribed by doctors. Inevitably, guesswork is a major element in this activity, and any good which comes from it is at least partly attributable to spontaneous drifts in the severity of illness and to non-specific processes in the treatment situation. Less attention has been given to the study of these important aspects of the treatment process than to the pharmacology and clinical utility of drugs used in treatment, but this carries the danger that the contribution of specific treatment techniques will be over-emphasized and the contribution of natural processes, both biological and social, overlooked. It may, of course, be argued that there is little point in trying to look further into these matters because the level of scientific understanding is not yet at a stage where improvements in these aspects of the treatment process can be obtained: trying harder only leads to disappointment. Yet continued study of the diagnostic process and how this leads to management decisions, of spontaneous changes and the day-to-day craft of drug therapy ought to lead to more effective delivery of what treatment is available.

Diagnosis is seldom formally studied in medical training although it is the principal intellectual skill of doctors. Philosophical and logical analysis probably goes against the grain of a predominantly empirical and practical profession, and neglect of it may not be a serious fault any more than lack of interest in the philosophy of scientific method prevents scientists from making important discoveries. Students probably learn almost informally through apprenticeship to experienced senior clinicians who have developed their own way of arriving at a diagnosis, presumably by discarding unconsciously methods which lead to error or take too long. It has been suggested that diagnosis is achieved by a variety of routes, from systematic step-by-step logical sequences as computers might do, to instant pattern recognition. The method called upon might well depend on the nature of the problem, its novelty, and the experience of the clinician. Naturalistic studies of clinicians in the act of making diagnoses suggests that they commonly generate hypotheses whilst information is being elicited from various sources and are ultimately left with one or two possibilities (Campbell 1987; Barrows and Feltovich 1987). This style is particularly adopted by experienced clinicians, beginners being more likely to follow an inflexible, structured interview evaluating information when it is all gathered in. No doubt there are penalties for either technique, the latter being ponderous and time-consuming, the former being at risk of ignoring or not seeking data which the various hypotheses do not require (evidence suggests that a firm diagnosis is reached within two minutes in psychiatric cases and is seldom changed thereafter (Kendell 1975)). The type of illness clearly has some influence on where emphasis is laid, the mental state examination being important in an acute psychotic breakdown, the psychiatric history in a neurotic disorder precipitated by stress. In psychiatry, probably more than in other branches of medicine, it is wise to develop the ability to view the patient and his problems from various perspectives, symptomatological, psychodynamic, behavioural, and social (Yager 1977). Such disciplined eclecticism permits switching models according to type of illness, stages of recovery, and therapeutic needs and it is probably better to do it explicitly and know where one is in the therapeutic process.

However, diagnosis is not the only purpose of the interview and examination. Whilst diagnosis is a factor in deciding treatment there are aspects of management which are determined by other factors. It has been shown repeatedly (see Williams 1979) that diagnosis is not a major factor in deciding whether a patient is referred to psychiatric specialist care, is admitted to hospital, nor what type of treatment, including which drug treatment, he gets. On reflection, this is not too surprising, because many other matters may be crucial: the ability of the patient to understand and his willingness to co-operate; his preferences and his social resources, particularly support from family and friends; the resources available to the doctor, the doctor's training, and the psychiatric 'school' to which he belongs. This probably reflects the fact that existing treatments are not so radical or efficient that the precise indications for a particular treatment and the best mode of its delivery are easy to determine.

Early contact with the patient during which the clinician's attention is focused on arriving at a diagnosis is also important in building the relationship between patient and doctor, which may well have powerful effects in treatment whether it be psychotherapy, behavioural management, drugs, or other physical methods.

Considerations of this kind suggest guidelines for the conduct of the initial interviews with a patient, particularly if treatment is subsequently to be embarked on. At the outset it is important to bear in mind that a trusting and supportive relationship must be developed, because not only may it be necessary to know the patient better, but it may be necessary to secure access to other sources of information and to obtain co-operation with treatment which may be unpleasant or tedious. On first acquaintance the patient should be allowed to talk about himself in his own way, because he needs to feel that he is being understood, and the manner in which he tells his story may also be instructive. A background history can then be obtained in which genetic factors, previous illness, education and social background, personality, and current stresses can be recorded. The presenting complaint can then be studied again in the light of this information and the pattern and duration of its development ascertained. Direct questioning can then be employed to help decide between emerging hypotheses which leads into a final 'menu-driven' enquiry to make sure than nothing important has been overlooked. It must be remembered that a patient's behaviour during an interview is a very small sample of his overall behaviour, and that his recall of events and his interpretation of them is conditioned by his feelings about himself and about the interview. It is therefore valuable to have the observations of a family member or close friend on the development of the illness, the personality of the patient, his relationships with others, social supports, stresses, and so on. A physical examination and laboratory investigations may in some cases be called for.

A diagnosis and preliminary management plan can then be made. At this point it is always wise to remind oneself of the dangers of making a diagnosis. There is a danger that the doctor's mind closes to other possibilities once he has made his mind up and new evidence, at variance with the original diagnosis, passes unnoticed. It is therefore better to have a differential diagnosis always in mind. Symptomatology evolves and diagnoses quite often need revision, and on longer acquaintance with the patient the understanding of his illness deepens as symptoms become less prominent and personality and background factors become better known. The clinician thus becomes aware of the individuality of the patient and begins to understand the development of the illness in the light of the patient's present and past circumstances. However, once a diagnosis has been made there is a danger that the patient will be viewed in the light of expectations generated by this 'label'. This is especially true of the schizophrenic psychoses and the personality disorders, and it becomes an obstacle to the individual's social recovery (Schiff 1966). It must be recalled that within a diagnostic group there is a wide variation in features of illness, quite apart from personality and social factors which constitute and sustain the individual.

The commencement of treatment

Having evaluated the illness and the circumstances of the patient and knowing the resources of the clinic, treatment begins. Unless there is intense distress there is no need to proceed with haste; indeed, evidence suggests strongly that factors other than specific treatment often achieve a great deal.

This has been clearly demonstrated in general practice, where minor illness improves as often following simple discussion and reassurance as after giving medicine which, amongst other things, may perhaps reinforce the patient's fear that a serious medical condition exists (Marsh 1977; Thomas 1978). Most psychiatric illness seen in general practice resolves within four weeks, usually with little treatment (Tennant *et al.* 1981) Studies of psychiatric out-patients show a 25 per cent reduction of symptoms after the initial interview (Uhlenhuth and Covi 1969), and out-patient attendance (Barrett and Hurst 1982) and brief hospitalization (Lieberman and Strauss 1986) are associated with symptom reduction and changes in insight and interpersonal adjustment. These effects have been so consistently observed that it is now commonplace for clinical trials of drug treatments of anxiety and depression to include a two week placebo run-in phase, at the end of which substantial numbers of patients no longer need treatment. Such improvements may not be sustained, and they are less likely in severe illness, but they do occur in patients sufficiently unwell to be referred to a psychiatric clinic and small samples of such cases have been intensively studied (Malan *et al.* 1975). The reasons for such 'spontaneous' recoveries are not often clear. They may sometimes occur when stress is removed, when circumstances have suddenly taken a turn for the better, when the patient has thought through his problems for himself—and, of course, the recurrent psychoses can remit suddenly. It is not surprising that much may happen at the time of the initial psychiatric consultation because people bring with them expectations, both hopeful and fearful, to which the doctor's sensitivity may be dulled by long clinical routine. Many patients may not realize that they are to see a psychiatrist, they may have erroneous ideas about what will take place (they will be hypnotized, interrogated on a couch, sent for electroconvulsive therapy), they may fear that the referring doctor suspects incipient insanity, they may fear and resent the social stigma, and so on (Skuse 1975). Clearly, it helps if these anxieties are dealt with during the first contact so that the patient feels he has been listened to and treated with respect. The process of declaring one's anxieties or despair and the release of feelings can in themselves be therapeutic. The giving of reassurance is important though not always easy (Kessel 1979). It must not be given too soon or it will seem insincere or inappropriate, it is often needed where the prognosis is not good, the doctor must be able to give time and be unruffled whatever the pressures on him, he must be positive and indicate that he, or a trusted colleague, is readily available. Inevitably, some doctors are therapeutic in themselves and others are not; again, a therapeutic ingredient demonstrated in clinical trials (see Chapter 7).

Having given these processes a chance to operate, the need of more specific treatment can then be determined. Psychological methods and social work investigation and support may be the techniques required, and they are not discussed further except to stress that gratuitous prescriptions of medicines should not be given if these methods are the main indication, since drugs may interfere with these other methods of management. For example, treatments based on learning theory or conditioning techniques may be disrupted by incidental medication because of state-dependent learning.

If treatment is thought necessary, the main indication of a particular class of drug is the leading syndrome concerned. Antipsychotic drugs are used in the schizophrenic psychoses and in mania, and in depressive and organic disorders where psychotic symptoms such as thought content disorder, hallucinations, marked agitation, or excitement are evident. Antidepressant drugs are chosen where there is a primary depressive disorder, mood stabilizers where there is mood disorder particularly of the bipolar kind, and anxiolytics in anxiety states. Hundreds of controlled trials have established this consistency between broad class of drug and wide diagnostic grouping, and studies of clinical practice show that diagnosis predicts treatment to this extent (Overall *et al.* 1972; Evenson *et al.* 1974). But not all schizophrenics respond to antipsychotic drugs (at least the first one or two tried), not all depressed patients respond to antidepressants or even electroconvulsive therapy, lithium salts have a substantial impact on only about half the cases of bipolar manic depression, and so on. Some reasons for these differences are known (poor compliance, extensive and rapid metabolism, intolerable unwanted effects) but in most cases there is no explanation. Sometimes, replacing the initial drug with a chemical congener or a drug within the same chemical class but with a different chemical structure and pharmacology may bring about improvement, but consistent predictors have not been uncovered. For example, the effect of different antipsychotic drugs on selective target symptoms in schizophrenic patients has not been consistently demonstrated (Galbrecht and Klett 1968; Goldberg *et al.* 1972), and the response of depressed patients to tricyclic antidepressants is not predicted by the relative potencies of these drugs in blocking the neural uptake of various monoamines. Nor is it possible to demonstrate why some depressed patients respond to tricyclic antidepressants whilst others respond to monoamine-oxidase inhibitors. In such a situation the clinician is obliged to try one drug after another and, since the choice available to him is considerable, he must make his own selection according to his own whims, because many studies of symptom patterns, of biochemical and pharmacological variables, and challenge tests have failed to discover reliable predictors of response. Properties incidental to the main therapeutic action may help in choosing a drug. If excitement or agitation are prominent, a sedative antipsychotic or sedative antidepressant can be selected or, conversely, drugs with stimulant properties may be preferred if there is retardation or lethargy. Having selected a drug as the main line of treatment this can be supplemented by others for the control of individual troublesome symptoms such as insomnia or anxiety.

Choosing the right drug for the individual patient is therefore not always easy. Response to previous episodes of the same illness is not always a guide, because the patient may be helped in one attack by a given drug which proves ineffective in a second episode. This may be because the initial response occurred at the time of spontaneous remission, but more probably it is due to each episode having slightly different pathology, evident sometimes by differences in symptoms (Young *et al.* 1987), perhaps indicating progression of the illness, especially in the schizophrenic psychoses.

The variation of treatment response with symptomatology or associated clinical factors can be illustrated by reference to depressive disorders. The classical 'endogenous' illness characterized by depressed mood, self-critical attitude, psychomotor slowing, early morning wakening with diurnal variation of symptoms which are at their most severe soon after waking, typically responds to tricyclic antidepressants. As pointed out by Kühn in his original description of the effects of imipramine (1958), 'the main indication is without doubt a simple endogenous depression' and 'every complication of the depression impairs the chances of success of treatment'. If the illness becomes more severe and retardation is marked and a self-critical attitude transmutes to delusional ideas, the illness is not likely to respond to a tricyclic but requires electroconvulsive therapy, or the addition of a neuroleptic (antipsychotic) drug to the tricyclic (Spiker *et al.* 1985). If the delusional ideas become more complex, bizarre, or not readily understood in terms of low mood (and such changes can occur within a single episode of illness) then improvement is more likely to be obtained with higher doses of antipsychotic, the antidepressant having less influence. If the depressive illness is not severe and does not have the clear characteristics of endogenous depression, and especially if symptoms include tension, fatigue, panics, and phobias, it may respond more fully to monoamine-oxidase inhibitors though tricyclics may still have some effect (Paykel 1987). Pre-existing personality disorder reduces the likelihood of response to existing antidepressants (Pilkonis and Frank 1988), as does brain damage associated with dementia or depression arising in a setting of serious or chronic physical disability. In the same patient, repeated episodes of depression may have different symptomatology and be considered different subtypes of depression (Paykel *et al.* 1976; Young *et al.* 1987): some inconsistency of treatment response is therefore not surprising.

Response to treatment may be conditioned by characteristics other than the nature of the psychiatric disorder. One aspect of the individual which clearly affects drug response is increasing age, mainly in relation to the tolerance of unwanted effects but also, perhaps, efficacy. The metabolism of most drugs is slowed by ageing, especially after the age of 65, so that therapeutic action and unwanted effects are seen at lower drug doses. Receptor changes undoubtedly occur with advanced age and any changes in the brain may well alter (both impair and facilitate) the effect of drugs on brain activity (see Chapter 15).

Concurrent physical illness should also be taken into account, especially any effect on drug distribution and metabolism. Clearly, patients with cardiac, renal, or hepatic impairment should be treated with caution. Weight gain, a common result of treatment with antipsychotics and antidepressants, is unwelcome in patients with cardiac, diabetic, and orthopaedic disorders. Tricyclic antidepressants are particularly dangerous to patients with cardiac conduction disorders (Roose *et al.* 1987). Interactions between psychotropic agents and drugs used in the management of medical conditions should be borne in mind especially the use of lithium salts in patients requiring treatment with diuretics. Nutritional status should be considered, especially where there has been considerable weight loss as is not uncommon in depressive disorders, anorexia nervosa, and old age, particularly in people with Alzheimer's disease (Singh *et al.* 1988). Body composition changes (especially reduced fat and reduced plasma proteins) will alter drug distribution, shortage of amino acids and vitamins may impair enzymic (particularly detoxification) activity (Williams 1978), and changes in the number of receptors (at least in blood platelets) occur (Goodwin *et al.* 1987).

The monitoring of treatment

Once treatment with a particular drug regime has been chosen it should be regularly reviewed, every day or every week at the start of treatment depending on the speed of change of the illness and the distress of the patient. Thereafter, once a response has been obtained the patient should be seen regularly until treatment is withdrawn. This may require prolonged contact, in the case of moderately severe depressive illness for six months and for schizophrenic psychoses many years. It is necessary to be clear about what the aim of a particular phase of treatment is: the suppression of an acute episode, continuation treatment to cover an attack until spontaneous remission occurs, prophylaxis against the next episode. In the acute phase the drug dosage is steadily increased until a response is obtained, the rate of increase depending on drug and illness including the latency between the onset of treatment or change of dose and clinical effects. For example, in the case of amitriptyline, treatment begins with a low dose of about 75 mg daily for the first 3–7 days because side-effects are then maximal and a therapeutic dose, usually 150 mg daily can then be instituted. The response can be evaluated between two and six weeks and the dose increased if necessary to 225 or 300 mg daily, if insufficient improvement has occurred and side-effects allow. If improvement is substantial on low doses there may be no need to increase it. If side-effects are severe it may be worth persisting with low doses because this intolerance may indicate slow metabolism and a therapeutic effect may be had on 50 mg daily. If an ill-sustained response has been obtained whilst increasing the dose it may be worth reducing it for a period because some drugs are only effective when their plasma concentrations lie within a certain range, high and low concentrations being without effect. There are few laboratory aids to monitoring treatment. The considerable individual variation in the extent and routes of metabolism, in plasma binding and other kinetic variables, renders plasma concentrations of little practical value in treatment with anxiolytics, antidepressants, and antipsychotics (Glassman 1985; Baldessarini *et al.* 1988). Serum concentrations of lithium salts may warn of impending accumulation but give little guidance about a therapeutic dosage, because low serum concentrations may be consistent with a prophylactic effect once treatment is well established.

Complex drug regimes should be avoided unless there are clear indications. Drug cocktails can easily and unwittingly develop in response to complaints of insomnia or tension or side-effects or because the abnormal behaviour requires acute control. Their removal may then be resisted by the patient through fear of a return of insomnia or dystonia or because relatives or nursing staff anticipate the return of disturbed behaviour. Changes in clinical state are difficult to judge if medication is constantly altered and side-effects and drug interactions are likely to be more common than if a single drug is used.

As much thought should be given to stopping treatment as starting it, and some estimate of the duration of treatment should be made in the initial treatment plans depending on the diagnosis, on the severity of the illness, on the duration of previous episodes, and published scientific evidence. Drug regimes should be dismantled carefully and the final doses reduced slowly, if necessary being given 2–3 times weekly. Withdrawal effects to anxiolytics and antidepressants, particularly if they are short-acting, will be lessened, the precipitation of an affective episode or schizophrenic relapse will be less likely, or it may develop more slowly so that treatment can be re-instituted before severe symptoms develop. It has to be borne in mind that if relapse occurs on discontinuing the treatment it may not respond to prompt re-establishment of that treatment. The patient should be assessed some weeks after treatment has ceased because drugs, especially if administered in depot form, may take weeks to leave the body and relapse may therefore not occur until 6–12 weeks later.

A wide range of drugs in each major psychotropic category is available in technologically sophisticated societies. In Great Britain at the time of writing there are 12 hypnotics, 14 anxiolytics, 21 antipsychotics, and 22 antidepressants. The individual clinician cannot acquire effective knowledge of so many drugs. It is better to know a few drugs well in order to become thoroughly familiar with individual variation in therapeutic response and unwanted effects and to be readily conversant with drug interactions likely to arise. (Specialists in other branches of medicine have similar problems: 13 beta-blockers, 17 non-steroidal anti-inflammatory drugs.) It is often better to use older, established drugs than newer products because efficacy and hazards are more certainly known and older drugs cost much less. Confusion is reduced if generic (scientific) names are used instead of brand names. For example, there are 8 branded products of diazepam, and the work of nurses and pharmacists is complicated by this. Generic names also have the advantage that they indicate the chemical class to which the drug belongs. The main disadvantage of using the generic name is that the patient may be dispensed a different brand when the prescription is repeated. Since different preparations of the drug often differ in shape, size, and colour this may lead the patient to think he has been given the wrong medication and may be particularly confusing to those taking several drugs. The quality of branded and generic products and their bioavailability are not usually different from each other, since licences from the Medicines Inspectorate to manufacturers are only granted if they match the brand leader.

Simplicity is therefore desirable in all aspects of drug treatment: progress and hazard are the more easily judged, experience in depth is more easily acquired, communication between doctors, nurses, pharmacists, and the patient is more reliable and the patient can co-operate with his treatment more easily and costs are minimized.

Treatment compliance

Many people do not take their medication as they should. Commonly they take too little, terminate the treatment too soon, or take none at all. They may take too much or take it at the wrong times. They may give it to others or exchange medicines. They may not take care of it and it may be accidentally ingested by children or they may take overdoses, perhaps with suicidal intent. Poor compliance with treatment advice has been extensively studied (Blackwell 1976; Becker and Rosenstock 1984) although it is difficult to do so with accuracy since most treatment is administered to out-patients whose privacy must be respected and because awareness of monitoring would almost certainly alter compliance. Nevertheless, even within hospital compliance is often poor, especially with long-term patients.

Compliance can be estimated by asking the patient about his drug taking, by counting tablets returned after a set period, by incorporating in the medication a marker substance which can be detected in the urine, or by identifying the drug in body fluids, usually by measuring the serum or plasma concentration. Non-compliance is probably more extensive than studies detect. Certainly, patients claim to have taken medication when chemical tests indicate that they have not, and they may improve compliance for a few days before they know that a blood sample will be taken. Even so, it is estimated that 25–50 per cent of out-patients omit sufficient of their medication to impair therapeutic efficacy.

There is no typical drug defaulter, but a number of factors or situations contribute to poor co-operation: unpleasant side-effects, lack of insight into the nature of the illness and its treatment, opposition to the use of medication to treat a nervous illness, the need to continue with medication for some time after symptoms have been suppressed, delay in the onset of relapse after the stopping of medication so that the patient thinks he or she is well without drugs, and complicated drug regimes. Many patients default to the extent that they do not even take their prescriptions to the pharmacist, and it has been estimated that up to 20 per cent of patients fail to do so within one month of issue (*Drug and Therapeutics Bulletin*, 1981). Undoubtedly many patients have genuine difficulty in remembering what they are told, especially if the advice is complex and beyond their medical knowledge. Ley and Spelman (1967) studied communication between patients and therapists and found that people remembered best what they are told first and what they consider important. Surprisingly perhaps, being old or anxious did not impair recall. It is therefore wise to give the patient essential information or advice only, to give it early in the consultation and to either give written advice or get the patient to write it down for himself. The *Drug and Therapeutics Bulletin* (1981) recommends telling the patient:

(1) the name of the medicine;

(2) whether it is meant to treat the disease or to relieve the symptoms, and therefore how important it is to take it;

(3) how to tell if it is working, and what to do if it appears not to be working;

(4) when and how to take it, before or after meals;

(5) what to do if a dose is missed;

(6) how long to take it;

(7) side-effects that are important for the patient, and what to do about them;

(8) possible effects on driving, on work, etc, and what precautions to take;

(9) interactions with alcohol and other drugs.

It has been suggested that non-compliance is not always a bad thing, particularly in patients sensitive to a drug who thereby prevent themselves developing toxic reactions, and it may lessen the chance of long-term toxicity or dependence in those requiring medication for lengthy periods. For many psychotropic drugs and particular psychiatric conditions the optimum dose, frequency of dosing, and duration of treatment are not well established so that the consequences for the patient of poor compliance are not really known. However, the consequence for the doctor is that he is getting inadequate feedback about his treatment and his experience is therefore misleading him.

A prominent category of misuse of medication is self-poisoning which is a major health problem (accounting for 11 per cent of all medical admissions to hospital and 30 per cent of emergencies in the Sheffield area over 20 years (Jones 1977). The drugs most commonly used are psychotropics, perhaps because they are among the most commonly prescribed of drugs or because they are given to people who have a high risk of suicidal behaviour. Skegg *et al.* (1983) found that only 3 per 1000 of patients prescribed psychotropic drugs in general practice in one year used them for self-poisoning, and conclude that this 'suggests that the frequency of self-poisoning with psychotropic drugs owes more to widespread prescribing of these drugs than to a special propensity of the patients receiving them'. Most self-poisonings are impulsive and usually involve women aged 15–29 years so it is clear where preventive action should be aimed.

Hazards of treatment

Most drugs have effects in addition to the main therapeutic action and these usually detract from any benefit derived from treatment. Unwanted effects are common with psychotropic drugs, particularly the older drugs, as would be expected from their multiple pharmacological actions, especially interactions with the receptors for acetylcholine and the biogenic amines. Anticholinergic effects are troublesome with the tricyclic antidepressants and some phenothiazines: dry mouth, constipation, delay in initiating micturition, and focusing difficulties can be severe, particularly in the elderly. They are most intense at the start of treatment and progressively decline with continued use. Extrapyramidal effects are prominent with antipsychotics, notably butyrophenones and phenothiazines with a piperazine side-chain in the molecular structure. Dystonic reactions occur early in treatment, often in a manner of days, and in the young: parkinsonism occurs usually after the first week and in older patients. The most distressing neurological effect is akathisia, an uncontrollable motor restlessness easily mistaken as an increase in psychotic agitation. Hypokinesis, perhaps the most common effect, is possibly the most socially damaging, since paucity of movement and facial expression can be easily mistaken for lack of interest and social dilapidation. These neurological reactions can be eased by anti-parkinson medication, although akinesis is not greatly relieved.

Antidepressants and phenothiazines frequently induce postural hypotension usually after about three weeks of treatment. This is particularly troublesome in the elderly whose ability to regain their balance is impaired, with consequent falls, injury, and occasional stroke. Weight gain occurs after some weeks of treatment with antidepressants, antipsychotics, and lithium salts and can be of the order of 10–15 kg and is clearly both inconvenient and a health hazard if treatment has to be continued for some years. The benzodiazepine anxiolytics and hypnotics are free from immediate unwanted effects apart from slight drowsiness or fatigue or slight impairment of psychomotor function. Their major hazard is dependence, which develops with continued use, although adaptive changes to their effects are detectable early in treatment (Lader and File 1987). Long-term hazards are associated with other drugs: tardive dyskinesia following the administration of antipsychotics, cardiac changes with antidepressants, and hypothyroidism in some patients treated with lithium salts. Psychotropic drugs are commonly used in self-poisoning attempts and tricyclic antidepressants are particularly dangerous because of their cardiac effects and tendency to induce epileptic convulsions. The older tricyclics (amitriptyline, dibenzepine, desipramine, doxepin) are the most dangerous, monoamine-oxidase inhibitors less so, and the newer drugs (mianserin, trazodone, lofepramine) are much safer (Cassidy and Henry 1987).

The monitoring and control of unwanted effects is a major element of therapeutics. It is usually wise to indicate to the patient that there may be some effects which have to be accepted in order to give relief from illness, but in general it is probably best to avoid detail because many patients are suggestible. It is important to give time to the discussion of any such effects so the patient can understand what is happening to him or her and is thereby given the opportunity to co-operate intelligently with treatment. Many unwanted effects derive from their recognized pharmacology and they are therefore predictable and dose-dependent. They should be managed initially by dosage reduction so long as this is compatible with continued efficacy. Should this not be possible, a different psychotropic drug should be substituted. For example, a patient who does not tolerate the anticholinergic effects of thioridazine may do better with chlorpromazine, trifluoperazine, or haloperidol whereas a patient with a similar illness who develops troublesome extrapyramidal effects with the latter drugs may be managed more comfortably with thioridazine. If a solution cannot be found in this way an antidote to the unwanted reactions might be added but is less desirable because all drugs have unwanted effects (for example, antiparkinson agents are anticholinergic) and the problems of polypharmacy develop. Most patients have to tolerate some unwanted effects and may adjust to them sufficiently to be surprised by their absence when treatment is eventually discontinued. Clearly, it is as important to monitor the patient regularly to minimize these effects as it is to assess efficacy. Unwanted effects unrelated to the characteristic pharmacological actions also occur but are much less common. Skin reactions are the most frequent, but pancytopenia and hepatotoxicity can occur. Drugs with complex pharmacology inevitably interact with other drugs. Monoamine-oxidase inhibitors require attention to diet, notably the avoidance of fermentation products and sympathomimetic amines, tricyclics impair the action of some drugs used in the treatment of hypertension, and thiazide diuretics should be avoided in patients receiving lithium salts.

Especial caution should be exercised when prescribing for women of reproductive age. Many psychotropic drugs induce enzymes implicated in the metabolism of steroid contraceptives so that impaired protection and breakthrough bleeding may occur. It is wise to enquire about the possibility of pregnancy and adequacy of contraception before prescribing drugs in order to avoid harm to any fetus which may be present. Drug transfer across the placenta to the fetus is similar to that of other natural lipid membranes in the body, mostly by simple diffusion especially for molecules of low molecular weight and high lipid solubility. (Active transport mechanisms are unusual in placental transfer unless the drug has structural similarities with natural substances transported in this way.) Drugs reaching the mother's brain and other tissues also reach the fetus and, since binding to plasma proteins is low in the fetus, most drugs quickly distribute from blood into the tissues. Some drugs concentrate in fetal tissue, such as phenothiazines which concentrate in the melatonin structures in the central nervous system. Despite this, psychotropic agents with the exception of lithium probably do not interfere with organogenesis. Treatment with lithium salts is associated with a fourfold increase in congenital malformations, mainly cardiovascular. Whether the development of finer neuronal structure or connectivity (expressed perhaps as changes in intellectual capacity or personality) is altered by these drugs is unknown but it would not be surprising if drugs which are known to have powerful interactions with many central neuronal receptors or enzyme systems such as monoamine-oxidase influence finer neuronal structure (Lewis *et al.* 1977). The use of drugs during pregnancy is therefore best avoided: if there are pressing indications, every effort should be made to find other methods of management during the first three months of pregnancy and the lowest effective doses only employed. Of course, a woman may not always be aware that she is pregnant, and this emphasizes the need for caution in women of reproductive age.

If drugs have been used during the later stages of pregnancy they may present problems for the child during the first hours or weeks of its life. Renal and hepatic functions are still grossly immature in the neonate, so that excretion and enzymic metabolism are slow and the body composition of the infant, particularly low plasma proteins, maintain high concentrations of drugs at receptors. Drug effects therefore persist in the neonatal period, benzodiazepines causing hypotonia and impaired respiration and suckling, phenothiazines cause central depression including defective temperature regulation, and tricyclic antidepressants cause persisting anticholinergic effects. Withdrawal symptoms (overactivity, tremor, tachypnoea) may occur 2–3 weeks after benzodiazepine withdrawal.

Drugs given to the mother can also reach the neonate through breast-feeding because the mechanisms of transfer across the epithelium of the mammary gland are similar to transfer across the placenta. Since drug prescription to nursing mothers is widely restricted, the accumulation of knowledge about effects on the fetus from this source is limited, but it seems that psychotropic drugs do not present a great problem. Benzodiazepines, antipsychotics, and antidepressants reach the neonate in small quantities, perhaps because of their extensive binding to plasma proteins in the mother.

Drugs can have effects unnoticed by patient or doctor or at least not often commented upon. It is always valuable to reflect on ways in which prescribed drugs may affect personal life. Drugs which cause sedation or impair visual acuity may impair the efficiency and safety of driving vehicles or work at machines or requiring close vision particularly in the first week of treatment (Betts *et al.* 1972; Brosan *et al.* 1986). Memory impairment and subtle cognitive effects may be caused by the drugs with anticholinergic effects and lithium salts (Haran *et al.* 1987). Drugs may interfere with sporting activities, and it is not uncommon to meet a middle aged marathon runner on tricyclic antidepressants or beta blockers regardless of their known cardiac activity! Despite the fact that an increasing proportion of the population is in receipt of medication of some kind the consequences for sporting activity is little studied (Powles 1981). Many drugs impair sexual function (potency, ability to achieve orgasm, spermatogenesis) particularly those with autonomic effects, but important though this is, it is also an area which has been little studied (Abel 1985; Drife 1987). The use of alcohol, caffeine in its various forms, and smoking, may alter drug action, especially if it is excessive as is often the case in emotional disorder and chronic illness. Following a heavy drinking bout, alcohol prolongs the elimination of many drugs due to competition for the same hepatic metabolic enzymes. Daily alcohol ingestion on the other hand has the reverse effect, due to the induction of the same enzymes. Hepatic cirrhosis will, of course, slow the clearance of drugs (Sellers and Holloway 1978). Large intakes of caffeine (coffee, tea, cola drinks, cocoa, chocolate) cause anxiety, irritability, insomnia, tremor, and cardiac arrhythmias and should therefore be considered when evaluating any patient with symptoms of anxiety, but caffeine also antagonizes benzodiazepines and tea interferes with alimentary absorption of phenothiazines (Ashton 1987). Smoking induces hepatic metabolizing enzymes.

Long term hazards are difficult to evaluate because they necessarily take time to develop and they may not be predictable from studies on animals other than man. Moreover, animals are not known to suffer from psychiatric disorder and the long-term adjustments of any underlying pathophysiology under the impact of treatment is unknown. However, there is some evidence that tricyclic antidepressants may induce rapid cycling in bipolar manic depression (Wehr and Goodwin 1987), that lithium withdrawal triggers psychosis (Mander and Loudon 1988), and that benzodiazepine withdrawal can precipitate anxiety symptoms more severe than those for which treatment was initiated (Lader and File 1987).

Treatments in combination

Treatments are often used together more often by chance than by design, particularly when several therapists or agencies are involved in management as, for example, when doctors change drug regimes during a course of treatment with psychological methods.

It is generally recognized that the use of several drugs simultaneously ('polypharmacy') is undesirable because it is not easy to decide which constituents of such combinations should be altered when a change in clinical state occurs, the incidence of unwanted effects and drug interactions increases, and patient compliance with treatment declines as it becomes more complex. Yet it is common for such cocktails to develop, often unwittingly, and a constant effort has to be made to prevent this happening: insomnia, constipation, headaches, drug-induced effects such as parkinsonism, create pressure to add to the drug regime and there is much less pressure to discontinue these additions when symptoms pass or even when the added treatments are ineffective. Clearly, this is a situation to be avoided. Unwanted effects may be better dealt with by modifying the original treatment, some symptoms, such as anxiety or insomnia may well ease as the main treatment becomes effective, and simple measures, including reassurance, may well ease other symptoms or increase the patient's capacity to cope with them. Sometimes very troublesome symptoms may require some, more complicated, re-arrangement of the primary regime. It may, for example, sometimes help to use two antipsychotic drugs, such as trifluoperazine or thioridazine, in the control of a paranoid illness in which the patient is anxious and develops severe extrapyramidal effects, since the central anticholinergic effects of thioridazine should offset parkinsonism caused by trifluoperazine, and the sedative effects of thioridazine counterbalance any tendency to activation by trifluoperazine. Again, in an acute psychotic illness with severe anxiety or panics, the use of a benzodiazepine in addition to an antipsychotic may prove to be the best method of controlling symptoms, perhaps allowing a reduced dosage of antipsychotic. Such combinations should be arrived at following close study of the patient and any addition to the regime should allow some compensation, such as a reduction in the dose of another drug, lessening of its unwanted effects, and so on. Occasionally, drug combinations have been found to have effects in combination which they do not have separately. In some cases (as with lithium salts, tryptophan, monoamine-oxidase inhibitors in depressive illness) a plausible neurochemical explanation exists, in some cases (amitriptyline with phenelzine in depression) it does not, and in some (for example, propranolol facilitation of antipsychotic response in schizophrenia) the explanation is a rather uninteresting pharmacokinetic interaction indicating that a higher dose of the original antipsychotic would suffice.

Electroconvulsive therapy is often given to patients who are receiving drug treatments, including psychotropic drugs, often because the drug regime has been established before the decision to employ electroconvulsive therapy has been made. Since many drugs alter seizure thresholds or alter the duration of a generalized seizure, it is likely that the efficacy of electroconvulsive therapy is affected. Whilst the effects of convulsive activity may be well studied in animals, the precise effects in humans of many commonly used drugs (including those employed primarily for their central nervous action) is unknown and it is therefore wise, once again, to use simple drug regimes if drugs are necessary at all. It is clearly wise to avoid, if at all possible, drugs which undoubtedly have anticonvulsant action such as benzodiazepines or anticonvulsants used in psychiatry such as carbamazepine. If electroconvulsive therapy is proving ineffective and, especially, if convulsions do not occur or are very brief, any drug regime should be reviewed. Tricyclic antidepressants and phenothiazines enhance seizure activity but, surprisingly perhaps, their concurrent use with electroconvulsive therapy does not improve its efficacy or reduce the number of applications of that treatment which are needed in the treatment of depression (Seager and Bird 1962; Imlah *et al.* 1965). Controlled trials of electroconvulsive therapy are not easy to carry out because blind evaluations are difficult and the use of 'mock' treatments (such as the administration of an anaesthetic and muscle relaxant without the electrical shock) meets ethical objections. There is, however, some fairly good evidence that electroconvulsive therapy combined with antipsychotic drugs is more effective in relieving acute schizophrenic episodes than electroconvulsive therapy or drugs alone (Taylor and Fleminger 1980). The interaction of electroconvulsive therapy and drug treatments remains unexplored territory. It seems likely that interactions exist but their importance for practical therapeutics is unknown.

It seems highly likely that drugs and psychological methods of treatment interact, because drug responses are undoubtedly influenced by placebo effects and drugs can alter mechanisms such as anxiety which are at the centre of interest of most psychological methods. Accessibility to psychological treatment might be improved if anxiety is reduced to tolerable levels (for example, anxiolytics in group psychotherapy, antipsychotics in instrumental conditioning procedures) so that that the patient can engage in the treatment he is being offered. Drugs can sometimes be helpful in promoting emotional abreaction or facilitating discussion of painful issues or events. Anxiolytics may also aid the desensitization treatment of phobias (Marks 1978). On the other hand, drugs may impair the psychotherapeutic process by directly affecting the neurological mechanisms involved or because changes developing during the drug state do not persist when the drugs are withdrawn ('state dependent learning'). Drugs may reduce the motive for psychological treatments which require time and commitment on the part of the patient and they may encourage authoritarian or distant attitudes in the doctor. Likewise, it is conceivable that psychological techniques have both positive and negative influences on drug treatments. Some conditions, such as endogenous depression or acute schizophrenic psychosis, may resolve so readily with drug treatment that probing psychological methods can only upset the patient unnecessarily, and in such cases any such enquiry that is necessary should be left until the acute illness has settled. On the other hand, psychological management may help aspects of illness which are not readily helped by drugs, such as interpersonal relations or the family's understanding or tolerance of the illness, but which affect the patient's illness, his symptoms, and need of medication (Weissman *et al.* 1974). Given the great variety of psychological techniques (psychodynamic, group, cognitive, behavioural) and the influence of such important variables as the social class of the patient and the experience and skill of the therapist, the task of unravelling the interactions, helpful and unhelpful, is enormous. It is difficult enough to establish the indications and efficacy of single treatments. The creation of a firm body of knowledge about which techniques can usefully be combined and which not, is for the future. The study of these interactions began soon after the modern drugs became available (Roth *et al.* 1964) and these difficult studies have been attempted by many since then but at the present time there is insufficient consistent evidence to make even general statements about a particular treatment combination for a particular psychiatric condition (Conte *et al.* 1986; Hollon and Beck 1978). There is therefore every reason to conserve resources and keep treatments simple.

Much has therefore to be considered when prescribing treatment for psychiatric disorder. Undoubtedly, the lack of specificity of treatment allows a fairly wide margin of error, but careful patient assessment and continued awareness of the 'present state of the art' allows the clinician to give each patient the most help with least hazard and discomfort. Whilst having at his disposal powerful pharmacological agents he should always actively consider the advantages of doing nothing, the consequences of loose prescribing by himself and colleagues on the population as a whole, the long-term consequences of treatment, and not only the good he expects but hazards as yet unknown. His transactions with the individual patient will then be informed, not only by scientific understanding, but by sound clinical judgement.

References

Abel, E.L. (1985). *Psychoactive drugs and sex*. Plenum Press, New York.

Ashton, C.H. (1987). Caffeine and health. *British Medical Journal* **295**, 1293–4.

Baldessarini, R.J. (1970). Frequency of diagnosis of schizophrenia versus affective disorders from 1944–1968. *American Journal of Psychiatry*, **127**, 759–63.

Baldessarini, R.J., Cohen, B.M. and Teicher, M.H. (1988). Significance of neuroleptic dose and plasma level in the pharmacological treatment of psychoses. *Archives of General Psychiatry*, 45, 79–91.

Barrett, J.E. and Hurst, M.W. (1982). Short-term symptom change in out-patient psychiatric disorders. *Archives of General Psychiatry* **39,** 849–54.

Barrows, M.H. and Feltovich, P.J. (1987). The clinical reasoning process. *Medical Education* **21,** 86–91.

Becker, M.H. and Rosenstock, I.M. (1984). Compliance with medical advice. In *Health care and human behaviour* (ed. A. Steptoe and A. Mathews) pp. 175–203. Academic Press, New York.

Betts, T.A., Clayton, A.B., and Mackay, G.M. (1972). Effects of four commonly-used tranquillisers on low-speed driving performance tests. *British Medical Journal* **iv,** 580–4.

Black, D.A.K. (1968). *The logic of medicine*. Oliver and Boyd, Edinburgh.

Blackwell, B. (1976). Treatment adherence. *British Journal of Psychiatry* **129,** 513–31.

Blashfield, R.K. and Draguns, J.G. (1976). Toward a taxonomy of psychopathology: the purpose of psychiatric classification. *British Journal of Psychiatry* **129,** 574–83.

Brosan, L., Broadbent, D., Nutt, D., and Broadbent, M. (1986). Performance effects of diazepam during and after prolonged administration. *Psychological Medicine* **16,** 561–71.

Campbell, E.J.M. (1987). The diagnosing mind. *Lancet* **i,** 849–51.

Cassidy, S. and Henry, J. (1987). Fatal toxicity of anti-depressant drugs in overdose. *British Medical Journal* **295,** 1021–4.

Conte, H., Plutchik, R., Wild, K.V. and Karasu, T.B. (1986). Combined psychotherapy and pharmacotherapy for depression. A systematic analysis of the evidence. *Archives of General Psychiatry* **43,** 471–9.

Crow, T.J. (1986). The continuum of psychosis and its implication for the structure of the gene. *British Journal of Psychiatry* **149,** 419–29.

Drife, J.O. (1987). The effects of drugs on sperm. *Drugs* **33,** 610–22.

Drug and Therapeutics Bulletin (1981). What should we tell patients about their medicines? *Drug and Therapeutics Bulletin* **19,** 73–4.

Evenson, R.C., Altman, H., Cho, D.W., and Slettin, I.W. (1974). The relationship of diagnosis and target symptoms to psychotropic drug adjustment. *Comprehensive Psychiatry* **15,** 173–8.

Faust, D. and Miner, R.A. (1986). The empiricist and his new clothes: DSM III in perspective. *American Journal of Psychiatry* **143,** 962–7.

Galbrecht, C.R. and Klett, C.J. (1968). Predicting response to phenothiazines. *Journal of Nervous and Mental Disease* **147,** 173–83.

Glassman, A.A. (1985). Tricyclic antidepressants—blood level measurements and clinical outcome: an APA task force report. *American Journal of Psychiatry* **142,** 155–62.

Goldberg, S.C., Frosch, W.A., Drossman, A.K., Schooler, N.R., and Johnson, G.F.S. (1972). Prediction of response to phenothiazines in schizophrenia. *Archives of General Psychiatry* **26,** 367–71.

Goldman, L.S., Sayson, R., Robbins, S., Elstein, A.S., Frazier, H.S., Neuhauser, D., Neutra, R.R., and McNeil, B.J. (1983). The value of the autopsy in three medical areas. *New England Journal of Medicine* **308,** 1000–5.

Goodwin, D.W. and Guze, S.B. (1974). *Psychiatric diagnosis*. Oxford University Press, Oxford.

Goodwin, G.M., Fraser, S., Stump, K., Fairburn, C.G., Elliott, J.M., and Cowen, P.J. (1987). Dieting and weight loss in volunteers increases the number of α_2-adrenoceptors and 5-HT receptors on blood platelets without effect on 3H-imipramine binding. *Journal of Affective Disorder* **12,** 267–74.

Guze, S.B. (1970). The need for toughmindedness in psychiatric thinking. *Southern Medical Journal* **3,** 662–71.

Haran, G., Karny, N. and Nachshon, I. (1987). Effect of lithium carbonate on lateralised cognitive functions. *Journal of Nervous and Mental Disease* **175,** 688–91.

Hollon, S.D. and Beck, A.T. (1978). Psychotherapy and drug therapy: comparisons and combinations. In *Handbook of psychotherapy and behavior change* (eds. S.L. Garfield and A.E. Bergin) pp. 437–90, 2nd edn. John Wiley, New York.

Howie, J.G.R. (1972). Diagnosis—the Achilles heel? *Journal of the Royal College of General Practitioners* **22,** 310–15.

Imlah, N.W., Ryan, E., and Harrington, J.A. (1965). The influence of antidepressant drugs on the response to electroconvulsive therapy and on subsequent relapse rates. *Neuropsychopharmacology* **4,** 438–42.

Jones, D.I.R. (1977). Self-poisoning with drugs: the past 20 years in Sheffield. *British Medical Journal* **i,** 28–9.

Judd, L.L. Hubbard, B., Janowski, D.S., Huey, L.Y., and Attenhill, P.A. (1977). The effect of lithium carbonate on affect, mood and personality of normal subjects. *Archives of General Psychiatry* **34,** 346–60.

Kahn, J.P., Puertollano, M.A., Schane, M.D., and Klein, D.F. (1988). Adjunctive alprazolam for schizophrenia with panic anxiety: clinical observation and pathogenetic implications. *American Journal of Psychiatry* **145,** 742–4.

Kendell, R.E. (1975). *The role of diagnosis in psychiatry* Blackwell, Oxford.

Kessell, N. (1979). Reassurance. *Lancet* **i,** 1128–33.

Koran, L.M. (1975). The reliability of clinical methods, data and judgements. *New England Journal of Medicine* **293,** 642–6, and 695–701.

Kramer, J.C. (1967). Treatment of chronic hallucinations with diazepam and phenothiazines. *Disease of Nervous System* **28,** 593–4.
Kühn, R. (1958). The treatment of depressive states with G22355 (imipramine hydrochloride). *American Journal of Psychiatry* **115,** 459–64.
Lader, M.H. and File, S. (1987). The biological basis of benzodiazepine dependence. *Psychological Medicine* **17,** 539–47.
Lazare, A. (1973). Hidden conceptual models in clinical psychiatry. *New England Journal of Medicine* **288,** 345–51.
Lewin, L. (1931). *Phantastica, narcotic and stimulating drugs*. Kegan Paul, London.
Lewis, P.D., Patel, A.J., Bendek, G., and Balazs, R. (1977). Do drugs acting on the nervous system affect cell prolification in the developing brain? *Lancet* **i,** 399–401.
Ley, P. and Spelman, M.S. (1967). *Communicating with the patient.* Staples Press, London.
Lieberman, P.B. and Strauss, J.S. (1986). Brief psychiatric hospitalisation: What are its effects? *American Journal of Psychiatry* **143,** 1557–62.
Macklin, R. (1973). The medical model in psychoanalysis and psychotherapy. *Comprehensive Psychiatry*, 14, 49–69.
Malan, D.H., Heath, E.S., Bacal, H.A., and Balfour, F.H.G. (1975). Psychodynamic changes in untreated neurotic patients. II. Apparently genuine improvements. *Archives of General Psychiatry* **32,** 110–26.
Mander, A.J. and Loudon, J.B. (1988). Rapid recurrence of mania following abrupt discontinuation of lithium. *Lancet* **ii,** 15–17.
Marks, I.M. (1978). Behavioural therapy in adult neurosis. In *Handbook of psychotherapy and behavior change* (eds. S.L. Garfield and A.E. Bergin) pp. 493–547, 2nd edn. John Wiley, New York.
Marsh, G.N. (1977). 'Curing' minor illness in general practice. *British Medical Journal* **2,** 1267–9.
Mayer-Gross, W., Slater, E. and Roth, M. (1954). *Clinical psychiatry*. Cassell, London.
Mayou, R. (1977). Psychiatric decision making. *British Journal of Psychiatry* **130,** 374–6.
Menninger, K., Ellensberger, H., Pruyser, P., and Mayman, M. (1958). The unitary concept of mental illness. *Bulletin of the Menninger Clinic* **22,** 4–12.
Overall, J.E., Henry, B.W., Markett, J.R., and Emken, R.L. (1972). Decisions about day therapy. I. Prescription for psychiatric out-patients. *Archives of General Psychiatry* **26,** 140–5.
Paykel, E.S. (1987). Depression, anxiety and antidepressant response. In *Anxious depression: assessment and treatment* (eds. G. Racagni and E. Smeraldi) pp. 171–9. Raven Press, New York.
Paykel, E.S., Prusoff, B.A., and Tanner, J. (1976). Temporal stability of symptoms patterns in depression. *British Journal of Psychiatry* **128,** 369–74.
Pilkonis, P.A. and Frank, E. (1988). Personality pathology in recurrent depression: nature, prevalence, and relationship to treatment response. *American Journal of Psychiatry* **145,** 435–41.
Powles, A.C.P. (1981). The effects of drugs on the cardio- vascular response to exercise. *Medicine and Science in Sports Exercise* **13,** 252–8.
Roose, S.P., Glassman, A.H., Giardina, E.G.V., Walsh, B.T., Woodring, S. and Bigger, J.T. (1987). Tricyclic antidepressants in depressed patients with cardiac conduction disease. *Archives of General Psychiatry* **44,** 273–5.

Roth, I., Rhudick, P.J., Shaskan, D.A., Slobin, M.S., Wilkinson, A.E. and Young, H.H. (1964). Long-term effects on psychotherapy of initial treatment conditions. *Journal of Psychiatric Research* **2,** 283–97.

Ryle, J.A. (1948). *The natural history of disease*, 2nd edn. Oxford University Press, Oxford.

Schiff, T.J. (1966). *Being mentally ill. A sociological theory.* Aldine, Chicago.

Seager, C.P. and Bird, R.L. (1962). Imipramine with electrical treatment in depression—a controlled trial. *Journal of Mental Science* **108,** 704–7.

Sellers, E.M. and Holloway, M.R. (1978). Drug kinetics and alcohol ingestion. *Pharmacokinetics* **3,** 440–52.

Shepherd, M. (1980). Psychotropic drugs and taxonomic systems. *Psychological Medicine* **10,** 25–33.

Singh, S., Mulley, G.P., and Losowsky, M.S. (1988). Why are Alzheimer patients thin? *Age and Ageing* **17,** 21–8.

Skegg, K., Skegg, D.C.G. and Richards, S.M. (1983). Incidence of self poisoning in patients prescribed psychotropic drugs. *British Medical Journal* **286,** 841–3.

Skuse, D.H. (1975). Attitudes to the psychiatric outpatient clinic. *British Medical Journal* **3,** 469–71.

Spiker, D.G., Weiss, J.C., Dealy, R.S., Griffin, S.J., Hanin, I. Neil, J.F., Perel, J.M., Rossi, A.J., and Soloff, P.H. (1985). The pharmacological treatment of delusional depression. *American Journal of Psychiatry* **142,** 430–6.

Stengel, E. (1959). Classification of mental disorders. *Bulletin of the World Health Organization* **21,** 601–63.

Taylor, P. and Fleminger, J.J. (1980). ECT for schizophrenia. *Lancet* **i,** 1380–3.

Temerlin, M.K. (1968). Suggestion effects in psychiatric diagnosis. *Journal of Nervous and Mental Disease* **147,** 349–53.

Tennant, C., Bebbington, P., and Hurry, J. (1981). The short-term outcome of neurotic disorders in the community: the relation of remission to clinical factors and to 'neutralising' life events. *British Journal of Psychiatry* **139,** 213–20.

Thomas, K.B. (1978). The consultation and the therapeutic illusion. *British Medical Journal* **1,** 1327–8.

Tyrer, P. (1985). Neurosis indivisible. *Lancet* **i,** 685–8.

Uhlenhuth, E.H. and Covi, L. (1969). Subjective change with the initial interview. *American Journal of Psychotherapy* **23,** 415–29.

Vaillant, G.E. (1984). The disadvantages of DSM III outweigh its advantages. *American Journal of Psychiatry* **141,** 542–5.

Weatherall, M. (1962). Tranquillisers. *British Medical Journal* **i,** 1219–24.

Wehr, T.A. and Goodwin, F.K. (1987). Can antidepressants cause mania and worsen the course of affective illness? *American Journal of Psychiatry* **144,** 1403–11.

Weissman, M., Klerman, G.L., Paykel, E.S., Prusoff, B., and Hanson, B. (1974). Treatment effects on the social adjustment of depressed patients. *Archives of General Psychiatry* **30,** 771–8.

Williams, P. (1979). Deciding how to treat—the relevance of psychiatric diagnosis. (1979). *Psychological Medicine* **9,** 179–86.

Williams, R.T. (1978). Nutrients in drug detoxification reactions. In *Nutrition and drug interactions* (eds. J.N. Hathcock and J. Coon) pp. 303–18. Academic Press, New York.

Wood, A.J. and Goodwin, G.M. (1987). A review of the biochemical and neuropharmacological actions of lithium. *Psychological Medicine* **17,** 579–600.

Yager, J. (1977). Psychiatric eclecticism: a cognitive view. *American Journal of Psychiatry* **134,** 736–41.

Young, M.A., Keller, M.B., Lavori, P.W., Scheftner, W.A., Fawcett, J.A., Endicott, J., and Hirschfield, R.M.A. (1987). Lack of stability of the RDC endogenous subtype in consecutive episodes of major depression. *Journal of Affective Disorder* **12,** 139–43.

3. Neuropharmacology

Introduction

Drugs are the mainstay of the biological treatment of a whole range of psychiatric disorders. Consequently, knowledge of some of the advances in neuropharmacology greatly aids the clinician in his day-to-day prescribing. This is so mainly for the unwanted effects rather than the main therapeutic effects, the scientific basis for the latter remaining empirical rather than rational.

Neuropharmacology has developed at a rapid rate. Within the lifetime of middle-aged, let alone elderly, clinicians and scientists, the first putative neurotransmitters were discovered in the brain, and the mechanisms for their synthesis and breakdown identified. Progress has been slower with respect to the physiological functions of the large number of neurotransmitters now believed to exist in the CNS. Recently, the availability of highly specific radioactively labelled biochemicals has resulted in the description of many different binding sites in the CNS; some of these sites have physiological significance. Finally, molecular biology has made an impact on CNS neuropharmacology, particularly with respect to the numerous peptides discovered in the brain. The most useful review of these aspects of neuropharmacology is that of Cooper *et al.* (1986).

The key to CNS function is the synapse, where electrical signals are transduced into chemical signals and back again (Siggins and Gruol 1986). Drugs can exert an influence at this junction through a variety of mechanisms relating to neurotransmitters—synthesis, release, breakdown, and effect on receptors (Iversen 1982). These will be outlined in turn.

Synthesis, storage, and release

The nucleus of the nerve cell contains deoxyribonucleic acid (DNA), which controls the synthesis of all proteins, including enzyme molecules. The enzymes which synthesize the neurotransmitter are themselves manufactured in the cell body and then migrate down the axon to the nerve terminal. The cell body and nerve terminals also have mechanisms for transferring into the neuron the appropriate precursor for synthesis of the particular neurotransmitter—choline, for example, in the case of those cholinergic nerves that release acetylcholine, tyrosine for dopaminergic and noradrenergic neurons, and so on.

The synthesized neurotransmitter is taken up into specialized synaptic vesicles, or granules, which electron micrographs reveal in large numbers inside the nerve terminals. Each nerve ending has thousands of vesicles that contain high concentrations of neurotransmitter, each granule containing several thousand molecules. Other substances are stored in the vesicles such as adenosine triphosphate (ATP).

After the neuronal membrane is depolarized by the nerve action potential, major fluxes of sodium, potassium and calcium occur. The last in particular is required to activate the storage vesicles, which then migrate to the cell boundary, where they fuse to the membrane. The vesicle contents are extruded into the synaptic cleft by a process of exocytosis.

Action on receptors

The synaptic cleft is narrow, so that very soon after release the neurotransmitter diffuses across to the postsynaptic membranes, where it binds to specific protein receptors. Binding of a substance to a brain-membrane preparation is insufficient evidence that receptors to that substance exist and fulfil some function. The binding should be (a) saturable, as only a limited number of receptor sites should exist, (b) specific—that is, related to only a few substances, (c) reversible, as transmitters act in a temporary manner, and (d) productive—that is, result in an appropriate physiological response. In Table 3.1 are listed several classes of receptors (see also later in this chapter).

Binding of the appropriate transmitter externally to the receptor alters the molecular configuration of the protein so as to cause changes in the postsynaptic neuron, either internally or within the cell membrane. Further biochemical events are set in train involving 'second messengers'. Ultimately a further electrical impulse is generated or on-going activity suppressed.

Receptor pharmacology is growing rapidly as the study of protein chemistry develops apace (Kito *et al.* 1984). Neurotransmitter receptors are now of clinical as well as pharmacological importance, with the finding that myasthenia gravis is an autoimmune disease in which a circulating antibody damages and antagonizes the acetylcholine receptor.

Inactivation and regulator mechanisms

Neurotransmission would be impossible if the transmitter were to activate the receptor permanently. The association of a transmitter to its receptor

Table 3.1. Classes of receptor

Subtype	Location/function	Agonist	Antagonist
Cholinergic			
Muscarinic	Widespread CNS	oxotremorine	atropine
Nicotinic	and neuro-muscular junction	nicotine	α-bungarotoxin
Dopaminergic			
D_1	Stimulates adenylate cyclase	SKF 38393 analogue	antipsychotics
D_2	Inhibits adenylate cyclase	quinperole	sulpiride
Adrenergic			
$Alpha_1$	Postsynaptic	phenylephrine	prazosin
$Alpha_2$	Mainly presynaptic	clonidine	idazoxan
$Beta_1$	Cardiac stimulation	isoprenaline	metoprolol
$Beta_2$	Bronchodilation	salbutamol	IPS-339
Serotonergic			
5-HT_1	5-HT-labelled	buspirone	—
5-HT_2	Spiperone-labelled	—	ketanserin
5-HT_3	—	—	ondansetron
GABAergic			
$GABA_A$	Affects chloride channels	muscimol (modulated by benzodiazepines)	bicuculline
$GABA_B$	?potassium channels	baclofen	
Opioid			
Mu	—	morphine	—
Delta	Receptor for enkephalins	—	—
Kappa	—	dynorphin	—
Sigma	—	phencyclidine	—

molecule is an equilibrium, with the transmitter molecules constantly dissociating and reassociating with the receptors. Mechanisms do exist, however, to remove the neurotransmitter from the vicinity of the receptors. One mechanism is the physical removal of transmitter from the synaptic cleft by diffusion away from and subsequent absorption into the circulation. Active re-uptake may occur through the presynaptic membrane back into the neuron, where the transmitter re-enters the storage granules. Another mechanism is enzymatic breakdown which transforms the neurotransmitter to inactive metabolites. Such enzymes are located either in the synaptic cleft or in the postsynaptic membrane itself. Finally, intracytoplasmic enzymes in the presynaptic neuron can break down any neurotransmitter that remains free in the cytoplasmic fluid. Important mechanisms regulate the synthesis of transmitters. One such 'feed-back loop' is intrasynaptic. Many neurotransmitter systems are believed to incorporate receptors on the presynaptic as well as on the postsynaptic membranes. Activation of these 'autoreceptors' is believed to initiate processes that ultimately inhibit further neurotransmitter synthesis and release. Consequently, excessive traffic across the synapse diminishes the amount of neurotransmitter available; this diminution tends to lessen trans-synaptic activity.

The demonstration of autoreceptors has markedly complicated psychopharmacology, because the effects of drugs are often different depending on whether the presynaptic or postsynaptic receptors are more sensitive.

A second synaptic regulator mechanism involves the postsynaptic receptors. Underactivity across the synapse results in a proliferation in numbers of receptors and perhaps an increase in sensitivity of the receptors. This is seen at its extreme in the peripheral phenomenon of 'denervation supersensitivity'. The converse also occurs to some extent: excessive trans-synaptic activity culminates in fewer available receptors ('down regulation').

Neuromodulators

The terms neuromodulators, neuroregulators, and neurohormones are used loosely to denote substances that, although not neurotransmitters in their own right, modify the actions of known neurotransmitters. Indeed, recent evidence indicates that a neuron can release more than one type of neurotransmitter simultaneously (Snyder and Goodman 1980). These co-transmitters are generally peptides which modulate the actions of the 'classical' transmitters such as GABA, acetylcholine and noradrenalin. For example, VIP and some other peptides alter the affinity of postsynaptic receptors for their nonpeptidic neurotransmitter molecules.

Sites of Drug Action

Drugs can act at several places and such effects may vary from species to species. First, drugs can interfere with synthesizing mechanisms by stimulating or blocking an enzyme in the synthetic chain. Drugs can also act as precursors, resulting either in increased amounts of the natural neurotransmitter or in the synthesis of a transmitter-like substance. Usually this 'false' transmitter is much less effective than the natural molecule, but it can be more active. The uptake and storage of neurotransmitters can be impeded resulting in depletion at the nerve endings.

The neurotransmitter can be released by a drug from storage granules, e.g. reserpine and dopamine-containing vesicles. Other drugs block the intracytoplasmic enzyme responsible for breaking down any transmitter that has leaked into the cytoplasmic fluid. Similarly, some drugs can act on the catabolic enzymes in the synaptic cleft, usually inhibiting them and thus prolonging the neurotransmitter's action. The re-uptake of the transmitter into the presynaptic neurone can also be blocked by some drugs.

Many important drugs act directly on transmitter receptors either activating them directly (agonists) or preventing the action of the natural neurotransmitter (antagonists). Some drugs have both properties, being either agonist or antagonist according to dose and conditions. These actions can be either competitive or non-competitive with the natural transmitter, but the two properties are more matters of degree than absolute distinctions. Some drugs act preferentially on presynaptic or postsynaptic receptors. The receptors can be 'sensitized' by some drugs so that neurotransmission is facilitated. Finally, some drugs may act directly on synaptic membranes, especially in altering ionophore permeability.

No drug has a single isolated effect and psychotropic drugs in particular have a multitude of actions.

Neurotransmitters

Acetylcholine

Synthesis, storage and release

Acetylcholine is synthesized from choline and acetyl radicals by the enzyme choline acetyltransferase (Table 3.2). Choline is synthesized in the liver and is then taken up into the axon by active transport from the extracellular fluid. The acetyl radical is provided by acetyl coenzyme A, which is derived from general metabolic functions.

Acetylcholine is sequestered in the synaptic vesicles. Small numbers of vesicles discharge spontaneously during resting conditions and are detected at the neuromuscular junction as minute spontaneous depolarizations—'miniature end-plate potentials'. However, when an axon potential arrives at the nerve ending (after a latent period of about 0.75 milliseconds), several hundred vesicles discharge simultaneously into the synaptic cleft. Calcium ions are essential for the process, which is antagonized by magnesium ions (Dunant and Israel 1985).

Inactivation

Body fluids and tissues contain cholinesterases that can split acetylcholine into choline and acetic acid (Massoulie and Bon 1982). Acetylcholine

Table 3.2 Synthesis and breakdown of acetylcholine

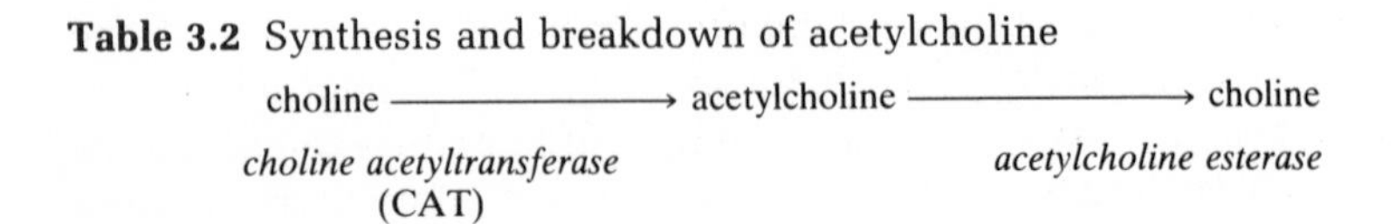

esterase, also called true or specific cholinesterase, is sited in neurons and neuroeffector junctions. Butyrylcholinesterase (pseudocholinesterase) is widely distributed throughout the body, including body fluids. True acetylcholinesterase hydrolyses acetylcholine more rapidly than it does any other choline ester; butyrylcholinesterase hydrolyses butyrylcholine with maximum velocity. Suxamethonium, a muscle relaxant, is rapidly hydrolysed by butyrylcholinesterase in the plasma, except in the one of 3000 persons in whom the enzyme is atypical (genetically determined) and has little affinity for suxamethonium. Consequently, neuromuscular blockade can last three hours or more.

Receptors

The acetylcholine receptors have been extensively studied, especially those at the neuromuscular junction. Classically the receptors have been divided into the muscarinic (activated by the alkaloid muscarine) and the nicotinic (activated and later blocked by nicotine) types. Muscarinic activation results in a rapid action, whereas nicotinic activation is rather slower and more sustained. Acetylcholine produces both effects, but many drugs are fairly specific to one or the other population of receptor. Further subdivision of both muscarinic and nicotinic receptors has been proposed.

Pathways

The cholinergic pathways have not generally been worked out in detail, mainly because of the lack of appropriate techniques. Instead, indirect evidence is used, such as the presence of synthetic and breakdown enzymes and uptake and binding mechanisms for choline and acetylcholine (Cuello and Sofroniew 1984).

Several cholinergic pathways have been proposed and may be interconnected by a major ascending tegmental–mesencephalic–cortical system (Fig. 3.1). One fairly well-defined pathway runs from the septum to the hippocampus, another from the habenular nucleus to the interpeduncular nucleus. Cholinergic neurons occur widely in the brain and spinal cord and hence influence many neuronal and behavioural functions. The diffuse activating system of the brain has important cholinergic components, being activated by cholinergic drugs and blocked by atropine and its analogues.

Drug mechanisms

Hemicholinium, a synthetic drug, interferes with the choline uptake system and thus lowers acetylcholine content in the brain. Botulinus toxin prevents the release of acetylcholine and kills by respiratory paralysis. Specific inhibitors of choline acetyltransferase have been developed, but little is known of their clinical actions.

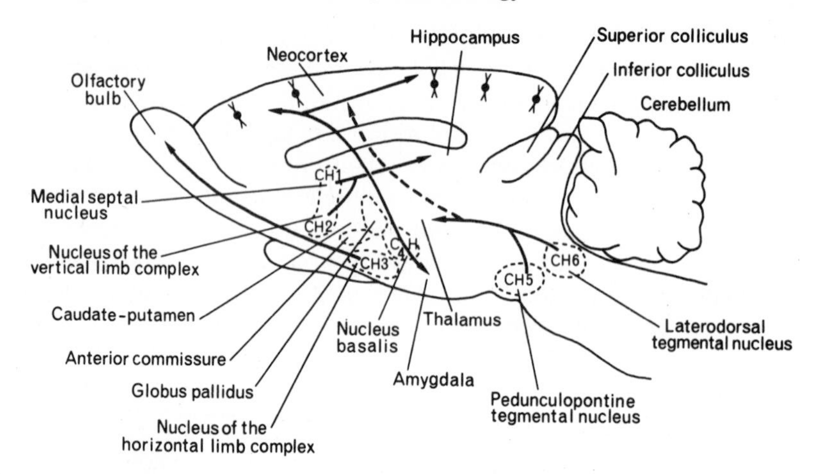

Figure 3.1. Schematic diagram of some ascending cholinergic pathways in the rat. (Modified from Cooper *et al.* 1986, with permission.)

A wide variety of drugs can block acetylcholinesterase, thereby increasing and prolonging acetylcholine actions. Physostigmine (eserine) is the prime example, and later members of this class include neostigmine, pyridostigmine, and edrophonium. Irreversible inactivators of acetylcholinesterase were developed as insecticides and nerve-gas poisons and include the organophosphates such as parathion. Physostigmine is the only therapeutic agent that penetrates the brain. It can be used in a dose of 0.5 to 2 mg intravenously to counteract many of the peripheral and central effects of poisoning by atropine and similar anticholinergic drugs and by psychotropic drugs with secondary anticholinergic actions such as amitriptyline.

Substances acting directly on cholinergic receptors, presynaptically and postsynaptically, include methacholine, carbachol, and the alkaloids, pilocarpine and muscarine. The most widely used cholinomimetic is nicotine from tobacco, but nicotine has complex actions.

The most important group, therapeutically, consists of the antimuscarinic agents, which directly block acetylcholine receptors. These agents include alkaloids such as atropine and hyoscine, synthetic drugs such as propantheline, and the antiparkinsonian drugs such as benztropine and trihexyphenidyl. Antipsychotic drugs such as chlorpromazine and thioridazine, and tricyclic antidepressants such as amitriptyline and prothiaden, also have powerful cholinoceptor-blocking properties.

Catecholamines

This category includes dopamine, an important neurotransmitter in the basal ganglia, limbic system, and other parts of the brain; noradrenalin

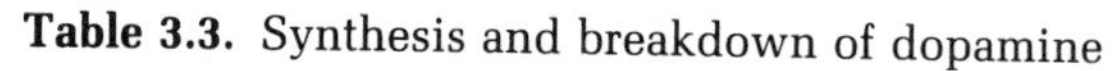

Table 3.3. Synthesis and breakdown of dopamine

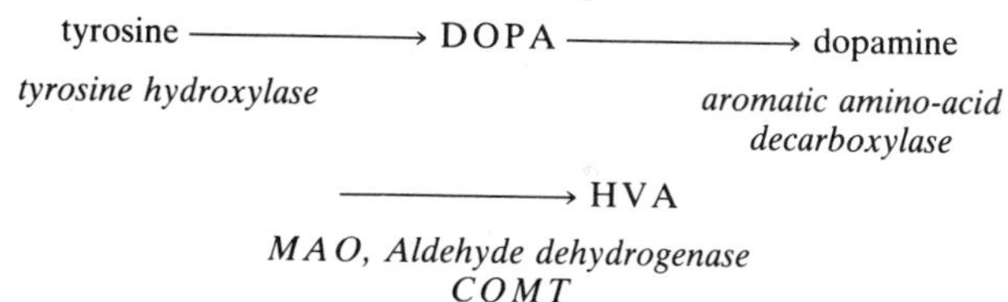

(norepinephrine), the transmitter in most sympathetic postganglionic fibres and certain tracts in the brain—especially the hypothalamus and the cerebral and cerebellar cortices; and adrenalin (epinephrine), the major hormone of the adrenal medulla, and also a probable central neurotransmitter. Because they share a common chain of synthesis, they will be dealt with together.

Synthesis, storage and release

The precursor is the amino acid tyrosine which is taken up into the nerve ending and hydroxylated to dihydroxyphenylalanine. The next step is the conversion of L-dopa to dopamine by the soluble enzyme L-aromatic amino acid decarboxylase (sometimes called dopa decarboxylase) (Table 3.3). Dopamine is then taken up into the vesicles, which in noradrenergic neurons contain dopamine-beta-hydroxylase, an enzyme that adds a hydroxyl group to the side chain (Table 3.4). Finally, in the adrenal medulla and in certain parts of the brain, noradrenalin is methylated to adrenalin by the cytoplasmic enzyme, phenylethanolamine *N*-methyltranferase.

The rate of synthesis of catecholamines depends on the amount of available tyrosine hydroxylase, i.e. it is the rate-limiting enzyme. Thus, only major manipulations of the other synthesizing enzymes would be expected to have any effect on the amount of catecholamine synthesized (Gibson 1985). The catecholamines are stored in granules that contain high concentrations (up to a fifth) of the substance, probably as a complex with adenosine triphosphate (ATP). Catecholamines are also found free in the cytoplasmic fluid and in the granules, thus forming two mobile pools as well as the intragranular reserve pool. Catecholamines move by active uptake from the cytoplasmic mobile pool into the granules.

Table 3.4. Synthesis and breakdown of noradrenalin

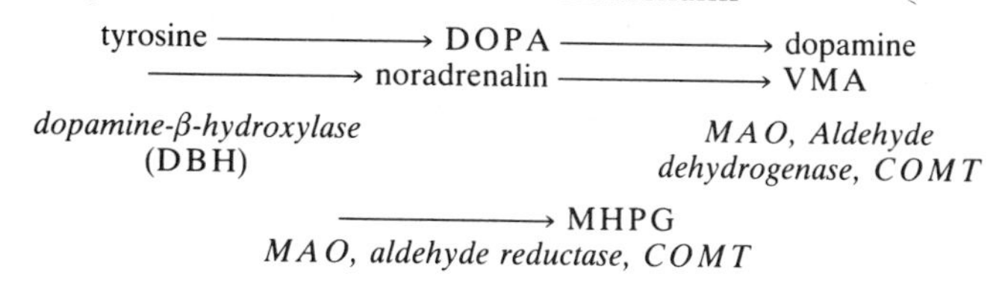

Inactivation

The most important mechanism whereby dopamine and noradrenalin are removed from the synaptic cleft and their influence on receptors is terminated is by re-uptake, first across the presynaptic membrane into the cytoplasm and thence into the storage vesicles. Simple diffusion also accounts for some transmitter inactivation.

Enzymatic breakdown requires several enzymes, both intracellular and extracellular. The two enzymes of major importance are monoamine oxidase (MAO) and catechol-ortho-methyltransferase (COMT). Both enzymes are widespread throughout the body, especially the liver and kidney. Monoamine oxidase is a mitochondrial enzyme that converts the catecholamine to its corresponding aldehyde by oxidative deamination.

The outcome of all these complex processes is that dopamine is converted mainly to its acidic derivative 3-methoxy-4-hydroxyphenylacetic acid [also called homovanillic acid (HVA)], and to a minor extent to dihydroxyphenylacetic acid (DOPAC).

The metabolites of noradrenalin are more complex. The main acidic metabolite is 3-methoxy-4-hydroxymandelic acid [also somewhat erroneously called vanillylmandelic acid, (VMA)]. In the rat and in the primate brain, the main metabolite is the alcohol derivative formed from the intermediate aldehydes by aldehyde reductase. This substance is 3-methoxy-4-hydroxyphenylglycol (MHPG), which is finally conjugated as the sulphate or glucuronide and is excreted. In the rat, most urinary MHPG derives from peripheral sources; in human beings, however, about two thirds of urinary MHPG stems from brain metabolism.

Receptors

Much work using radioactive-isotope-labelled agonists and antagonists has been carried out to characterize catecholamine receptors. Dopamine receptors have been identified and are most sensitive to dopamine and less sensitive to noradrenalin, adrenalin, and isoprenaline.

Some receptors (D1) are in close association with the enzyme adenylate cyclase, which when activated will increase the amount of cyclic adenosine monophosphate (cyclic AMP) in the cytoplasmic fluid. Others (D2) seem to inhibit adenylate cyclase. More complex classifications for dopamine receptors have been suggested, but no generally accepted schema has emerged.

The noradrenergic receptors are divisible into alpha and beta categories. The alpha-adrenoceptors are activated more potently by adrenalin and noradrenalin, whereas the beta-adrenoceptors are maximally activated by isoprenaline. The latter receptors can be further divided into beta$_1$, chiefly at cardiac sites, and beta$_2$, which occur elsewhere, including the bronchi. Alpha-adrenoceptors have also been subclassified, but alpha$_1$-adrenoceptors are postsynaptic and alpha$_2$-adrenoceptors are presynaptic. Both alpha- and beta-adrenoceptors can be excitatory or inhibitory, depending on the location. The brain appears to possess both alpha- and beta- adrenoceptors, but their characteristics are not always entirely typical.

Pathways

Dopamine receptors and, possibly, dopaminergic neurons are found in the vomiting centre (area postrema). Thus, dopaminergic blockade exerts an antiemetic effect. In the brain stem, dopaminergic neurons emanate from what are termed the A8- and A9-region cell bodies in the pars compacta of the substantia nigra. These dopamine cell bodies merge imperceptibly with the A10-region cells located in the medial region above the interpeduncular nucleus (Horn *et al.* 1979) (Fig 3.2).

The axons of A8 and A9 cells form the nigrostriatal pathway, which runs in the crus cerebri and internal capsule to innervate the caudate nucleus, putamen, globus pallidus, and, possibly, the amygdala. This is the pathway that degenerates in idiopathic parkinsonism and those forms of the disorder that follow exposure to toxic substances such as carbon monoxide and MPTP. Antipsychotic drugs produce the parkinsonian syndrome by competitively blockading the dopamine receptors on the cholinergic interneurons in the striatum. The motor abnormalities such as stereotyped movements induced by amphetamines are mediated through excessive dopaminergic activity in the basal ganglia.

The A10 cell bodies form the mesolimbic projection system, which runs

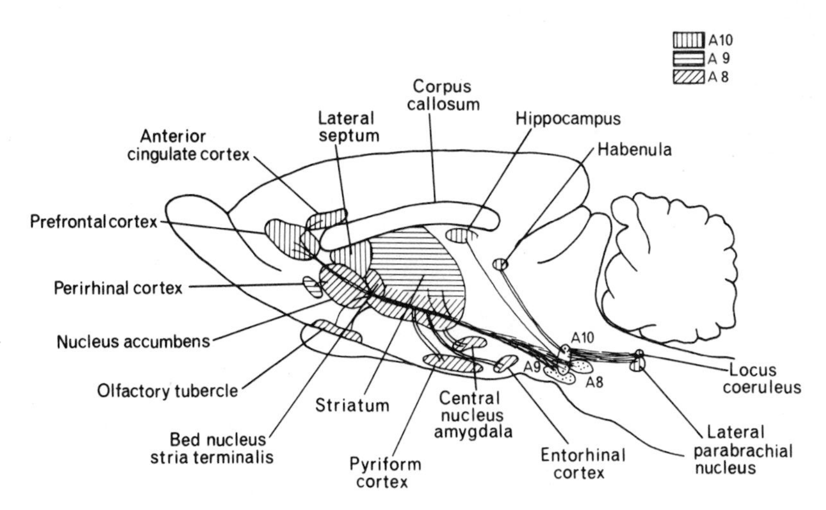

Figure 3.2. Schematic diagram of main dopaminergic pathways emanating from cell groups A8, A9, and A10. (Modified from Cooper *et al.* 1986, with permission.)

more medially to terminate in the nucleus accumbens just anterior to the caudate, the olfactory tubercle, the septum, and related areas. This tract is believed to act in the regulation of emotional behaviour, especially its motor components. Axons from A10 neurons and from the medial part of the A9 group also project to the frontal, cingulate, and entorhinal cortices. Thus, dopaminergic synapses influence the highest levels of cerebral function.

Several short dopaminergic pathways run close to the midline from the central grey area to various nuclei in the thalamus and hypothalamus (Fig 3.3). The best-defined short tract is the tuberoinfundibular, with its cell bodies in the arcuate nucleus and its axons running into the median eminence and pars intermedia of the pituitary. The tuberoinfundibular tract inhibits the release of prolactin from the anterior pituitary. Thus, dopamine agonists decrease prolactin concentrations whereas dopamine antagonists such as antipsychotic drugs elevate them. Other short dopaminergic pathways are the incertohypothalamic, which links the hypothalamus and lateral septum, and the medullary periventricular, in the periaqueductal grey matter. Dopamine is found also in the retina and olfactory bulb.

All noradrenergic cell bodies are confined to the hindbrain, in the pons and medulla. A1, A2, and A5 cells are located in the ventral medulla and project both to the spinal cord and rostrally.

The clearest cell-body grouping is the locus coeruleus, the 'blue site,' situated in the floor of the fourth ventricle. It constitutes A6 cells, with A7 cells located ventrolaterally to it and A4 cells just caudally. The locus coeruleus contains the most abundant noradrenergic cell population. It receives input from the periphery (Svensson 1987), and is responsible for noradrenergic innervation of all the cortices, geniculate bodies, colliculi, thalamus, and all parts of the hypothalamus (Moore and Bloom 1979) (Fig. 3.4).

The rostral projection pathways are the dorsal and the ventral. The dorsal

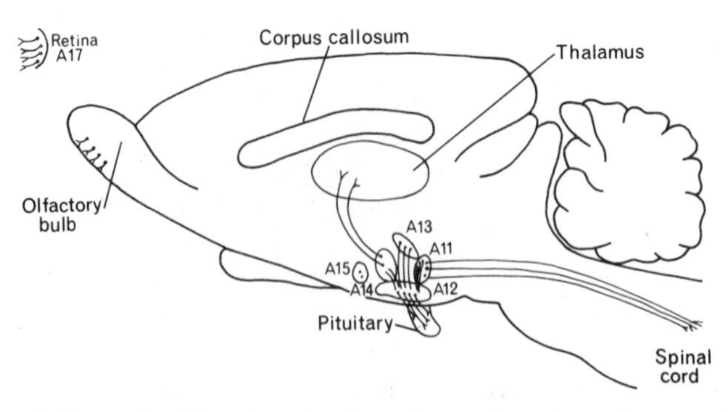

Figure 3.3. Schematic diagram of other dopaminergic pathways. (Modified from Cooper *et al.* 1986, with permission.)

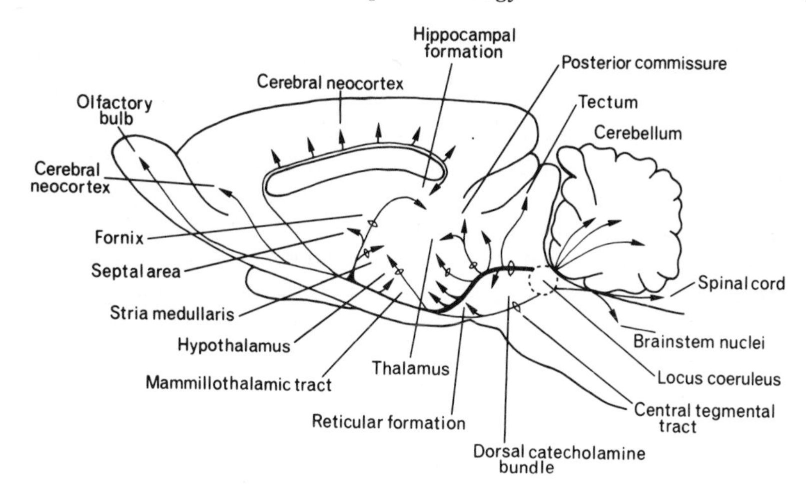

Figure 3.4. Schematic diagram of main noradrenergic pathways. (Modified from Cooper *et al.* 1986, with permission.)

pathway starts in the locus coeruleus and projects ventrolaterally to the central grey area. Its main component runs in the medial forebrain bundle to innervate all the cortices, the thalamus, geniculate bodies, colliculi, habenula, some hypothalamic nuclei, and the olfactory bulb. The ventral pathway is formed from A1, A5, and A7 cell bodies and runs through the medullary reticular formation, the pons, and mesencephalon, gradually overlapping the dorsal bundle. It extends through the cuneate nucleus and the A8 cell region to innervate the septal area, preoptic area, hypothalamus, periventricular area, mammillary bodies, and substantia nigra. A4 cells caudal to the locus coeruleus probably project to the cerebellum. Yet another tract runs down into the spinal cord. At their terminals, the fibres of the locus coeruleus pass vertically towards the cortical surface and then form T-shaped branches that run parallel to the surface. Most amine release takes place away from synapses.

Drug mechanisms

Drugs that interact with the synthetic enzyme tyrosine hydroxylase profoundly alter catecholamine function. Tyrosine analogues such as alpha-methyl-*p*-tyrosine impair the synthesis of dopamine and noradrenalin by blocking this enzyme.

Precursor administration increases catecholamine synthesis, provided that tyrosine hydroxylase is bypassed. Thus, administration of L-dopa increases the synthesis of dopamine in dopaminergic neurons and of noradrenalin in noradrenergic neurons. Concomitant administration of a peripherally acting dopa decarboxylase inhibitor such as carbidopa or benserazide results in even higher brain concentrations of dopamine. Large doses of L-dopa also affect other neurotransmitters by swamping uptake mechanisms and enzymes. Conversely, the administration of alpha-methyldopa results in the synthesis of alpha-methylnoradrenalin, which acts as a false transmitter to diminish central noradrenergic function, with hypotension and sedation. The storage of catecholamines is disrupted by reserpine and tetrabenazine, which interfere with the mechanism whereby catecholamines are transported from the cytoplasmic pool into the granules.

Many sympathomimetic agents act indirectly by displacing noradrenalin from its granule stores without impairing synthesis. Ephedrine and amphetamine are important examples. Tyramine also releases noradrenalin, but probably by displacement from the mobile pool. These drugs exhibit tachyphylaxis, that is, their effects diminish on repeated administration as the catecholamine pools become depleted.

The major inactivation pathway, re-uptake, is blocked by the tricyclic antidepressants and related drugs. These compounds affect the catecholamines and serotonin to varying extents: the re-uptake of dopamine is usually least impaired. Cocaine and amphetamine can also inhibit re-uptake whereas lithium may facilitate it.

Monoamine oxidase inhibition results in a failure to catabolize catecholamines in the cytoplasmic pool. The catecholamines are therefore available for uptake into the stores and subsequent release. Monoamine oxidase exists in two forms, A and B. Noradrenalin is inactivated mostly by type A, and dopamine by both types. No known drugs effectively block COMT.

Many drugs act directly on catecholamine receptors. Dopamine agonists include apomorphine, piribedil, and bromocriptine, whereas the antipsychotic drugs are very effective dopamine antagonists, acting by blockade of the receptors. Agonists on the alpha-adrenoceptor include noradrenalin and the directly acting sympathomimetic agents, phenylephrine and phenylpropanolamine; beta-adrenoceptor agonists include isoprenaline, terbutaline, isoxsuprine, and salbutamol. The alpha-adrenoceptors are blocked by phenoxybenzamine, phentolamine, some ergot alkaloids, and some antipsychotic agents such as chlorpromazine and haloperidol. Beta-adrenoceptor blockade is the main action of the large and important group of drugs such as propranolol. Some beta-adrenoceptor blocking agents preferentially affect beta$_1$- or beta$_2$-receptors. Similarly, specificity is shown by alpha$_1$- and alpha$_2$-receptor agonists and antagonists.

5-Hydroxytryptamine (serotonin)

It was known for a long time that a vasoconstrictor substance was present in the plasma; the substance, named serotonin, was identified over 30 years ago as 5-hydroxytryptamine (5-HT) and found to be widely distributed in the body.

Synthesis, storage, and release

The precursor of 5-HT is the essential amino acid tryptophan, an indolic compound. Tryptophan is the only amino acid bound largely to plasma albumin, and it is taken up into the brain by an active transport process. Plasma concentrations of tryptophan fluctuate diurnally, and the diurnal rhythms may affect synthesis of 5-HT in the brain. Hydroxylation by the enzyme tryptophan hydroxylase to 5-hydroxytryptophan then takes place. This is the rate-limiting step, and concentrations of tryptophan are normally below maximal so that the availability of tryptophan and the extent of its binding to plasma proteins govern the amount of neurotransmitter synthesized. The 5-hydroxytryptophan is decarboxylated by L-aromatic amino acid decarboxylase to 5-HT (Table 3.5).

Like the catecholamines, 5-HT is taken up and stored in granules at the presynaptic ending. The storage is in association with adenine nucleotides, mainly ATP. Some 5-HT probably exists in a mobile extragranular pool. Other tissues such as blood platelets can take up and store 5-HT. The discharge of 5-HT into the synaptic cleft is by ionic activation and exocytosis.

Inactivation

Re-uptake into nerve terminals is the primary route of inactivation of 5-HT. The process is energy dependent and can work against a considerable concentration gradient. Similar uptake mechanisms exist in the blood platelet, which has been proposed as an accessible model in man of central serotonergic processes.

Intracytoplasmic 5-HT can form a substrate for monoamine oxidase, especially type A. The substrate converts 5-HT into 5-hydroxyindoleacetaldehyde, which can then be oxidized by aldehyde dehydrogenase to the acidic metabolite, 5-hydroxyindoleacetic acid (5-HIAA). Like those of HVA and VMA, the egress of 5-HIAA from the cerebrospinal fluid can be blocked by probenecid, thus giving a rough measure of 5-HT turnover.

Table 3.5. Synthesis and breakdown of 5-HT

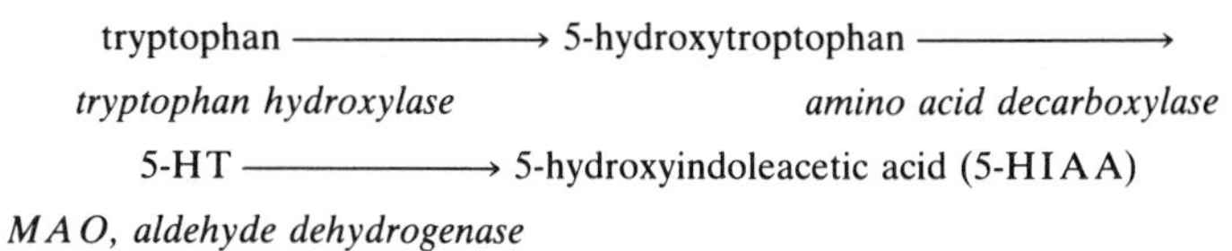

Receptors

There is some evidence that different types (5-HT_1 and 5-HT_2 and 5-HT_3) or at least different configurations of receptor exist (Tricklebank 1987). Yet further subdivisions, e.g. 5-HT_{1a}, 5-HT_{1b} etc., have been proposed. The physiological roles of some of these receptors are unclear (Conn and Sanders-Bush 1987).

Pathways

The serotonergic pathways stem from cell bodies designated groups B1 to B9, situated mainly in the midline raphe nuclei (Fig 3.5). B3, B6, and B9 are situated a little more laterally to the raphe nuclei. The rostral projections are not clearly known, but diffuse innervation to the forebrain, possibly through a projection in the medial forebrain bundle, has been shown. Serotonergic fibres project from the raphe to the limbic system (hippocampus and amygdala), lateral geniculate, and superior colliculus (Molliver 1987). Another serotonergic pathway runs caudally from midline regions in the brain stem to innervate the spinal cord (Baumgarten and Schlossberger 1984).

Drug mechanisms

The synthesizing enzyme tryptophan hydroxylase can be blocked by *p*-chlorophenylalanine, thus decreasing concentrations of 5-HT. Conversely, L-tryptophan can be administered and will increase 5-HT concentrations in the brain. However, large doses are needed to attain this, possibly interfering with the brain uptake of other amino acids. The administration of 5-hydroxytryptophan can also increase 5-HT synthesis. As it does with the catecholamines, reserpine depletes the nerve endings of 5-HT and prevents its storage (Fuller 1980).

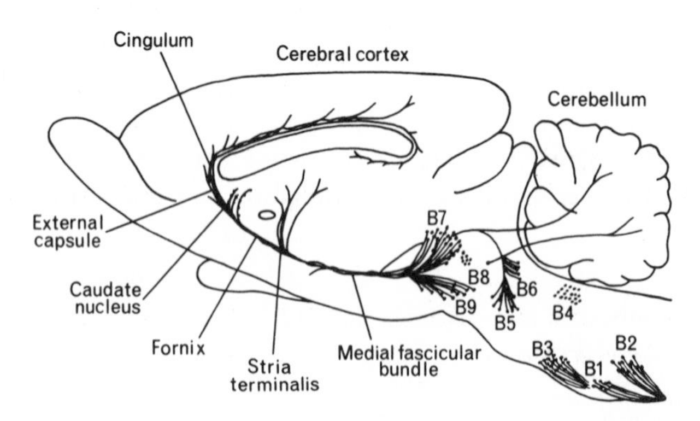

Figure 3.5. Schematic diagram of main serotoninergic pathways. (Modified from Cooper *et al.* 1986, with permission.)

The re-uptake of 5-HT into the presynaptic endings and vesicles can be blocked by some of the tricyclic antidepressants such as clomipramine and amitriptyline. Monoamine oxidase inhibitors increase 5-HT concentrations by preventing the breakdown of the intracytoplasmic pool.

Hallucinogens such as LSD and mescaline have complex actions on 5-HT systems. These drugs inhibit serotoninergic cell firing, probably by blocking autoreceptors on these cells. Hallucinogens have much less effect on tryptaminergic postsynaptic receptors. Non-hallucinogenic analogues such as methysergide show no such selectivity, blocking both types of receptor. Cyproheptadine is a potent 5-HT (and histaminic) receptor antagonist. Recently, several different types of anxiolytic or putative anxiolytic have been developed which act on one or other of the 5-HT receptor subtypes.

Gamma-aminobutyric acid (GABA)

GABA was identified first as an important constituent of the crustacean nervous system and later of the mammalian central nervous system. GABA eventually proved to be a powerful inhibitor and has fulfilled most of the criteria for a neurotransmitter (Tapia 1983). Progress in research has been slow because of the lack of drugs acting specifically on GABA mechanisms. It has been estimated that 40 per cent of synapses in the brain are 'GABAergic', making GABA the most ubiquitous neurotransmitter.

Synthesis, storage, and release

GABA is synthesized by decarboxylation of the amino acid glutamic acid by the enzyme glutamic acid decarboxylase (GAD) (Table 3.6). GAD seems to be localized exclusively in neurons that contain GABA. GABA appears to be apportioned into several 'pools', with newly synthesized GABA being released preferentially over stored GABA. The release of GABA in response to electrical stimulation is dependent on calcium ions.

Inactivation

Like the monoamine transmitters, GABA is taken back into the presynaptic nerve endings by a high-affinity uptake mechanism. Enzymic breakdown

Table 3.6. Synthesis and breakdown of GABA

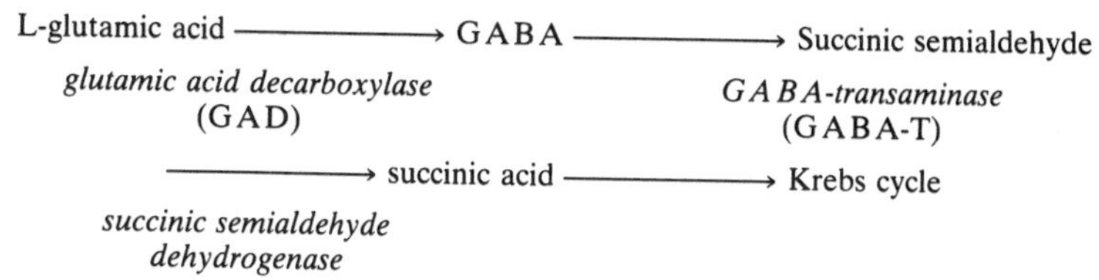

entails transamination to succinic semialdehyde by GABA: glutamate aminotransferase. This mitochondrial enzyme is widespread in the central nervous system in both neurons and glial cells. The next step is oxidation to succinic acid by succinic semialdehyde dehydrogenase, the succinic acid then entering the Krebs cycle.

Receptors

The brain contains many short interneurons, many of which appear to be inhibitory in function. GABA is the neurotransmitter in many instances. Postsynaptic GABA receptors have been detected in brain extracts and in the spinal cord. GABA may act as well on presynaptic receptors to inhibit the release of some other neurotransmitters. GABA receptors have been classified as $GABA_A$ and $GABA_B$. It is believed that $GABA_A$ receptors are close to chloride ionophore channels and that GABA influences their opening. Thus, GABA would stabilize the resting membrane potential near the choride equilibrium level, producing inhibition.

Pathways

GABA nerve endings are active in both presynaptic and postsynaptic inhibition in the spinal cord. These pathways seem in part to descend from the medulla and short interneurons also participate. The Purkinje cells of the cerebellum are GABA neurons and are themselves under inhibitory influences from other short GABA interneurons in the cerebellar cortex. The entire output of the cerebellar cortex is through the GABA inhibitory axons of the Purkinje cells to the deep cerebellar and vestibular nuclei. Another GABA pathway originates in the caudate nucleus and terminates in the substantia nigra, exerting an inhibitory influence on the nigrostriatal dopaminergic neurons. GABA neurons are widespread throughout the brain, including the cortices. Inhibitory influences are believed to be exerted more specifically on the noradrenergic locus coeruleus cells and the serotoninergic cells of the raphe nuclei. Dopaminergic (mesolimbic) and cholinergic projection pathways are also thought to be influenced by GABA inhibition.

Drug mechanisms

Some convulsants are believed to inhibit GABA synthesis, and many other drugs interfere with the GABA uptake mechanism. The anticonvulsant drug sodium valproate may slow GABA breakdown by inhibiting succinic semialdehyde dehydrogenase.

The research alkaloid muscimol is a specific receptor agonist, whereas bicuculline and picrotoxin are receptor antagonists. The benzodiazepines potentate the actions of GABA in a complex way.

Other neurotransmitters

The amino acid glycine is a strong candidate as an inhibitory neurotransmitter in the spinal cord (Daly and Aprison 1983). One of strychnine's actions is powerful antagonism of glycine receptors.

Glutamic acid and aspartic acid, both dicarboxylic amino acids, have widespread excitatory functions in the crustacean and mammalian nervous systems and fulfil many of the criteria for a neurotransmitter role (Cotman *et al.* 1981; Foster and Fagg 1987).

There has been much interest in the possible neuroregulatory functions of polypeptides (Krieger 1983). Some, such as oxytocin, vasopressin, luteinizing-hormone-releasing hormone (LH-RH), thyrotropin-releasing hormone (TRH), and growth-hormone-release-inhibiting hormone (somatostatin), are released by the hypothalamus and transported by the hypophyseal portal system to the anterior pituitary, where they regulate endocrine secretions. However, these releasing factors are found in other areas of the brain and may 'modulate' neurotransmission, i.e. modify neuronal responses to other neurotransmitters. ACTH also seems to have functions in the central nervous system and is distributed in the hypothalamus and limbic system. Substance P has a definite distribution in the brain and spinal cord and may be implicated in pain transmission. In Huntington's chorea, substance P concentrations in the substantia nigra are decreased. Other peptides found in the central nervous system include neurotensin, vasoactive intestinal peptide (VIP), cholecystokinin, bradykinin, and angiotensin II. The central nervous system functions of these peptides, many of which were originally discovered in the gut, remain unclear. Some may have antipsychotic properties (Verhoeven and Van Ree 1987).

Finally, one of the most important developments in recent years has been clarification of the mechanisms of narcotic drugs. Specific binding sites for opioids have been found in the central nervous system, particularly in sites known to be associated with pain transmission. Specific narcotic antagonists such as naloxone also bind to these receptor sites with high affinity.

The endogenous ligand or neurotransmitter eluded identification for about a year and was then reported by Hughes and Kosterlitz to be two pentapeptides that they termed 'enkephalins'. It was noted that the amino acid sequence of one of the enkephalins occurred in fragments of beta-lipotropin, a pituitary polypeptide believed to be the precursor of beta-melanocyte-stimulating hormone.

The fragments were termed 'endorphins', to indicate any endogenous substance having the pharmacologic properties of morphine. Three endorphins were identified: alpha-, beta-, and gamma-. The primary stored product in the brain is beta-endorphin. Other endorphins containing the amino acid sequence of the other enkephalins have also been described (Bloom 1983).

The next steps entailed the use of highly sophisticated research techniques developed by protein chemists and molecular geneticists. Pituitary cells were found to contain a large peptide that seemed to be a combined precursor to both beta-endorphin and ACTH. The peptide, termed pro-opiocortin (or 31K, its molecular weight), is apparently processed by corticotrophs in the pituitary to form ACTH and an inactive form of beta-endorphin and by intermediate lobe cells to form an inactive corticotropin and beta-endorphin.

The structure of 31K was then identified through the use of now-standard molecular genetic techniques to analyse the nucleic acid sequence of the DNA by which 31K is synthesized. Such work revealed the presence in 31K of yet a third polypeptide, gamma-MSH (melanocyte-stimulating hormone).

This example of the use of techniques derived from molecular biology and genetics will undoubtedly be the harbinger of a major shift in emphasis of a substantial proportion of neuropharmacology away from classical biochemical pharmacology towards molecular studies. Because of the importance of peptide molecules in influencing neuronal function, such a change can have an immediate impact and highly specific compounds can be synthesized to modify neuronal function. These techniques are currently being extensively applied and it should not be too long before the findings can be translated into practical therapeutic advances.

References

Baumgarten, H.G. and Schlossberger, H.G. (1984). Anatomy and function of central serotonergic neurons. In *Progress in tryptophan and serotonin research* (eds. H.G. Schlossberger, W. Kochen, B. Linzen, and H. Steinhart) pp. 173–88. Walter de Gruyter, Berlin.

Bloom, F.E. (1983). The endorphins: a growing family of pharmacologically pertinent peptides. *Annual Review of Pharmacology and Toxicology* **23,** 151–70.

Conn, P.J. and Sanders-Bush, E. (1987). Central serotonin receptors: effector systems, physiological roles and regulation. *Psychopharmacology* **92,** 267–77.

Cooper, J.R., Bloom, F.E., and Roth, R.H. (1986). *The biochemical basis of neuropharmacology* (5th edn). Oxford University Press, New York.

Cotman, C.W., Foster, A.C., and Lanthorn, T. (1981). An overview of glutamate as a neurotransmitter. *Advances in Biochemical Psychopharmacology (New York)* **27,** 1–27.

Cuello, A.C. and Sofroniew, M.V. (1984). The anatomy of the CNS cholinergic neurons. *Trends in Neuroscience* **7,** 74–7.

Daly, E.C. and Aprison, M.H. (1983). Glycine. In *Handbook of Neurochemistry* (ed. A. Lajtha) Vol. 3, pp. 467–99. Plenum Press, New York.

Dunant, Y. and Israel, M. (1985). The release of acetylcholine. *Scientific American* **252,** 58–66.

Foster, A.C. and Fagg, G.E. (1987). Taking apart NMDA receptors. *Nature* **329,** 395–6.

Fuller, R.W. (1980). Pharmacology of central serotonin neurons. *Annual Review of Pharmacology and Toxicology* **20,** 111–27.

Gibson, C.J. (1985). Control of monoamine synthesis by precursor availability. In *Handbook of neurochemistry* (ed. A. Lajtha) Vol. 8, pp. 309–24. Plenum Press, New York.

Horn, A.S., Korf, J. and Westerink, B.H.C. (eds.) (1979). *The neurobiology of dopamine*. Academic Press, New York.

Kito, S., Segawa, T., Kuriyama, K., Yamamura, H.I. and Olsen, R.W. eds. (1984). *Neurotransmitter receptors*. Plenum Press, New York.

Krieger, D.T. (1983). Brain peptides: what, where, and why? *Science* **222,** 975–85.

Iversen, L.L. (1982). Neurotransmitters and CNS disease. *Lancet* **2,** 914–18.

Massoulie, J. and Bon, S. (1982). The molecular forms of cholinesterase and acetylcholinesterase in vertebrates. *Annual Review of Neuroscience* **5,** 57–106.

Molliver, M.E. (1987). Serotonergic neuronal systems: what their anatomic organization tells us about function. *Journal of Clinical Psychopharmacology* **7,** 3S-23S.

Moore, R.Y. and Bloom, F.E. (1978). Central catecholamine neuron systems: anatomy and physiology of the dopamine systems. *Annual Review of Neuroscience* **1,** 129–69.

Siggins, G.R. and Gruol, D.L. (1986). Synaptic mechanisms in the vertebrate central nervous system. In *Handbook of physiology, intrinsic regulatory systems of the brain*, Vol. IV (ed. F.E. Bloom). American Physiological Society, Bethesda, MD.

Snyder, S.H. and Goodman, R.R. (1980). Multiple neurotransmitter receptors. *Journal of Neurochemistry* **35,** 5–15.

Svensson, T.H. (1987). Peripheral autonomic regulation of locus coeruleus noradrenergic neurons in brain: putative implications for psychiatry and psychopharmacology. *Psychopharmacology* **92,** 1–7.

Tapia, R. (1983). γ-Aminobutyric acid: metabolism and biochemistry of synaptic transmission. In *Handbook of neurochemistry*, 2nd edn. (ed. A. Lajtha) Vol. 3, pp. 423–66. Plenum Press, New York.

Tricklebank, M.D. (1987). Subtypes of 5-HT receptors. *Journal of Psychopharmacology* **1,** 222–6.

Verhoeven, W.M.A. and Van Ree, J.M. (1987). Antipsychotic properties of neuroleptic-like neuropeptides in schizophrenia: a clinical review. *Human Psychopharmacology* **2,** 137–49.

4. Behavioural Studies in Animals and Humans

As well as providing techniques for use in the development of new drugs and other therapies, psychopharmacology has used those techniques to derive a large body of knowledge concerning the effects of drugs (Sudilovsky *et al.* 1975). This chapter will focus on the former and outline behavioural methods used in the assessment of psychotropic drugs in animals and man.

Studies in animals

Behaviour is the product of a host of internal and external factors and it is not surprising that it has proved difficult to develop valid models of abnormal behaviour in animals (Horovitz 1975). Two kinds of animal model of mental illness can be distinguished. The first attempts the daunting task of trying to create in animals a behavioural disorder akin to that in man. Such models must possess, in common with the human disorder similar inducing conditions, behavioural states produced, underlying neurobiological mechanisms, and reversal by effective treatments. As many of these factors are poorly understood for the human condition, it is inevitable that few models of this type exist.

The second type is more distantly related to the human condition and is established empirically. In general, these animal models are selectively sensitive to treatments effective in one particular human disorder. Examples of the latter type of model will be presented with respect to psychosis, depressive disorders, and anxiety.

Models of psychotic behaviour

As described in the previous chapter, antipsychotic drugs affect dopamine disposition, and the search for newer compounds has concentrated on tests designed to detect such effects. One set of tests, the pharmacological, use the known action of drugs as the baseline and investigate the new compound with respect to its interactions. Other tests are more neuroanatomical in that they exploit the known effects of interfering with specific dopaminergic pathways (Iversen 1987).

Prime examples of the former are tests which measure various aspects of amphetamine-induced behaviour. In the intact rat small doses of amphetamine induce running; larger doses produce a characteristic pattern of motor behaviour, termed stereotypy in which isolated elements of motor behaviour, e.g. grooming, are monotonously repeated. All antipsychotic drugs block stereotypy.

An example combining pharmacological and anatomical techniques is the nigro-striatal lesioned preparation. When this tract is cut on one side of the brain, the animal will respond to amphetamine by turning towards the side of the lesion, and to apomorphine by turning away. There is by and large a good correlation between the potency of antipsychotic drugs in biochemical terms and their ability to prevent turning behaviour.

However, these models are probably more relevant as models of the motor disorders induced by antipsychotic drugs than any effects on higher functions. Lesions of the mesolimbic cortical dopamine system can be induced with the neurotoxin, 6-hydroxydopamine, resulting in supersensitivity of the dopamine receptors as assessed behaviourally. A variety of drugs can be tested using this preparation.

Serotonin pathways have also been evaluated. A hyperactivity syndrome can be induced by treatment with tryptophan in combination with a monoamine oxidase inhibitor. The behavioural picture includes exploration, head weaving and circling movements, together with piloerection, proptosis, salivation, and shivering. Inhibitors of 5-HT synthesis, but not of catecholamines, block this syndrome. However, dopaminergic mechanisms are also involved, probably downstream of the 5-HT pathways. Another hyperactivity syndrome follows lesions in the ventral tegmental area of the rat, and again, both dopamine and 5-HT are involved.

Models of depressive syndromes

A wide range of approaches has been popular in setting up models of depression (Willner 1984; Jesberger and Richardson 1985). Work on maternal deprivation in monkeys stems from clinical observations that in children removal of the mother induces three behavioural stages in the child—hyperactivity, despair, and withdrawal. An extensive literature, mainly ethological, has developed describing the effects of separation from the mother on infant monkeys. Social influences on the severe psychological disturbances which ensue were an especial focus of research. Rats also show behavioural abnormalities if reared from weaning in social isolation. Although there is general agreement that such developmental models are of relevance to clinical conditions, it is probable that the clinical conditions modelled are child psychoses and autism rather than adult depressive disorders.

Another model which excited much attention was the 'learned helplessness' model of Seligman (1975). Dogs exposed to unavoidable electric shock could not learn to avoid shocks later; instead they remained still and appeared helpless. However, marked species differences exist and one form of unavoidable punishment may generate data different from other forms. However, in rats at least, antidepressant drugs reduce the severity of the learned helplessness syndrome.

Other models include the well-known biochemical technique using amine depleters such as reserpine, and studies of diurnal rhythms in endocrine and other physiological functions.

The olfactory bulbectomy model of depression in the rat has the interesting property of only detecting antidepressant activity after chronic administration of the drug (Leonard and Tuite 1981). Some GABA-ergic compounds are active in this model but may have antidepressant activity in the clinic. Trazodone is the only antidepressant compound established clinically which is inactive in this model.

Models of anxiety

One set of models evaluate the decrease in behavioural responding when animals are punished (Treit 1985). Refinements of these techniques involve operant conditioning. For example, in the Geller–Seifter procedure, rats lever-press for a reward. Once established, such responses can be suppressed by electric shocks and the suppression reversed by anxiolytic drugs. Most antipsychotic drugs fail to increase punished responding, and pain-suppression is not the mechanism as opioids are ineffective.

No other behavioural test matches the predictive ability of the Geller–Seifter test. Other paradigms were studied such as the conditioned emotional response. In this behavioural situation, an animal is trained to respond for food. Then a discriminating stimulus is introduced and its termination marked by the presentation of an electric shock. Under these conditions, responding is markedly reduced during the discriminative stimulus and this suppression is interpreted as due to anxiety associated with anticipation of an unavoidable shock. This model has not proved very useful.

Another test of greater predictive validity is the social interaction test (File 1980). This involves placing two male rats in situations where familiarity with the test box and level of illumination can be varied independently. Active social interactions decrease as unfamiliarity or light level is increased. This effect is reversible by anxiolytic drugs.

Recently, anxiolytic substances have been used to induce models of anxiety. The beta-carbolines provide fairly convincing states of anxiety in primates and these states are prevented by benzodiazepines. Whether this reversal is a property of non-benzodiazepine anxiolytics as well has not been established.

Studies in humans

As the above sections show, behavioural studies in animals have attempted to set up empirical models which bear some validity to mental illness with respect to prediction of treatment response. In general, behavioural studies in humans have not sought such goals, except perhaps in models of anxiety and, recently, drug-induced models of memory impairment. Rather, test batteries have been assembled to quantify the effects of psychotropic drugs on psychological functioning (Hindmarch 1980). Generally those effects are unwanted side effects, and normal subjects have been used to evaluate such effects without the complicating factor of change related to any psychiatric illness. Of course, use of normal subjects raises questions about the generalizability of the information to patient populations but, as a general rule, quite good predictions can be made concerning the type, severity, and persistence of side effects.

There are literally hundreds of different types of psychological tests and some of them are widely used. Most have been well standardized, yet maverick researchers alter the parameters without proper justification. This is unfortunate, as it prevents close comparisons between the data from different centres. Naturally, each test has to be evaluated for its sensitivity to drug response if it is being used as a correlate of drug action, but this is quite straightforward: dose–effect curves provide powerful tools of drug sensitivity.

Many considerations govern the choice of test procedures. It is important that the test be within the capabilities of the individual to be tested, not only when drug-free but particularly when under the influence of a depressant drug; otherwise a 'floor' effect is attained. Conversely, too easy a test or one performed normally at maximal capacity will fail to show stimulant drug actions because of a 'ceiling' effect. Tests which are time-consuming may be inappropriate because they cannot be incorporated into an already lengthy battery and are not suitable for short-acting drugs. Tests may interfere with each other. Thus, a vigilance task may prove so soporific that subsequent motivation is reduced.

Many tests involve learning, in that performance improves with repeated administration. Training to a plateau of achievement can be time-consuming. Or a test may require elaborate training on the part of the researcher or the provision of expensive equipment.

It is wise to construct a battery of tests and not to rely on one or two old favourites. Equally, tests which repeatedly fail to show drug effects should be discarded since they merely add 'noise' to the test system. Various types of behavioural assessment will now be briefly reviewed.

Assessment of sensory function and processing

Sensory thresholds are not very susceptible to psychotropic drug effects. More complex sensory functions are affected. Detection, perception, and recognition of a stimulus are three aspects which have been extensively studied. Tests include a continuous attention task in which subjects have to press a key which matches a number display, and one in which subjects have to detect one letter in random sequences of letters presented at a constant rate. Both errors and latency to response are quantifiable. However, these tests, despite their apparent simplicity, do involve higher mental functions, because of the use of numbers or letters. More basic sensory tests use simple auditory tones as discriminative stimuli.

Cancellation tests which involve the minimum of motor response are also sensitive to drugs. One such task involves cancelling forty 4s randomly set within a block of 400 numbers. More complex tasks, e.g. cancelling 4s only when they precede 3s, seem if anything less sensitive.

One sensory test which has been widely used is the Stroop Test, in which letters of one colour are formed into the name of another colour. For example, RED is printed in blue. A long delay can be induced in subjects calling out the colour. However, this test is more used as a stress-inducing task rather than as a psychopharmacological one.

Staring at ambiguous figures with two distinct perspectives such as the 'falling staircase' or Necker cube produces spontaneous reversals, the rate of which can show psychotropic drug effects. Subjective estimates of the elapse of time are also affected by some drugs.

Assessment of central processing ability

One of the most widely-used and sensitive tests of this type is the Digit Symbol Substitution Test, a subtest of the Wechsler Adult Intelligence Scale. In this, the subject is provided with a key of numbers and simple symbols. Then he is given 90 seconds in which to code as many numbers as possible into symbols. Some control for the motor component can be provided by asking the subject merely to copy as many symbols as possible within that time.

A frequently used test which assesses the level of integration ability of the CNS is the critical flicker fusion threshold (CFFT). The frequency of a flickering light is increased until the subject reports seeing it continuously. It is then slowed until flickering resumes. The flicker frequency provides a measure of control integration or 'arousal', the higher the frequency, the more the arousal. An auditory equivalent (flutter fusion) is less popular.

Central processing can be assessed in several ways. Simple arithmetic, serial subtraction, and concept identification tasks have all been used.

Memory and learning tasks have been extensively developed recently because of interest in the amnestic effects of many psychotropic drugs (Curran 1986) and the growing importance of dementia. Although many theoretical debates continue on the 'organization' of memory, the distinction between long- and short-term memory is still widely acknowledged. A wide range of tasks has been developed or adapted for use in psychopharmacological studies, and includes work recall, learning of nonsense syllables, digit span, logical memory, reproduction of geometric figures, and cued recall.

Assessment of motor function

Simple repetitive tapping is quite sensitive to both depressant and stimulant drugs. But, like several other tests of apparent simplicity, motivation and even practice effects can exert an influence. Gross body movement can be assessed by steadiness tests: the stabilometer comprises a balanced platform on which the subject stands, and the ataxiameter comprises a transducer which measures the excursions of a string clipped to the subject's belt. Localized unsteadiness can be assessed by holding a stylus in an opening or by measuring tremor with an accelerometer transducer attached to an extremity.

Handwriting, an overlearned skill, can be assessed in terms of length of a standard passage or height of standard letters. It is particularly sensitive to the extrapyramidal effects of antipsychotic drugs.

A variety of tests measure motor manipulation abilities. These include placing pegs in a peg board and picking up ball-bearings with tweezers. Practice effects are common.

Assessment of sensorimotor performance

Some of the above tests sample selected aspects of behavioural functioning whose relevance to everyday tasks is not immediately apparent. Tests of sensorimotor function assess complex integrative 'input–processing–output' abilities. One of the simplest is reaction time to a stimulus, usually auditory or visual. However, as perusal of the reaction time literature shows, this is a deceptively simple task which can be elaborated into choice and multiple reaction time tasks with fore periods, and so on. It can be combined with EEG evoked potential studies. Generally speaking, reaction time tasks are drug-sensitive.

Another task which combines sensory, central and motor components is card-sorting into categories. Although conventional playing cards are often used, it is possible to use cards with 2, 4, or 8 spots which accordingly contain 1, 2, or 3 'bits' of information, i.e. quite complex abilities can be assessed. The Gibson spiral maze and the pursuit rota task seem less drug-sensitive than does the card-sorting task.

Among the more complex, 'real-life' tasks is car-driving ability. This can be assessed by using car simulators in the laboratory, by driving on private roads such as a disused aerodrome, or by taking subjects out in dual-control cars. Various aspects of driving performance can be assessed, including steering, braking, and risk-taking. An even more complex task is assessment of flying ability in pilots using flight simulators. Of course, all these tests give only partial indications of how the drugged driver or pilot would react in a 'real' emergency.

Assessment of subjective states

A large literature is extant concerning scales for measuring clinical psychopathological states (Burdock *et al.* 1982; Hamilton 1986). However, surprisingly few scales have been developed to assess mood in normal subjects. Visual analogue scales are popular (e.g. Bond and Lader 1974). The subject is presented with a 100-mm line labelled at the extremes, e.g. 'anxious' – 'calm', and marks how he or she feels at the moment somewhere along the line. Other functions which can be assessed include bodily feelings, side effects, and sleep variables (Aylard *et al.* 1987).

Other techniques include adjective check lists, which are ticked 'yes' or 'no', and more elaborate questionnaires often derived from personality inventories (Glass *et al.* 1987).

Physiological measures

These are divisible roughly into the peripheral, central, and neuroendocrine (Lader 1975). Tests of autonomic function are essential in quantifying the side effects of many psychotropic drugs and may also give information concerning effects on neurotransmitter amines. Cardiovascular system function can be measured by recording heart rate, blood pressure, superficial hand vein pressure, skin temperature, baroreflex activity, and so on. Complex electrocardiographic techniques are becoming increasingly used. The blood pressure rise in response to intravenous tyramine gives an estimate of the integrity of catecholamine uptake mechanisms, because tyramine is an indirectly acting sympathomimetic amine.

Salivary gland activity can be assessed by measuring secretory volume with a suction cup over the orifice of the parotid duct or by measuring the increase in weight of dental rolls placed in the mouth. Gastric and colonic motility are feasible measures of gastrointestinal function. Pupil diameter, assessed photographically or by matching to a series of calibrated discs, is a useful measure. Accommodation and intraocular pressure are other measures of drug effects on the eye. Finally, sweating can be assessed by recording the number of active sweat glands or the electrical conductance in a standard area of skin.

Great activity has surrounded measures of central physiological functioning. The EEG has become easily quantifiable using laboratory computers, and can provide very sensitive measures of drug effects. For example, doses of benzodiazepine undetectable on behavioural tests increase fast-wave activity to a significant extent. The EEG is invaluable as an empirical indicator of drug actions of various types, enabling dose– and time–effect curves to be constructed. The interpretations of these actions is more problematical. Characteristic patterns in the EEG tend to be produced by various groups of psychotropic agents, but untypical patterns are encountered. Another aspect of the EEG which can be quantified is the evoked responses to discrete stimuli such as auditory tones or visual pattern reversals. Again, quite sensitive drug effects can be detected. Since much is known of the behavioural correlates of various components of the evoked responses, drug actions can be analysed.

Neuroendocrine measures are relevant to two aspects of drug effects, side effects and effects on neurotransmitter disposition (see also Chapter 5). The development of sensitive hormonal assays has led to the routine evaluation of psychotropic drugs in terms of their effects on such hormones as cortisol, prolactin, and growth hormone.

References

Aylard, P.R., Gooding, J.H., McKenna, P.J., and Snaith, R.P. (1987). A validation study of three anxiety and depression self-assessment scales. *Journal of Psychosomatic Research* **31,** 261–8.

Bond, A. and Lader, M.H. (1974). The use of analogue scales in rating subjective feelings. *British Journal of Medical Psychology* **47,** 211–18.

Burdock, E.I., Sudilovsky, A., and Gershon, S. (eds.) (1982). *The behavior of psychiatric patients. Qualitative techniques for evaluation*. Marcel Dekker, New York.

Curran, H.V. (1986). Tranquillizing memories: a review of the effects of benzodiazepines on human memory. *Biological Psychology* **23,** 179–213.

File, S.E. (1980). The use of social interaction as a method for detecting anxiolytic activity of chlordiazepoxide-like drugs. *Journal of Neuroscience Methods* **2,** 219–38.

Glass, R.M., Uhlenhuth, E.H., and Kellner, R. (1987). The value of self-report assessment in studies of anxiety disorders. *Journal of Clinical Psychopharmacology* **7,** 215–21.

Hamilton, M. (1986). Assessment of psychopathology. *Human Psychopharmacology* 1 (eds. I. Hindmarch and P.D. Stonier). John Wiley, Chichester.
Hindmarch, I. (1980). Psychomotor function and psychoactive drugs. *British Journal of Clinical Pharmacology* **10,** 189–209.
Horovitz, Z.P. (1975). Problems in predicting new psychotropic agents through studies in animals. In *Predictability in psychopharmacology: preclinical and clinical correlations* (eds. A. Sudilovsky, S. Gershon, and B. Beer) pp. 179–87. Raven Press, New York.
Iversen, S.D. (1987). Is it possible to model psychotic states in animals? *Journal of Psychopharmacology* **1,** 154–76.
Jesberger, J.A. and Richardson, J.S. (1985). Animal models of depression: parallels and correlates to severe depression in humans. *Biological Psychiatry* **20,** 764–84.
Lader, M.H. (1975). *The psychophysiology of mental illness*. Routledge & Kegan Paul, London.
Leonard, B.E. and Tuite, K. (1981). Anatomical, physiological and behavioural aspects of olfactory bulbectomy in the rat. *International Review of Neurobiology* **22,** 251–86.
Seligman, M.E.P. (1975). *Helplessness*. Freeman, San Francisco.
Sudilovsky, A., Gershon, S., and Beer, B. (eds.) (1975). *Predictability in psychopharmacology: preclinical and clinical correlations*. Raven Press, New York.
Treit, D. (1984). Animal models for the study of anti-anxiety agents: a review. *Neuroscience and Biobehavioral Reviews* **9,** 203–22.
Willner, P. (1984). The validity of animal models of depression. *Psychopharmacology* **83,** 1–16.

5. Biological Aspects of Psychiatry

This is in itself a huge topic. Reference should be made to the *Handbook of Biological Psychiatry* (van Praag *et al.* 1979) for a full, earlier account. Here we shall concentrate on areas within the larger topic which are most relevant to therapeutics.

Each of the main biological hypotheses of the mechanisms of psychiatric disorders—affective illness, schizophrenia, and anxiety—relies to a substantial extent on data accruing from therapeutic trials. However, it must be borne in mind constantly that the modes of action of most psychotropic drugs are still poorly understood. Consequently, elaborating hypotheses on the pathophysiology of disorder based on mechanisms of drug action is little more than attempting to explain one unknown in terms of another. Nevertheless, establishing such hypotheses has proved heuristic, at least in stimulating studies incorporating careful clinical observations. Developments in the symptomatology of chronic schizophrenia and in the nosology of the anxiety disorders owe much to observations made in the course of therapeutic studies.

The emphasis on biological processes in psychiatric disorders in this chapter should not lead to the impression that other influences, social, psychological, etc., are unimportant. Rather, it is the interaction between these various factors that would best repay careful analysis (Kidman 1985).

Biological hypotheses of affective disorders

The initial impetus to such theories was the clinical observation in the early 1950s that reserpine, a drug that depletes monoamines in nerve endings, often produced a depressive illness, or at the very least, definite psychomotor retardation. The idea arose that perhaps depression was due to a deficiency in biogenic amines (Silverstone and Cookson 1982). Conversely, mania was believed to be related in some way to a surfeit of these amines (Silverstone and Cookson 1982). Further support for this notion was forthcoming when it was discovered that both major groups of antidepressant drugs—the tricyclics and the monoamine oxidase inhibitors—increased the availability of the amines in the brains of animals. The former did this by blocking re-uptake, the latter by disrupting a major breakdown pathway (Potter 1984). Finally, some amine precursors have antidepressant properties (van Praag 1984).

The subsequent problem was demonstrating these presumed amine abnormalities in depressed patients. Technical difficulties abound, such as distinguishing between central and peripheral amine metabolites, controlling for mode of death in studies of patients committing suicide, taking into account concomitant medication, and so on. By and large, no convincing, reproducible biogenic amine abnormalities have been uncovered in depressed patients (Curzon 1988). Perhaps the most robust finding has been the demonstration that a subgroup of depressed patients with low CSF 5-HIAA concentrations are prone to show suicidal and perhaps aggressive behaviour (Editorial 1987). Even more limited objectives using amine measures, such as predicting which patient will respond to which antidepressant, have been unsuccessful.

More recently, elaborations of the simple biogenic amine hypothesis have been put forward. One suggests that subtypes of depression exist related to deficiencies in noradrenalin (catecholamine hypothesis) and 5-HT (serotonin hypothesis) respectively. Such speculations have prompted major research endeavours by the pharmaceutical industry with the development of selective NA and 5-HT reuptake blockers. No evidence has accrued regarding identifiable selectively responsive subgroups of depressives. Nor is efficacy improved over the standard tricyclics, although side effects and cardiotoxicity are generally much reduced.

Indeed, the whole value of re-uptake blockade and inhibition of amine metabolism as sufficient mechanisms to explain the mode of action of antidepressants has been questioned: (1) some clinically effective antidepressants have minimal effects on amine disposition; (2) biochemical effects rapidly supervene following administration of antidepressants yet clinical response is gradual or even delayed; (3) some effective uptake inhibitors, e.g. cocaine, are not effective antidepressants.

The search for more gradual biochemical effects of antidepressants led to the finding that postsynaptic beta-adrenergic receptors in the brain diminish in number following antidepressant treatment whether tricyclics, atypical compounds, MAOIs or even ECT. This 'down-regulation' is accompanied by a loss of sensitivity of adenylate cyclase to stimulation with a beta-sympathomimetic. In parallel, 5-HT_2 receptors are sensitized to 5-HT (Blier *et al.* 1987). Furthermore, close links seem to exist between noradrenergic and serotonergic systems; for example, the integrity of 5-HT systems is necessary for down-regulation of beta-receptors. Thus, the neurotransmitter receptor hypothesis has emerged which postulates that depressive illness is related to an abnormality in the regulation of neurotransmitter receptors (Stahl and Palazidou 1986). As the receptors are complex proteins, links to molecular biology are clear. The antidepressant drugs are postulated to correct this abnormality by regulating the number of receptors. Of course, many objections can be proferred to this hypothesis relating to the dangers of extrapolating from rat to human brain, the problems of assessing receptor function in humans, and the ease with which associations are viewed as cause and effect. Nevertheless, a number of interesting approaches to assessing receptor number and function have been adopted.

Post-mortem studies from patients who have committed suicide suggest that 5-HT uptake sites are decreased whereas 5-HT_2 binding sites are increased. However, clinical diagnosis and drug treatment are often unclear. Direct assessment in life of 5-HT binding using positron emission tomography (PET scan) is still in its infancy.

Neuroendocrine studies have attempted to assess receptor function in patients. This approach has been vaunted as a 'window into the brain', by measuring pituitary hormone release to a variety of probes (Roy *et al.* 1984). Some findings are replicable:

(1) some, but by no means all or exclusively, depressives show decreased sensitivity to the suppression of cortisol secretion by dexamethasone (Braddock 1986); drugs interfere with this response (Kraus *et al.* 1988);

(2) many depressives show decreased sensitivity to the stimulation of thyroid stimulating hormone (TSH) secretion by thyrotropin releasing hormone (TRH); and

(3) and decreased sensitivity to $beta_2$-adrenergic stimulation by clonidine of growth hormone secretion.

The level at which these decreased sensitivities are mediated is unclear, both primary mechanisms in the pituitary itself or secondary mechanisims in the monoaminergic pathways controlling hormone release being possible.

Because of difficulties investigating brain receptor function directly, models have been set up using circulating platelets and lymphocytes. This presupposes that receptor abnormalities occur throughout the body and implies a genetic mechanism. Human platelets have several receptor types such as $beta_2$-adrenergic and 5-HT, both uptake and 5-HT_2 sites. The 5-HT uptake receptor site seems to be significantly reduced in depressed patients but no consistent findings have emerged concerning the other types of receptor (Healy and Leonard 1987). Human lymphocytes possess $beta_2$-adrenergic receptors whose responsivity but not total number may be reduced in depression.

The search for amine and amine receptor changes in depression has led to a series of empirical findings which have suggested abnormalities in depression. To date, no coherent hypothesis has emerged. Nevertheless, these changes have suggested a whole series of therapeutic strategies for the treatment of depression which are still at the research stage. These include the use of beta-adrenergic agonists to directly down-regulate the beta-receptors, the use of drugs such as rolipram that interfere with second messenger systems beyond the receptors, combinations of drugs acting on both 5-HT and NA mechanisms (so much for the logic behind selective re-uptake inhibitors!), and adjuvant hormone therapies such as ACTH, ovarian hormones, and TSH.

The impression should not be left that only noradrenalin and 5-HT have been researched and are relevant to the biochemical pathogenesis of depression. Attention has also focused on acetylcholine, with respect to both depression and mania. It has been postulated on the basis of much data that a state of increased cholinergic muscarinic activity occurs in patients with primary affective disorder, both when ill and in remission (Sitaram *et al.* 1984).

Dopamine hypothesis of schizophrenia

This is another major hypothesis in biological psychiatry which stems from clinical observations, namely the efficacy of antipsychotic medication in controlling the symptoms of schizophrenia. That these drugs were at least as effective in controlling the symptoms of many other conditions such as mania, agitation, and organic states was glossed over, as were observations that some symptoms of schizophrenia were fairly unresponsive to antipsychotic medication.

An additional problem concerns the mode of action of antipsychotic drugs. The initial observation was that antipsychotic drugs enhanced the turnover of dopamine in rat brain in proportion to their clinical potencies. This augmented dopamine turnover was postulated as arising from dopamine receptor blockade interfering with inhibitory feedback mechanisms. Later studies confirmed this suggestion but only with respect to D_2 receptors, which were found to be blocked by both phenothiazines and butyrophenones with binding affinities proportional to clinical potencies. However, D_1 receptors did not seem relevant, as butyrophenones bound only weakly to them.

Antipsychotic drugs are fairly non-selective and block cholinergic, beta-adrenergic, serotonergic, and histaminergic receptors. However, binding affinities to these receptors do not correlate with clinical potencies.

Other drugs which lessen dopaminergic activity also have antipsychotic properties. They include reserpine which depletes nerve endings of dopamine and other amines, low doses of apomorphine which inhibit dopamine release, and alpha-methyl-para-tyrosine, which inhibits dopamine synthesis.

By contrast, dopaminergic agents worsen psychotic symptoms of overactivity (Cesarec and Nyman 1985). Amphetamines activate psychoses or induce schizophrenic states in abusers or volunteers given large amounts. Levodopa, which acts almost entirely through increasing dopamine levels, also can worsen schizophrenic symptoms.

The dopamine hypothesis of schizophrenia developed from these observations and suggested that dopamine mechanisms may be overactive in schizophrenia. Direct assessments of this have been tried. Dopamine turnover assessed by HVA concentrations in CSF was normal in schizophrenics. However, small elevations in dopamine levels in post-mortem schizophrenic brains have been reported, mainly confined to the nucleus accumbens and caudate nucleus. The most reproducible finding in post-mortem studies has been an increase in the number of D_2 receptors in caudate, nucleus accumbens, and olfactory tubercle. However, antipsychotic drug treatment 'up-regulates' D_2 receptors, so much discussion has revolved around the issue as to whether increased D_2 receptors in schizophrenics represents a disorder- or a treatment-related abnormality. A few apparently drug-free schizophrenic patients who came to post-mortem had increased levels of D_2 receptors but to a lesser extent than drug-treated patients. This question remains unresolved (Owen *et al.* 1978; Mackay *et al.* 1982).

A further complication concerns the brain changes seen in some chronic schizophrenics. Computer tomography (CT scans) confirmed earlier air encephalograms in the finding of loss of brain tissue in some patients. The relationship of such changes to cognitive deficits, symptom patterns, and response to antipsychotic treatment is being actively pursued.

Some attention has been focused on possible abnormalities of noradrenergic function in schizophrenic patients. Some antipsychotic drugs (e.g. clozapine) are more potent alpha-adrenergic antagonists than dopamine antagonists. Further, response to clonidine, an alpha$_2$-agonist, is attenuated in schizophrenics as compared with normals. Yet another system exciting attention is the sigma opioid receptor; phencyclidine is believed to act on this mechanism (Deutsch *et al.* 1988).

Monoamine oxidase has been extensively evaluated in many different types of psychiatric patient. Decreased MAO levels have been reported in the platelets of schizophrenics. However, as brain levels are apparently normal, the meaning of this finding is unclear.

Thus, several neurotransmitter systems have been studied in the context of psychosis and schizophrenia (Snyder 1982). The most consistent findings implicate dopaminergic mechanisms but no compelling evidence has yet been produced to suggest that such abnormalities constitute anything other than biochemical correlates of overactive behaviour. It may well be that fundamental abnormalities in the different types of psychosis are all mediated through a final common dopaminergic pathway.

Hypotheses of anxiety

Biological theories of anxiety and related states have ranged more widely than those for affective disorders and schizophrenia (Judd *et al.* 1985). Recently, however, interest has been rekindled in drug models of anxiety and panic and this section will concentrate on those models (Lader and Bruce 1986; Dorow and Duka 1986).

For many years, the adrenergic systems in the body, peripheral and then central, were the focus of experimental interest. Many adrenergic agents such as adrenalin and isoprenaline were found to induce physiological responses in both anxious patients and normal volunteers. In the former, perception of these bodily changes tended to induce genuine feelings of anxiety, whereas in normal volunteers the emotion produced had an artificial 'as if' quality. These sympathomimetic amines do not penetrate into the brain and the model of anxiety produced is unconvincing.

Centrally-acting sympathomimetic drugs such as yohimbine provide more convincing models. At low dose, yohimbine blocks alpha$_2$-adrenoceptors, thereby enhancing neuronal release of noradrenalin. At higher doses it blocks alpha$_1$-adrenoceptors, resulting in an adrenolytic action. Administration of yohimbine causes subjects to feel uncomfortable, restless and irritable and to appear tense and anxious; heart rate and systolic blood pressure are raised. Plasma free MHPG, a noradrenalin metabolite, is elevated. Yohimbine can precipitate panic attacks in patients diagnosed as suffering from a panic disorder.

Both tricyclic antidepressants and some benzodiazepines such as alprazolam can lessen or even prevent panic attacks. Longterm imipramine treatment diminished plasma MHPG levels but did not alter yohimbine-induced increases in these levels or patient ratings of anxiety. This suggests a decrease in noradrenalin turnover (Charney and Henninger 1985*b*). Alprazolam significantly reduced both resting MHPG and yohimbine-induced rises in MHPG suggesting a more complex mode of action (Charney and Henninger 1985*a*).

Patients with an anxiety state have a less efficient exercise response than normal controls. From this observation, Pitts and McClure (1967) speculated that perhaps lactate might induce anxiety in susceptible individuals. A whole series of studies have established the capabilities of lactate infusions to produce anxiety states and panic attacks. Over 80 per cent of patients with panic disorder but less than 20 per cent of normal subjects experience a panic attack when given lactate. Nevertheless the mechanism of action of the lactate remains unclear. Lactate-induced panics can be prevented by the prior administration of imipramine.

Another substance known to be anxiogenic in man is pentylenetetrazol but no systematic work has been carried out. This substance may provide a model of the anxiety experienced in the aura by some temporal lobe epileptics. Carbon dioxide inhalations have also been claimed to be anxiogenic.

The development of adrenalin- and yohimbine-induced models of anxiety stemmed from the well-known sympathomimetic concomitants of anxiety such as tachycardia and tremor. Another starting point has been the benzodiazepines and the discovery of specific high-affinity receptors for them in the brain. In the search for endogenous substances binding to these receptors, a class of compounds, chemically beta-carbolines, was studied. In animals, these compounds are proconvulsant, lowering the dose of a convulsant such as pentylenetetrazol needed to induce convulsions, and antagonizing the anticonvulsant actions of the benzodiazepines. The beta-carbolines also antagonize the sedative actions of benzodiazepines and prolong sleep latency. In primates, several of the beta-carbolines induce syndromes resembling anxiety: Rhesus monkeys become agitated, and heart rate, blood pressure, and plasma cortisol and catecholamines become raised. Very few administrations have been carried out in man, but marked anxiogenic properties have been claimed (Dorow *et al.* 1987). These anxiety and panic attacks occur in waves and can be aborted by giving a benzodiazepine.

Another substance known to induce anxiety is caffeine. High doses of this methylxanthine derivative can produce insomnia, tremor, irritability, nausea and diarrhoea, and palpitations. Anxious patients apparently are more sensitive than normal subjects to the anxiogenic properties of caffeine, and panic attacks can be induced. Caffeinism has been described and the difficulty of distinguishing it from spontaneously occurring anxiety states has been emphasized (Greden 1974).

All these drug-induced models suggest that fairly crude and widespread biochemical changes may underlie the states of anxiety and panic rather than highly specific mechanisms (Hoehn-Saric, 1982). This evidence is unsupportive of more focused models of anxiety which implicate specific regions of the brain such as the limbic system (Gray 1982). As a general rule non-specific mechanisms are preferable to specific mechanisms as explanations, because far fewer assumptions need to be made. Consequently, viewing anxiety as an emotional state associated with diffuse overactivity in the brain is the most economical strategy. Indeed, many neurotransmitters may be involved in anxiety, 5-HT recently attracting more attention (Iversen 1984; Kahn *et al.* 1988).

Biochemical mechanisms in dementia

Our final example is one in which therapeutics has not played an important role—indeed, some would say it has been signally unsuccessful. Although many drug treatments have been claimed to help demented patients (and some of these claims have been allowed by licensing authorities), most specialists in psychogeriatrics remain sceptical.

In Alzheimer's dementia and senile dementia of Alzheimer's type, characteristic morphological changes are seen such as numerous senile plaques and neurofibrillary tangles. A progressive deterioration of dendrites in cortical and hippocampal pyramidal cells takes place. There is also a loss of cells in the locus coeruleus. In Alzheimer's disease of early onset (type 2), cell loss is much greater than late-onset type (type 1). In both types, a biochemical deficit in the presynaptic nerve cells of the cholinergic systems is seen and reflected by a deficiency of choline acetyl transferase. In late onset dementia, this deficit is confined to the temporal lobes. This cholinergic deficit provides a convincing rationale for the memory impairments seen in Alzheimer patients. In type 2 disease, other biochemical abnormalities have been described such as deficits in noradrenergic, serotonergic and dopaminergic systems. However, the most consistent evidence implicates an abnormality in somatostatin disposition in the cerebral cortex.

From these established biochemical abnormalities, it would seem logical to attempt to increase cholinergic function. A similar strategy underlies the use of L-dopa in parkinsonism. The first approach was to use precursors such as choline or lecithin. This has been largely unsuccessful and it is doubtful whether increasing precursor concentrations in the body actually affects central cholinergic activity. The second approach was to block cholinesterases, but the available pharmacological tools such as physostigmine are unsatisfactory. The third tactic was to use muscarinic agonists but, again, available substances are few and unimpressive in practice.

Thus, biochemical observations have furnished some rationale for therapeutic strategies but the lack of appropriate drugs has limited progress.

References

Blier, P., de Montigny, C., and Chaput, Y. (1987). Modifications of the serotonin system by antidepressant treatments: implications for the therapeutic response in major depression. *Journal of Clinical Psychopharmacology* **7,** 24S-35S.

Braddock, L. (1986). The dexamethasone suppression test. *British Journal of Psychiatry* **148,** 363–74.

Cesarec, Z. and Nyman, A.K. (1985). Differential response to amphetamine in schizophrenia. *Acta Psychiatrica Scandinavica* **71,** 523–38.

Charney, D.S. and Heninger, G.R. (1985*a*). Noradrenergic function and the mechanism of action of antianxiety treatment. I. The effect of long-term alprazolam treatment. *Archives of General Psychiatry* **42,** 458–67.

Charney D.S. and Heninger, G.R. (1985*b*). Noradrenergic function and the mechanism of action of antianxiety treatment. II. The effect of long-term imipramine treatment. *Archives of General Psychiatry* **42,** 473–81.

Curzon, G. (1988). Serotonergic mechanisms of depression. *Clinical Neuropharmacology* **11,** Suppl. 2, S11–S20.

Deutsch, S.I., Weizman, A., Goldman, M.E., and Morihisa, J.M. (1988). The sigma receptor: a novel site implicated in psychosis and antipsychotic drug efficacy. *Clinical Neuropharmacology* **11,** 105–19.

Dorow, R. and Duka, T. (1986). Anxiety: its generation by drugs and by their withdrawal. In *Advances in biochemical psychopharmacology* Vol. 41 (eds. G. Biggio and E. Costa), pp. 211–25. Raven Press, New York.

Dorow, R., Duka, T., Höller, L. and Sauerbrey, N. (1987). Clinical perspectives of β-carbolines from first studies in humans. *Brain Research Bulletin* **19,** 319–326.

Editorial (1987). *Lancet* **2,** 949–50.

Gray, J.A. (1982). *The neuropsychology of anxiety*. Clarendon Press, Oxford.

Greden, J.F. (1974). Anxiety or caffeinism: a diagnostic dilemma. *American Journal of Psychiatry* **131,** 1089–92.

Healy, D. and Leonard, B.E. (1987). Monoamine transport in depression: Kinetics and dynamics. *Journal of Affective Disorders* **12,** 91–103.

Hoehn-Saric, R. (1982). Neurotransmitters in anxiety. *Archives of General Psychiatry* **39,** 735–42.

Iversen, S.D. (1984). 5-HT and anxiety. *Neuropharmacology* **23,** 1553–60.

Judd, F.K., Burrows, G.D. and Norman, T.R. (1985). The biological basis of anxiety. *Journal of Affective Disorders* **9,** 271–84.

Kahn, R.S., van Praag, H.M., Wetzler, S., Asnis, G.M., and Barr, G. (1988). Serotonin and anxiety revisited. *Biological Psychiatry* **23,** 189–208.

Kidman, A. (1985). Neurochemical and cognitive aspects of depression. *Progress in Neurobiology* **24,** 187–97.

Kraus, R.P., Grof, P., and Brown, G.M. (1988). Drugs and the DST: need for a reappraisal. *American Journal of Psychiatry* **145,** 666–74.

Lader, M. and Bruce, M. (1986). States of anxiety and their induction by drugs. *British Journal of Clinical Pharmacology* **22,** 251–61.

Mackay, A.V.P., Iversen, L.L., Rossor, M., Spokes, E., Bird, E. *et al.* (1982). Increased brain dopamine and dopamine receptors in schizophrenia. *Archives of General Psychiatry* **39,** 991–7.

Owen, F., Cross, A.J., Crow, T.J., Longden, A., Poulter, M., and Riley, G.J. (1978). Increased dopamine-receptor sensitivity in schizophrenia. *Lancet* **2,** 223–26.

Pitts, F.N. and McClure, J.N. (1967). Lactate metabolism in anxiety neurosis. *New England Journal of Medicine* **227,** 1329-36.

Potter, W.Z. (1984). Psychotherapeutic drugs and biogenic amines. Current concepts and therapeutic implications. *Drugs* **28,** 127-43.

Roy, A., Pickar, D. and Paul, S. (1984). Biologic tests in depression. *Psychosomatics* **25,** 443–51.

Silverstone, T. and Cookson, J. (1982). The biology of mania. In *Recent advances in clinical psychiatry*, Vol. 4 (ed. K. Granville-Grossman), pp. 201–41.

Sitaram, N., Gillin, C., and Bunney, W.E. (1984). Cholinergic and catecholaminergic receptor sensitivity in affective illness: strategy and theory. In *Neurobiology of mood disorders* (eds. R.M. Post and J.C. Ballenger) pp. 629–51. Williams & Wilkins, Baltimore.

Snyder, S.H. (1982). Neurotransmitters and CNS disease. *Lancet* **2,** 970–74.

Stahl, S.M. and Palazidou, L. (1986). The pharmacology of depression: studies of neurotransmitter receptors lead the search for biochemical lesions and new drug therapies. *Trends in Pharmacological Sciences* **7,** 349–54.

van Praag, H.M. *et al.* (eds.) (1979). *Handbook of biological psychiatry*, Vols. 1–6. Marcel Dekker, New York.

van Praag, H.M. (1984). Studies in the mechanism of action of serotonin precursors in depression. *Psychopharmacology Bulletin* **20,** 599–602.

6. The evaluation of treatment

The evaluation of treatment accounts for much of the decision making of everyday clinical practice. It combines naturalistic observation of the individual patient with past personal experience, general clinical consensus, and that fraction of accumulated scientific information known to the clinician. In psychiatry it is not as straightforward or efficient as in many other branches of medicine, partly because of the intricacies of the treatment process described in Chapter 2. The biological and social forces acting on the patient quite independently of his attendance at the clinic, his expectations and reaction to contact with the clinic, the intimacies of the interaction between patient and doctor, and the expertise of the latter are all potent forces at work before pharmacological agents are introduced into the transaction. The drug is therefore one element in a complex interacting system. There is no calculus which uniquely predicts the outcome of such intervention. It would not be wholly surprising if drug effects were swamped by everything else, especially since existing pharmacological agents do not have actions which are so precise and intense that they can be detected with certainty amongst a cacophony of other changes.

Nevertheless, doctors have usually been confident about the value of their treatments even though they are often aware that what is in vogue in one generation is forgotten by the next.

> The history of therapeutic modes in psychiatry reveals a general pattern in the waxing and waning of specific somatic and psychotherapeutic methods. New therapies are characteristically introduced amid tremendous enthusiasm accompanied by the reporting of remarkable cure and improvement results. In time, this initial enthusiasm declines and evaluation of results becomes increasingly conservative. Finally, the treatment is either rejected or is accepted into the general psychiatric armamentarium with decidedly more limited applicability than its early proponents claimed for it. (Tourney 1967).

How can such a situation be controlled? Clearly it is necessary that those prescribing psychotropic drugs should be fully conversant with the complexity of the pharmacology of the substances they use, be more overtly aware of how that knowledge is derived, and understand the psychosocial pressures on themselves and on their patients which bias them to take one course of action rather than another. It should then be possible to make out the 'commanding heights' of the therapeutic landscape which can then be firmly established by scientific enquiry: more minor features can thereafter be explored if research resources allow, but many of the decisions of day-to-day clinical practice will depend heavily on 'clinical judgement' based on reasoned deductions from a firm knowledge base.

This chapter will be concerned mainly with three aspects of treatment evaluation: the complexity of pharmacological responses, the assessment of efficacy when drugs are used in therapeutics and finally, some of the broader sociopolitical consequences of chemotherapeutics. Similar considerations apply to other methods of treatment, including older 'physical methods' such as electroconvulsive therapy or psychosurgery, but since chemotherapy is, and is likely to remain, the dominant mode of biological treatment techniques, these other treatments will not receive further attention.

The pharmacological response

In thinking through a pharmacological problem, whether in a research investigation or in the treatment of an individual patient, it is helpful to consider systematically a series of factors which condition drug activity.

Multiple effects

No drug has a single action except in experimental preparations designed to reveal isolated effects. Even in a microscopic system such as the synapse, drugs may interact with a number of processes including enzymes, uptake mechanisms, and pre- and postsynaptic receptors. In the conscious human, existing psychotropic agents have multiple effects in the brain and other organs, usually covertly recognized as a main therapeutic effect and a series of 'unwanted' effects. For example, in considering actions in the central nervous system alone, chlorpromazine can have an antipsychotic action, cause sedation, cause Parkinsonism and other extrapyramidal reactions, lower the seizure threshold or act as an antiemetic. Many so-called unwanted effects may be apparent to the patient and cause much discomfort (e.g. the anticholinergic effects of tricyclic antidepressants), some may be important in toxic doses (e.g. the cardiac effects of tricyclic antidepressants) or reveal themselves after some delay (e.g. tardive dyskinesia induced by neuroleptics). Others may be subtle and apparent only on special testing (e.g. central anticholinergic effects on memory). These individual effects may have different dose thresholds, may have different latent periods and may be more or less prominent in different individuals. In prescribing a drug, one is therefore exposing a person to a series of changes which may outweigh the benefit of a chosen therapeutic action and it is important to bear this constantly in mind.

Dose effects

The effect of a drug varies with dose. Usually, increasing the dose increases the effect (the effect is commonly linearly related to the logarithm of the dose) but below and above a certain range there is little change with dose or 'paradoxical' effects may appear. For example, in the anaesthetized cat, the response of the blood pressure or nictitating membrane to intravenous noradrenalin or stimulation of the cervical sympathetic nerves is potentiated by low doses of chlorpromazine and blocked by higher doses (Thoenen *et al.* 1965). Or again, the behavioural effects of amphetamine in mice are potentiated by small doses of chlorpromazine and blocked by higher doses: tricyclic antidepressants have similar effects, but potentiation is dominant throughout most of the dose range (Lapin 1962). Between certain doses the drugs are without effect. Such apparent vagaries are probably due to multiple actions of these drugs at adrenergic synapses, causing blockade of re-uptake and presynaptic release in low doses with postsynaptic blockade and inhibition of presynaptic release in higher doses. Such processes may account for the fact that some tricyclic antidepressants, notably nortriptyline, show antidepressant action over a restricted dose range: either side of this 'therapeutic window' the therapeutic action weakens and disappears. The pharmacological profile of any drug therefore changes with the dose and if a therapeutic action depends on a number of processes this may only be seen within a certain range of doses.

Initial level effects

The effect of a drug is also conditioned by the instantaneous ongoing activity of the system being treated, the so-called initial level effect (Wilder 1958). If sheep mesenteric artery, cut into spiral strips, is stretched the tension in the muscle increases, an almost linear relation. If the tissue is exposed to noradrenalin and the experiment repeated, high levels of tension cause relaxation rather than contraction. At high levels of tension therefore noradrenalin has paradoxical effects (Speden 1960). There are many such examples in animal physiology and psychology—the blood pressure response of sympathomimetic drugs in conscious dogs (Korol and Brown 1967), or the effects of phenothiazines on the treadmill activity of mice (Irwin *et al.* 1958). Experimental studies of emotional reactions in humans have demonstrated similar phenomena. Gardos *et al.* (1968) rated student volunteers according to their habitual anxiety measured by self-rating questionnaire. Their responses to placebo and to the benzodiazepines, oxazepam and chlordiazepoxide, were then studied. Subjects who were very anxious experienced a considerable reduction in anxiety following the drugs, those who were moderately anxious had a smaller reduction, and those who were calm became anxious after receiving benzodiazepines. Interestingly, those whose anxiety was greatly relieved by chlordiazepoxide experienced increased anger and aggressiveness. Obviously, in clinical practice, one would not knowingly give an anxiolytic to someone who was not anxious, but histrionic display might be mistaken for anxiety and benzodiazepines might also be given for another purpose, e.g. to ease muscle spasm. Aggressiveness was an early reported behavioural 'side-effect' of the benzodiazepines and has been demonstrated, along with other 'paradoxical' effects, in many experimental studies.

Time effects

Another factor to be considered is the time a tissue, organ, or patient has been exposed to a drug. Does a drug have the same effect on acute administration as it does on long term use? Clearly it may not, because it may take time for a drug to penetrate to its site of action in effective concentration, the early effects may be those at the more accessible receptors, the receptors may become more or less sensitive, the metabolism of the drug may produce a product with a greater or different activity, and so on. A striking clinical example of these changes is provided by the tricyclic antidepressants. During the first week or so of treatment these are fairly poisonous remedies causing drowsiness, dry mouth, difficulty in focusing, and hand tremor, but these lessen with continued prescription. The mood elevating effect does not declare itself for about two weeks and may then take four to six weeks to develop fully. Similarly, the antipsychotic action of the neuroleptics takes about six weeks to develop fully and, if treatment is stopped, relapse may not occur for several weeks (Clark *et al.* 1963) even though chlorpromazine has mostly left the tissues by this time. Other long term changes in clinical practice are evidenced by physical dependence on alcohol or benzodiazepines and by the development of tardive dyskinesia in patients exposed to neuroleptics. Hypnotics and many other drugs suppress rapid-eye-movement sleep and when discontinued the rebound increase in this phase of sleep may last many weeks (Dunleavy *et al.* 1972). Rebound phenomena occur when many drugs are discontinued, especially if they are eliminated quickly from the tissues, common examples being alcohol and some hypnotics (Kales *et al.* 1978). Animal experiments have dissected and documented such changes in greater detail than is possible in human studies showing that drug effects on different behaviours in the same animal may decline, or intensify with time or remain unchanged (Irwin 1961) and they repeatedly confirm the longevity of many drug effects. For example, a single injection of pentobarbitone to rats influences the response to a second injection thirty days later (Aston 1966), a lengthy period for an animal with a life expectancy of about three years! Therefore the patient exposed to psychotropic drugs is never quite the same again, a point worth considering when selecting patients for controlled trials or when switching a patient from one treatment to another in the course of ordinary clinical work.

Drug interactions

When prescribing, it is therefore important to bear in mind any treatment that patient has received in the recent past and also any concurrent treatment. Drug interactions have been extensively documented and they are usually of clinical interest because they are a source of adverse effects, but drug combinations may be therapeutically useful as in the treatment of chronic depression. It is important to note that two drugs may interact through a number of physiological systems so that the outcome may depend on a number of parameters. For example, if rats are given chlorpromazine intraperitoneally and at varying intervals thereafter are given pentobarbitone, also intraperitoneally, the duration of narcosis is prolonged if the interval is less than 12 hours (due to a central, neuronal interaction) and reduced if the interval is between 12–72 h (due to the induction of hepatic microsomal enzymes) (Kato and Chiesara 1962). The implications for human therapeutics of the habit of drinking alcohol are fairly obvious.

Individual variation

Individuals vary considerably in their response to most drugs (Smith and Rawlins 1973). Such variation may arise from differences in the sensitivity of the target organ or structure or in the distribution of the drug, including hepatic metabolism: these in turn are influenced by many factors such as age, body composition, nutrition, degree of physical activity and so on. Such variation was illustrated by an early study determining the dose of sodium amylobarbitone causing light narcosis in pregnant women: it ranged between 4–19 mg/kg (Paxson 1932). A more recent study of the plasma concentrations of nortriptyline in 25 patients receiving a standard oral dose found a thirty-fold range (Alexanderson *et al.* 1969). With such variation what is one man's meat can easily be another's poison. Illness also affects response to drugs. This is obvious where there is impaired cardiac, hepatic, or renal function but psychiatric states also alter the response. Brain damage often reduces the tolerance to centrally acting drugs and may unleash paradoxical agitation and disinhibition to sedative agents, or tranquillization when amphetamine is given to hyperkinetic children. Increased tolerance to anxiolytics or sedative neuroleptics in severe anxiety or hypomania is readily understandable because the systems on which they presumably operate are highly driven, but some physical accompaniments of nervous illnesses such as changes in pituitary-adrenal function documented in the major psychoses, or acid–base shifts in panic, or malnutrition and body-composition changes associated with anorexia may well influence the kinetics and dynamics of many drugs in ways which are not readily predictable.

Milieu effects

Drugs are not usually given to individuals in isolation, but in hospital wards, within a family setting or other social grouping. The importance of 'social' factors was discovered early in the development of behavioural pharmacology by Chance (1946) who found that the dose of amphetamine required to kill half of a batch of rats was much less if the animals were housed together than if they were housed singly. Brown (1960) found that a dose of pentobarbitone which produced full hypnosis in mice housed in isolation caused marked stimulation and overactivity when they were grouped together. It is a common, social observation that the effects of alcohol can be very different when it is taken in quiet solitude than when taken in a social group and the effects are conditioned by what is going on in the group. A 'sedative' agent can readily become a 'stimulant' leading to overactivity, gregariousness and social disinhibition. Some benzodiazepines, particularly chlordiazepoxide, lower the threshold for hostile feelings which may only become manifest in social interactions (Salzman *et al.* 1974). Such phenomena are difficult to study in a controlled way, but the following experiment (Starkweather 1959) in normal volunteers illustrates the subtlety of the processes involved. They were tested individually on a simple psychomotor task immediately before and immediately after working in pairs on a similar task requiring their co-operation, on seven separate occasions at weekly intervals. For three of the sessions both partners were given placebo. On other occasions they were both given phenobarbitone, or both given amphetamine, or one was given phenobarbitone and the other amphetamine. The analysis of the changes which occurred was rather complex but the outcome was clear. Changes in performance after each 'social interaction' were related, not to the drug the subject had taken himself, but to the drug his partner had taken. The partner who took amphetamine consistently slowed the person he worked with, whilst the partner taking phenobarbitone consistently speeded up his partner whatever drug the latter had taken. Clearly, the situation might well be much more complicated in a ward where psychotic patients were treated with neuroleptics but these interactions have been studied: they demonstrate that particular features of ward atmosphere have a noticeable effect on certain symptoms, and their response to neuroleptics, but not others (Kellam *et al.* 1967).

Such social or 'milieu' effects were the subject of a great deal of debate when antipsychotic drugs were first introduced into clinical practice, partly because sceptics felt that patient improvement was not due to any specific pharmacological effect of the new drugs, but to the greater interest, confidence and optimism of staff who now had new treatments to believe in and who were involved in a new mental health policy with which to manage the mentally ill outside hospital (Shepherd *et al.* 1961; Klerman 1963). In an interesting attempt to evaluate the contribution of drugs and 'moral therapy' (intensive social and psychological treatment), Hamilton *et al.* (1963) compared trifluoperazine, prochlorperazine, and placebo in 126 chronic schizophrenic patients, half of whom also received this 'moral treatment' and half of whom received usual 'routine care'. In men, moral treatment with placebo was as effective as either drug with routine care: there was no further improvement when moral treatment was combined with drugs. In women, the results were rather different. Moral treatment had a slightly deleterious effect when combined with placebo, the modest improvement on prochlorperazine was enhanced by moral treatment and the more powerful effect of trifluoperazine was reduced when combined with moral treatment. The interaction between the environment and drug effects was therefore different in the two sexes. In men, moral treatment did not enhance the drug: in women, it enhanced the weaker drug and counteracted the more powerful drug. Such environmental interactions have been detected in schizophrenic patients treated at home where the emotional atmosphere has an important effect on the relapse rate and the effectiveness of antipsychotics. In families with high 'expressed emotion' relapse is more frequent and the protective effect of maintenance antipsychotics can be demonstrated. In more equable families relapse is much less common and the ability of these drugs to prevent it (compared with placebo) is not apparent (Vaughn and Leff 1976). In rodents and man, therefore, the social milieu conditions the response to certain psychotropic agents and, perhaps, other drugs as well.

Therapist effects

The social interaction at the focus of treatment is, of course, the doctor–patient relationship and it would not be surprising if this affected the response to drug treatment. Obviously, many factors could be involved, such as the doctor's enthusiasm for the treatment, his capacity to encourage and support the patient, the degree of psychotherapeutic involvement, and so on. Clinical trials in which these have been measured, albeit rather crudely, have shown some influence on the activity of anxiolytic, antidepressant and antipsychotic drugs (Joyce 1962; Rickels *et al.* 1971; Shader *et al.* 1971). Inevitably perhaps, in view of the subtle changes in treatment settings, the effect of the therapist is not easily replicated even by the same investigators. Enthusiastic therapists may be found to augment drug effects in one study and to reduce them in another. This will-o'-the wisp character makes it difficult to harness such forces, but it is unwise not to recognize their presence.

Placebo effects

Clearly, milieu and interpersonal influences can modify the actions of drugs which have known effects. It is therefore not too surprising that inert substances, 'dummies', or placebos can produce changes. Indeed, placebos have many of the 'pharmacological' properties already described (Wolf 1959; Shapiro and Morris 1978; Joyce 1982) including dose effects, time effects, unwanted effects, they may cause dependence and their use may be accompanied by relevant bodily changes: e.g. endorphin release probably mediates placebo-induced analgesia (Levine *et al*. 1978). Placebo effects are determined by many interacting factors in the treatment situation and it is not possible to state what factors on their own will be consistently associated with response to placebo. There is, for example, no evidence that placebo reactors have a particular type of personality or that they will consistently react. Placebo reactions may occur even though the individual knows that he is receiving an inert substance and accepts that to be the case and, perhaps against common-sense expectation, relief from physical and emotional discomfort is more likely with a placebo the more intense it is. The hopes, fears and expectancies of the individual patient are critical and in most societies much is expected of pills and potions. Placebo reactions may involve any organ system and relief has been documented in many physical conditions including angina pectoris, rheumatoid arthritis, peptic ulcer, hypertension, the common cold and most psychiatric disorders. To take a dramatic example as illustration, a study of surgery for angina pectoris involved a 'sham' operation for some patients. The sham or placebo operation was as effective as the operation under scrutiny and patients who received it experienced subjective improvement, increased exercise tolerance, used nitroglycerine less often and their ECGs were improved. Since so much can happen, placebo reactions deserve further study and analysis (Grunbaum 1986) and more use in clinical practice (Benson and Epstein 1975). Clearly, in the evaluation of any new treatment, placebo factors must be taken into account.

Controlled trials

Given the multiplicity of forces operating on a patient at the time he is treated, how is it possible to be certain that any change, good or bad, is due to the specific treatment itself? During the past three decades or so it has become increasingly accepted that some kind of formal clinical experimentation is required to establish at the very least the main tenets of clinical psychopharmacology. The commonest therapeutic experiment is the comparative clinical trial in which the treatment which is the focus of interest is compared with a standard treatment whose efficacy is known, or to placebo, or to no treatment at all. Each treatment is given to a group of subjects and it is argued that random, coincidental factors will average out within each group but that any treatment effect, supposing it to be fairly substantial in most subjects and to have a uniform latency, will summate and be detectable. The way treatments are given is constrained by a number of requirements which allow a logically sound evaluation of the results.

Patients are allocated at random and prospectively to treatments. It is assumed that the new treatment is no more effective than those against which it is to be compared. Differences between such treatments could still occur because the many factors involved will occasionally converge to cause changes in favour of or against one of the treatments. Statistical theory allows, on the basis of certain assumptions, the calculation of the likelihood of such 'chance' occurrences, and so it is possible to state whether a particular outcome is likely, say 1 in 20 or 1 in 100 experiments. The effect of the new treatment can then be compared with this and if it is of such magnitude that it would occur by chance less often than 1 in 20 times (or 1 in 100 times or whatever chance occurrence is considered important) it is judged to be a 'real' effect or 'statistically significant'.

In principle, this may appear simple and clear-cut but in practice there are many obstacles to obtaining reliable results. Extensive discussion of these issues is to be found in monographs dealing with clinical trials and with statistics in medical research (Armitage 1981; Pocock 1983) and only some of the more important issues are considered further, taking first the randomized controlled comparative trial outlined above.

One must, first of all, decide on the basis of available information, what dose-ranges are to be compared, how quickly doses are to be increased, whether all patients are to receive standard doses, or whether dosage is to be individualized according to tolerability. The duration of the trial must be decided bearing in mind that the response of most psychiatric conditions to known treatments requires several weeks. It is not uncommon for initial trials of new drugs to use dosages which are too small (for good, toxicological reasons) for too short a time (drop-outs increase as length of treatment increases), and it is not easy to get these conditions right at the beginning of the assessment of a new drug.

The kind of patient or subject to be included in the trial must be decided and clearly defined. It should be explicitly stated at the outset who is to be excluded not only with respect to age, sex, or diagnosis, but any other factor considered to be important, such as the source of the referral. It is then possible to state that the patients included are a sample of a particular population. One can then generalize results from the experimental sample to the parent population as a whole. For example, if the patients entered into the trial were of both sexes, aged 18–65, attending a psychiatric clinic suffering from a primary depressive disorder with certain stated characteristics, the results of that trial could only be generalized to patients of that type. They could not be applied safely to elderly patients, patients with secondary depressions or patients seen in general practice. Further trials with such patients would be necessary to test whether their treatment responses were similar (there is, of course, evidence to indicate that this is unlikely).

Patients are randomly allocated to treatment groups to ensure that, so far as is possible, the patients comprising each group are similar in all important respects. Randomization is only likely to achieve this if large numbers of patients are studied. Smaller numbers are vulnerable to freak runs of male, elderly, or good prognosis patients in one treatment group. This can to some extent be overcome by various techniques of restricted randomization such as entry of patients in pairs matched for important variables or randomising within categories such as sex or prognosis. Such subgroups can then be analysed separately assuming that they are of sufficient size to allow reliable statistical analysis.

The expectations and prejudices of patients or doctors participating in the trial can be minimized if neither knows what treatment the patient is receiving, the so-called double-blinded technique. Also, others involved in the trial, including those carrying out the analyses, should also be blind so far as is possible and should remain so until the analysis of the trial is completed. Since even rats involved in experiments have been shown to comply with the investigators unstated biases (Rosenthal 1967) the need for such stringent regulations is obvious! Clearly, drugs should be formulated so that all drugs look and taste alike and have similar side-effects, otherwise any differences may become apparent when patients talk amongst themselves or to doctors. Often, drugs cannot be so formulated and blindness may then be preserved if those taking one drug take matching dummies of the other drugs being studied so that whatever active treatment is administered the drugs taken together look the same ('double-dummy technique'). Drugs may differ in unwanted effects and this can sometimes be obscured by adding a drug, psychopharmacologically inactive, which contributes the necessary side-effects: e.g. in comparing tricyclic antidepressives with placebo in the treatment of depression the placebo could be atropine. Usually, with care, comparative treatments can be assembled so that blindness is, in most cases, achieved. If it cannot, or if there is some ethical objection to a particular arrangement, blindness of assessment, but not of treatment administration, can be obtained by video-taping interviews, removing clues which might indicate which treatment the patient was on, and getting the assessment or ratings made by an assessor who has nothing to do with the administration of treatment or those involved in it. At the start of the trial explicit rules must be set down about breaking the code to discover which treatment a patient is actually receiving should his condition cause concern. The code should be kept by someone not involved in the administration, assessments, or analyses. Clearly, frequent code-breaking would imperil the blindness of the trial.

Methods of assessment should be valid (measuring whatever one is interested in measuring), reliable (particularly between raters) and they should be sensitive to change (Cronholm and Daly 1983). They may be ratings made by the doctor of the patient's symptoms and mental state or they may be assessments made by the patient himself. It is often valuable to have both kinds of rating since patient and observer may not always agree or the patient may find it easier to rate himself without pressure from an interlocutor. With repeated assessments it is preferable that the same rater sees a particular patient through his treatment. If a number of raters are involved in a trial they should arrange sessions throughout the trial to compare their methods of rating: this will help prevent drift as the trial proceeds. On each occasion rating should be made without reference to preceding ratings, though if they are frequent it may be possible to remember from one occasion to the next. By observing a few rules of this kind measurement error is minimized, an important matter since there is so much 'noise' from other sources in treatment trials. Other kinds of measurements can also be taken. Social performance can be assessed by rating methods perhaps using evidence from families. In some situations psychomotor tests or physiological measurements may be valuable.

The number of patients entered into a trial should be sufficiently large to allow valid use of the appropriate statistical tests. If a difference between treatments is obtained it must be large enough compared to the variation in each treatment group to be unlikely to have occurred by random, 'chance' factors alone. Equally, if only small differences between treatments are found it cannot be concluded that the treatments are equally efficacious unless sufficient numbers of patients have been tried to ensure, to a given likelihood, that a difference is not hidden by random variation. Of course, false conclusions are unlikely to be drawn if the treatment differences are large. For example, treatment groups would not need to be large to decide that intravenous thiopentone sodium is a more powerful anaesthetic than saline: larger groups would be necessary to demonstrate that aspirin is better than placebo in relieving headache and much larger still to demonstrate whether or not a new antidepressant is better than amitriptyline. If one is only interested in larger treatment differences or not concerned about missing small ones, fewer patients may suffice. Often the treatment decisions of clinical practice are of this type and the smaller, less sensitive, clinical trial is valuable (Powell-Tuck *et al.* 1986). The numbers of patients required to achieve the result at a particular level of statistical significance can be estimated when a trial is planned provided something is already known of the variation of treatment response to established drugs and the likely differences in potency of the drugs being compared.

The effort involved in recruitment, assessment, and analysis is lost if patients do not take trial medication or secretly take other medicines during the trial. Compliance with trial medication can be estimated by tablet counts, by measuring plasma concentrations of the trial drugs, or by detecting in the urine chemicals included in the pharmaceutical formulation of trial drugs. Patients may deliberately deceive investigators by returning the correct numbers of pills but without ingesting them, or by taking them only for a few days prior to assessment so that blood and urine samples will contain at least some of the appropriate agents. Many patients will not be drug-free at the start of the trial and it often improves the sensitivity of a trial to include a placebo pre-trial washout phase which will allow the detection of those who improve quickly without the use of active medication and who can then be withdrawn from the study. This however, may give an exaggerated estimate of the superiority of the active drug with respect to placebo.

There are many other experimental designs which can be used in clinical drug research. Some are particularly useful where the number of patients available for a study is small either because the condition is uncommon or because limited resources or ethical considerations make it imperative to terminate the trial as soon as possible. In a sequential trial, patients are entered in pairs, one patient receiving, blind, the experimental treatment, the other the standard or controlled treatment. The superiority of one treatment over the other, or the absence of a difference, is tallied for each pair and where, as pairs accumulate, superiority in one direction or the other reaches beyond chance expectations, the trial is stopped. A trial can also be ended when it is deemed unlikely that one of the treatments will prove better because, up to that point, pairs have either not differed or one treatment is better as often as the other. Sequential trials are vulnerable to an atypical run favouring one treatment early in the trial.

In cross-over trials, troublesome interindividual variation can be contained by submitting each patient to each treatment in turn, either randomly assigned or given in balanced order, Each patient therefore acts as his own control. Such trials are difficult to carry out and interpret where a drug lingers in the tissues long after treatment is discontinued (as is the case for most psychotropic drugs) or where changes occur after a latent period (as for example with antidepressant drugs). Washout periods between active drug phases are therefore necessary and this may present management and ethical problems in clinical situations.

Single cases can be the subject of clinical trials, the patient being given a sequence of treatments (including placebo or no treatment) and changes in mental state and behaviour monitored. Again, lags in treatment response and drug elimination can be a problem but with careful design and appropriate statistical methods the relation between treatment and response can be determined. It is, of course, important that patient and assessor are blind to when treatment switches occur. Single case designs mimic the clinical treatment situation more than other designs and evidence of groups of patients can be built up from individual cases (Murphy *et al.* 1974). Treatment-response subgroups can also be neatly detected by this approach. All designs have problems of organization, design and interpretation and many modifications of the basic designs have been developed to meet particular needs of pharmacology, clinical populations, ethics, and so on (Byar *et al.* 1976).

Ethical objections are often raised against clinical trials mainly on the grounds that an individual patient may be denied the most effective treatment for his particular condition. There would, of course, be little point in submitting a patient to an inferior treatment since clinical trials are usually motivated by the need to find improvements in treatment. Anxiety often arises because a patient may be denied a standard treatment whose reputation rests on the fact that it has been accepted by custom without ever having its efficacy adequately tested. These treatments are sometimes subsequently found to be inadequate or ineffective and there is a case for trials to be carried out on accepted treatments comparing them against placebo. It has also to be recognized that any treatment is a clinical experiment and is based on accumulated experience on previous patients both in trials and in ordinary clinical work: every patient is therefore the beneficiary of the risks taken by his predecessors. It is clearly better that risks are taken within a clinical trial where they can be reliably evaluated and it is also important that new treatments are assessed as early as possible so that untried, but ineffective, treatments are not persisted with for too long. When these aspects are considered participation in a clinical trial often guarantees an individual patient the best care, particularly since clinical trials these days involve careful assessment of physical health. Trials should be carried out with the patient's fully informed consent (Helmchen 1983).

Controlled trials and clinical practice

Clinical trials can never provide answers to all the varied therapeutic problems of everyday clinical life, but they can help to establish the main skeleton of knowledge from which it should be possible to reach out to a particular problem with rather less than total ignorance (Herxheimer *et al.* 1986). Even if a trial is technically sound it may give a 'freak' result because of some unusual concatenation of factors important to its outcome. Replication of trials is therefore important and there are techniques, including meta-analysis, which allow the results of several trials to be combined so long as sufficient information is published about each of them and so long as they are broadly similar in design. Such procedures have been employed to confirm the value of imipramine (Rogers and Clay 1975) and ECT (Janicak *et al.* 1985) in the treatment of depressive illness. Nevertheless, even where the outcome of several trials is consistent, they need to be interpreted with care: dissonance between the verdict of trials and clinical consensus is not uncommon, as in the case of early trials of antidepressant treatments (Overall *et al.* 1962; Medical Research Council 1965) which showed the monoamine oxidase inhibitors phenelzine and isocarboxazid to be less effective than placebo. One of the reasons for this early disagreement (the other was probably that the doses of the monoamine oxidase inhibitor were too low) is that treatment comparisons were made within a fairly heterogenous population of depressives and, although there has never been clear agreement on who is likely to respond to the monoamine oxidase inhibitors, the efficacy of these drugs in depressive illness has subsequently been established. The broad heterogeneity of the patients entered into larger trials reduced their relevance to individual patients within the target population. This gap can be bridged by 'focused' trials on particular subgroups of patients identified by subset analysis of larger trials or suggested by clinical observation. Such studies move nearer to actual clinical practice and should help to reduce disagreements between the outcome of clinical trials and general clinical experience.

It is important not to let such disagreements lead to disillusionment with trials because there are many factors contributing to 'clinical experience' which can also lead practitioners away from reality. There is a natural tendency for clinicians to attribute any improvement to the treatment being used at the time or to themselves: if the patient does not improve or deteriorates, poor compliance, defects in the patient's personality or the natural history of the illness are accepted explanations. Inevitably the effectiveness of treatments is overestimated. Clinical trials which reduce such magnification are therefore disturbing, the more so since they may question long-established practice or accepted authority. Controlled trials give a less enthusiastic verdict of treatments, old and new, than uncontrolled studies. This has been well documented in psychiatry since the reviews of Foulds (1958) and Fox (1961) showed that about 85 per cent of scientifically unacceptable studies reported benefit from treatment whereas for scientifically acceptable reports the proportion was about 40 per cent. Any change, anything new is good for both doctor and patient as in most walks of life, the classical example being a series of experiments (at the Hawthorne Works at Western Electric Company, Chicago) in which working conditions were varied with a view to increasing productivity and each proved to be beneficial including the final one which involved reverting to the original conditions! (Whitehead 1938). (In former days regular movement of long term patients through different wards was a recognized way of provoking some change, hopefully beneficial, if only temporary.) The perceptive and shrewd clinician has some in-built defences against therapeutic illusions but it is a historical fact that doctors have had great faith in worthless or dangerous remedies and have persisted in their use despite warnings from sceptical voices, for example, radical mastectomy for breast cancer, diethylstilboestrol for habitual abortion, and deep insulin coma therapy for schizophrenia (Bourne 1953). It is therefore important to initiate controlled trials when a new treatment is introduced: if they are delayed there is resistance to carrying them out because of ethical objections to withholding 'established' treatments.

The development of new treatments

Controlled trials test therapeutic hypotheses: they do not initiate them. The rational and organized development of new treatments, including drugs, is especially difficult in psychiatry because there are no secure cornerstones on which to build. The psychiatric equivalents of beta-blockers or H_2-antagonists are a distant prospect. There are no clear uncontested models of psychiatric disorder, symptoms are heavily conditioned by cultural factors, little is known of aetiology, and there are no clearly equivalent disorders in animals. One therefore has to be content with any approach which organizes existing knowledge and has heuristic value.

Drug treatments have been developed mainly in relation to the 'medical' or 'disease' models of psychiatric disorder. In outline these postulate a pathological process which manifests itself in phases of activity of variable duration which may leave residual damage or functional deficits. The afflicted mind is not a passive recipient of these insults but reacts to accommodate acute changes and to adjust to permanent deficits. Personality, social, and cultural factors are not therefore left out in such a model and the relative contribution of disease process and adaptations will vary: in some conditions, such as the milder neuroses adaptive or reactive processes probably dominate whereas in the psychoses, most clearly in those of organic aetiology, the disease process itself is a major determinant of the clinical abnormalities. Clearly it is desirable to have measures of these components of the illness in each individual patient but, apart from some organic conditions, these have not been developed. Treatments can be fashioned to modify any of the various processes involved, the most potent treatment being the one which eliminates the central pathological process. The historically important paradigm of major psychiatric disorder is neurosyphilis, where understanding of the complex clinical presentation was advanced by discovery of the neuropathology and then of the causative infective agent. Management at this stage consisted mainly of nursing and custodial support. The advent of arsenical and fever therapies still required considerable attention to psychosocial aspects, but with the introduction of penicillin, which has a radical effect on the primary aetiological agent in the early stages of the illness, other factors in the illness became much less important. The problem with functional disorders is that single, major aetiological factors may not exist and it is not currently possible to define processes against which treatment should be targeted. Treatments may, of course, affect both the postulated disease processes and individual reactions to that process but they may themselves constitute a threat or stress to the patient not only in the organic sense, but also by effects on psychological adaptations or defence mechanisms (Sarwer-Foner 1960).

Inevitably, therefore, attempts to understand treatment mechanisms, to develop techniques and to refine existing ones have sprung from many disciplines: genetics, biochemistry, pharmacology, electrophysiology, behavioural techniques in humans, both normal and ill, and in experimental animals (see Chapters 4 and 5). Essentially, one can begin from two starting points, (a) aberrant behaviour, and (b) known psychotropic agents.

Aberrant behaviour can be studied, either as it occurs naturally in human illnesses or in normal people who may differ in their habitual anxiety, depression, cognition, or whatever, or in response to stress. Questionnaires measuring subjective state or symptoms, biochemical, physiological, or behavioural measurements can then be made and their modification by drugs documented. In the case of putative disease states, 'markers' such as the dexamethasone suppression test, changes in the production of 5-hydroxyindole acetic acid in the cerebrospinal fluid, or platelet uptake of 5-hydroxytryptamine, may prove useful, in this case for depressed patients. Abnormal behaviour in animals considered equivalent to that seen in humans can similarly be studied with the added advantage that intracerebral changes can also be documented. For example, separation of young animals from their mothers or peers induces behaviours redolent of human depression and there is some evidence that these can be reversed by chronic treatment with imipramine, monoamine oxidase inhibitors, and ECT but not by antipsychotic drugs or anxiolytics. The condition induced in animals therefore shares many of the important characteristics of depressive reactions in humans and may therefore be an appropriate model for neurochemical study and therapeutic experiment. Non-invasive neuropharmacological techniques currently being developed may, of course, render much animal experimentation unnecessary.

Known psychotropic drugs sometimes initiate non-transient states which mimic natural disease, amphetamine-induced schizophreniform psychosis and reserpine-induced depression being two examples. Each of these has allowed some understanding of the underlying neurochemical changes and has provided, respectively, major support for the dopamine theory of schizophrenia and the monoamine theories of depression. Another approach starting with drugs already known to have major psychotropic actions is to measure their 'profile' of activity on a series of laboratory tests. Changes in the profile can then be studied following systematic modification of the drug molecular structure using existing knowledge of structure–activity relations (Loew and Taeschler 1968). Such a technique led to the development of haloperidol from morphine analogues (Janssen 1965). Unfortunately, none of these strategies has produced drugs with really novel actions although the spectrum of pharmacological effects can be transmuted to yield compounds with very different overall effects.

Disappointingly, none of this considerable effort matches the achievements of clinicians whose chance but astute observations led to the detection of novel agents during the first decade of the modern psychotropic era beginning in 1953. The calming effects of chlorpromazine were recognized during its use in surgery to prevent shock, elevation of mood was noted when iproniazid was introduced in the treatment of tuberculosis and when imipramine was given to schizophrenics as a neuroleptic, the anxiolytic effects of meprobamate were observed during the study of muscle relaxants such as mephenesin whose properties had in turn been noticed during the toxicological testing of antibacterial glycerol ethers (Ayd and Blackwell 1970)! Clinical observation should not therefore be despised: indeed, Kuhn's description of the indications and clinical actions of imipramine cannot be improved upon. Such 'serendipity' has been strangely muted during the ensuing quarter of a century.

Unwanted effects, adverse reactions, selective toxicity

Drugs owe their place in therapeutics in one or more main effects which control or eliminate some pathological process or physiological system, but they have other actions which are undesirable. Clearly, the aim is to increase the former and minimize the latter. Completely 'clean' drugs do not exist, though they are in principle possible and may, before too long, be available through improved methods of drug delivery (Gregoliades 1977; Urquhart 1982). Unwanted effects tend to be played down and it is a useful corrective to think of chemotherapeutics as 'selective toxicity' (Albert 1951). It then becomes clear that toxicity as well as efficacy requires careful evaluation. This is not as simple as it might at first appear because adverse effects may produce symptoms or physical changes similar to the illness being treated (Kupfer and Detre 1971) or other intercurrent illness: for example, dry mouth, hand tremor, and lethargy occur in anxiety, and minor involuntary movements are not uncommon in schizophrenia or the elderly. Also any treatment, especially new treatment, may lead to greater self-monitoring particularly if a doctor shows interest in untoward effects, as is evidenced in studies of placebos. On the other hand, some effects may not be at all obvious to the patient or to others, but they may nevertheless be important, especially the subtle behavioural changes which may be caused by psychotropics and other drugs. Such 'behavioural toxicity' can be detected in psychomotor tests in the early phases of treatment (Wittenborn 1980; Hindmarch 1980) and whilst there may be some readjustment with continued use, impairments are likely to persist and may be subtly disabling. Just how important behavioural effects are in ordinary life, in the home, at work, is virtually impossible to measure but since up to 20 per cent of adults receive psychotropic drugs in any one year (Skegg *et al.* 1977) serious consequences could in absolute terms be quite common. There is, for example, evidence that the use of psychotropic agents increases the chances of a road traffic accident (Skegg *et al.* 1979; Honkanen *et al.* 1980). Subtle effects in interpersonal interactions, particularly the tolerance of frustration, could have effects in the immediate social environment which would not obviously be related to treatment. Some adverse effects appear years after drug use: they may then be striking and even life-threatening or they may develop imperceptibly and, though obvious, may not be noticed for some years (e.g. tardive dyskinesia associated with antipsychotic use).

Social monitoring of innovation and safety

Clearly, it is necessary to monitor both the efficacy and safety of treatments. If this is not apparent from the evidence presented in this chapter one has only to recall that, until the past two decades or so, treatment in psychiatry (and not only psychiatry) was heavily influenced by fashion, that many of these treatments were ineffective, and that the therapeutic catastrophe which had such an impact on the subsequent regulation of drug development involved a psychotropic drug, thalidomide. Technologically advanced countries have regulated the manufacture and supply of medicines since the late nineteenth century but with the growth of pharmacology and the pharmaceutical industry, statutory control over these activities has grown to the point where bureaucratic stultification of innovation and development may have been reached. In the UK the government introduced, in 1968, the Medicines Act which established the Medicines Commission to advise it on how the supply and use of drugs for therapeutic purposes should be controlled. It also set up the Committee on the Safety of Medicines to collect information on adverse drug reactions and to issue clinical trial certificates and product licences to intending manufacturers. The Licensing Authority also has a number of other advisory committees including the Committee on the Review of Medicines, established to review all products on the market before the Medicines Act came into force and to decide which should continue to hold a product licence. Such committees require a great deal of sound information on which to base decisions. Manufacturers are required to produce detailed information on synthesis, pharmacology, kinetics, formulation, toxicology, safety in human volunteers, and evidence of efficacy and safety from clinical trials (Sneader 1986). Not surprisingly, it now takes at least ten years from the synthesis of a new compound to the issuing of a product licence.

These legislative developments have been a logical and perhaps inevitable consequence of the growing biological technologies which bring new possibilities to the management of disease, deviant behaviour, and emotional suffering. They have also given some urgency to issues which have smouldered for some decades. How much should the decision of the individual clinician be constrained by the verdict of clinical trials? Is clinical freedom dead, especially where expensive methods of investigation and treatment (not only by drugs) are being considered? 'The medical profession has always preferred to travel hopefully rather than to arrive because arrival is often so disappointing. This habit leads to oscillating fashions, and fashions in treatment are something that we neither can nor should afford' (Hampton 1983). Clearly, if these habits are to be contained by clinical trials they need to be properly designed and well-executed, and this requires skilled investigators with the necessary time, facilities, and organizational backing and also suitable patients who may be required in large numbers. Resources are likely to be available for only major therapeutic issues and the construction of a 'shopping list' of these has been proposed (Herxheimer *et al.* 1986). Ideally such trials should commence soon after the introduction of a new technique or treatment because this is not only economically efficient but abolishes the ethical dilemma of witholding an 'effective' or 'established' treatment. Clinical trials thus become an essential component of a continuously developing technology rather than something done for academic interest. The public needs to understand that this is the only responsible way to introduce new methods.

The monitoring of adverse events is rather more difficult than establishing efficacy because their nature and latency are not easily predicted. Toxicity studies on animals and man, including 'behavioural toxicity' are usually carried out early in drug development and are necessary for a product licence application, but thereafter the detection of adverse effects, especially idiosyncratic, is more difficult. Minor adverse reactions to established drugs are common (about 40 per cent of treated patients in general practice, Martys 1979) especially for drugs acting on the central nervous system, and the acceptability of a new preparation would have to be judged with this in mind. During initial clinical trials when the patient is inevitably under close scrutiny unwanted effects can be recorded as spontaneously reported or in response to checklists, and appropriate clinical tests such as haematology, liver function tests, or electrocardiogram can be carried out as indicated by the known pharmacology. Thereafter, when the drug is available for general prescription, monitoring is obviously more difficult. The reporting of the more serious adverse effects by doctors working in hospital or general practice to a central national agency (the 'yellow card' system to the Committee on the Safety of Medicines in the UK) depends on the interest and initiative of those concerned, but it has been fairly effective in their early detection (Venning 1983). That such reactions are due to a particular drug then needs confirmation either by re-challenging the patient with the drug, assuming that to be safe, or by controlled studies of larger numbers of patients such as retrospective case control studies in which the drug history of those affected is compared with that of a group of unaffected controls. In order to obtain an accurate picture of the incidence of unwanted effects, including the more serious reactions, 'post-marketing surveillance' of the first 10 000 patients to receive a new drug in general practice is probably necessary (Inman 1981).

Obviously, much effort and expense is involved and such an investment obliges those who prescribe drugs to critically assess what they are doing, to participate in peer review, to be aware of the pattern, efficacy and cost of the treatment programmes in which they participate ('pharmacoepidemiology', Zito *et al.* 1987), and to recognise in themselves emotional and ideological barriers to the acceptance of clear evidence (Dykes 1974; Spodick 1982). It is therefore necessary to evolve ways of getting accurate information through to practitioners and to ensure that this is free from sponsor bias and the tendency not to publish or to ignore negative trials (Vere 1988). The techniques of the advertising industry should be adopted with care! Such matters can themselves be the subject of controlled trials. For example, in a study of the use by general practitioners of three groups of drugs, including cerebral vasodilators, doctors were divided into three 'treatment' groups, those given printed information, those given face-to-face tutorials by a pharmaceutical expert, and a control group who were ignored. The prescribing habits of those given face-to-face instruction were changed but printed information was without effect (Avon and Southeria 1983).

Scientific and technological innovation is increasingly expensive and in therapeutics it also involves the use of large numbers of animals and human beings. It must therefore also be efficient. The study of innovation is no longer an entirely academic pursuit (Mosteller 1981) and it is not only interesting but valuable to review the 'natural history' of how drugs were developed (Ayd and Blackwell 1970) and how adverse effects were detected (Venning 1983) so that the process may be improved upon. Real originality probably cannot be planned but conditions which foster it might be sought. What leads one individual to see important significance in data which another dismisses as being of no interest has been the subject of a case study

(Barber and Fox, 1958) which is of particular import to psychopharmacology because of the serendipitous discoveries which initiated the modern psychotropic era. The price of discovery is probably eternal vigilance.

References

Albert, A. (1951). *Selective toxicity*. Methuen, London.

Alexanderson, B., Price-Evans, D.A. and Sjoqvist, F. (1969). Steady-state plasma levels of nortriptyline in twins: influence of genetic factors and drug therapy. *British Medical Journal* **4,** 764–8.

Armitage, P. (1987). *Statistical methods in medical research*, 2nd edn. Blackwell, Oxford.

Aston, R. (1966). Latent hypersensitivity to pentobarbital in the rat. *Proceedings of the Society for Experimental Biology and Medicine* **121,** 623–6.

Avorn, J. and Southeria, S.B. (1983). Improving drug-therapy decisions through education outreach: a randomised controlled trial of academically based 'detailing'. *New England Journal of Medicine* **308,** 1457–63.

Ayd, F. and Blackwell, B. (1970). *Discoveries in biological psychiatry*. Lippincott, Philadelphia.

Barber, B. and Fox, R.C. (1958). The case of the floppy-eared rabbits: an instance of serendipity gained and serendipity lost. *American Journal of Sociology* **64,** 128–36.

Benson, H. and Epstein, M.D. (1975). The placebo effect. A neglected asset in the care of patients. *Journal of the American Medical Association* **232,** 1225–7.

Bourne, H. (1953). The insulin myth. *Lancet* **ii,** 964–8.

Brown, B.B. (1960). CNS drug action and interaction in mice. *Archives Internationales de Pharmacodynamie et de Thérapie* **128,** 391–414.

Byar, D.P., Simon, R.M., Friedewald, W.T., Schlesselman, J.J., Demets, D.L., Ellenberg, J.H., Gail, M.H., and Ware, J.H. (1976). Randomised clinical trials. Perspectives in some recent ideas. *New England Journal of Medicine* **295,** 74–80.

Chance, M.R.A. (1946). Aggregation as a factor influencing the toxicity of sympathomimetic amines in mice. *Journal of Pharmacology and Experimental Therapeutics* **87,** 214–9.

Clark, M.L., Ray, T.S. and Ragland, R.E. (1963). Chlorpromazine in chronic schizophrenic women: rate of onset and rate of dissipation of drug effects. *Psychosomatic Medicine* **25,** 212–7.

Cronholm, B. and Daly, R.J. (1983). Evaluation of psychiatric treatment. In *Methodology in evaluation of psychiatric treatment* (ed. T. Helgason) pp. 3–32. Cambridge University Press, Cambridge.

Dunleavy, D.L.F., Brezinova, V., Oswald, I., Maclean, A.W., and Tinker, M. (1972). Changes during weeks in effects of tricyclic drugs on the human sleeping brain. *British Journal of Psychiatry* **120,** 663–72.

Dykes, M.H.M. (1974). Uncritical thinking in medicine. The confusion between hypothesis and knowledge. *Journal of the American Medical Association* **227,** 1275–7.

Foulds, G.A. (1958). Clinical research in psychiatry. *Journal of Mental Science* **104,** 259–65.

Fox, B. (1961). The investigation of the effects of psychiatric treatment. *Journal of Mental Science* **107,** 493–502.

Gardos, G., Dimascio, A., Salzman, C., and Shader, R.I. (1968). Differential actions of chlordiazepoxide and oxazepam on hostility. *Archives of General Psychiatry* **18,** 757–60.

Gregoliades, G. (1977). Targetting of drugs. *Nature* **265,** 407–11.

Grunbaum, A. (1986). The placebo concept in medicine and psychiatry. *Psychological Medicine* **16,** 19–38.

Hamilton, M., Hordern A., Waldrop, F.N., and Lofft, J. (1963). A controlled trial on the value of prochlorperazine, trifluoperazine and intensive group treatment. *British Journal of Psychiatry* **109,** 510–22.

Hampton, J.R. (1983). The end of clinical freedom. *British Medical Journal* **287,** 1237–8.

Helmchen, H. (1983). Ethical and practical problems in therapeutic research in psychiatry. In *Methodology in Evaluation of Psychiatric Treatment* (ed. T. Helgason) pp. 251–64. Cambridge University Press, Cambridge.

Herxheimer, A., Zentler-Munro, P., and Winn, D. (1986). *Therapeutic trials and society. Making the best use of resources.* Consumer's Association, London.

Hindmarch, I. (1980). Psychomotor functions and psychoactive drugs. *British Journal of Clinical Pharmacology* **10,** 189–209.

Honkanen, R., Ertama, L., Linnoila, M., Alha, A., Lukkari, I., Karlsson, M., Kiviluoto, O., and Puro, M. (1980). Role of drugs in traffic accidents. *British Medical Journal* **281,** 1309–12.

Inman, W.H.W. (1981). Postmarketing surveillance of adverse drug reactions in general practice. *British Medical Journal* **282,** 1131–2; 1216–7.

Irwin, S. (1961). The actions of drugs on psychomotor activity. In *Extrapyramidal system and neuroleptics*, (ed. J.M. Bordeleau) pp. 143–54. Editions Psychiatrique, Montreal.

Irwin, S., Sablok, M., and Thomas, G. (1958). Individual differences. Correlation between control locomotor activity and sensitivity to stimulant and depressant drugs. *Journal of Pharmacology and Experimental Therapeutics* **123,** 206–11.

Janicak, P.G., Davis, J.M., Gibbons, R.D., Eriksen, S., Chang, S., and Gallagher, D. (1985). Efficacy of ECT: a meta-analysis. *American Journal of Psychiatry* **142,** 297–302.

Janssen, P.A.J. (1965). The evolution of the butyrophenones, haloperidol and trifluperidol, from meperidine-like 4-phenylpiperidines. *International Review of Neurobiology* **8,** 221–63.

Joyce, C.R.B. (1962). Differences between physicians as revealed by clinical trials. *Proceedings of the Royal Society of Medicine* **55,** 776–8.

Joyce, C.R.B. (1982). Placebo and other comparative treatments. *British Journal of Clinical Pharmacology* **13,** 313–8.

Kales, A., Scharf, M.B., and Kales, J.D. (1978). Rebound insomnia: a new clinical syndrome. *Science* **201,** 1039–41.

Kato, R. and Chiesara, E. (1962). Increase of pentobarbital metabolism induced in rats pre-treated with some centrally acting compounds. *British Journal of Pharmacology* **18,** 29–38.

Kellam, S., Goldberg, S.C., Schoolar, N.R., Berman, A., and Schmelzer, J. (1967). Ward atmosphere and outcome of treatment of acute schizophrenia. *Journal of Psychiatric Research* **5,** 145–63.

Klerman, G.L. (1963). Assessing the influence of the hospital milieu upon the effectiveness of psychiatric drug therapy: problems of conceptualisation and of research methodology. *Journal of Nervous and Mental Disease* **137,** 143–54.

Korol, B. and Brown, M.L. (1967). The influence of the existing arterial pressure on autonomic drug responses in conscious dogs. *Archives Internationales de Pharmacodynamie et de Therapie* **170,** 371–8.

Kupfer, D.J. and Detre, T.P. (1971). Once more—on the extraordinary side-effects of drugs. *Clinical Pharmacology and Therapeutics* **12,** 575–82.

Lapin, I.P. (1962). Qualitative and quantitative relationships between the effects of imipramine and chlorpromazine on amphetamine group toxicity. *Psychopharmacologia* **3,** 413–22.

Levine, J.D., Gordon, N.C., and Fields, H.L. (1978). The mechanisms of placebo analgesia. *Lancet* **ii,** 654–7.

Loew, D.M. and Taeschler, M. (1968). Profiles of activity of psychotropic drugs. A way to predict therapeutic effects. *International Pharmacopsychiatry* **1,** 1–20.

Martys, C.R. (1979). Adverse reactions to drugs in general practice. *British Medical Journal* **ii,** 1194–7.

Medical Research Council (1965). Clinical trial of the treatment of depressive illness. *British Medical Journal* **i,** 831–6.

Murphy, D.L., Baker, M., Goodwin, F.R., Miller, H., Kotin, J. and Bunney, W.E. (1974). L-tryptophan in affective disorders: indoleamine changes and differential clinical effects. *Psychopharmacolgia* **34,** 11–20.

Mosteller, F. (1981). Innovation and evaluation. *Science* **211,** 881–6.

Overall, J.E., Hollister, L.E., Porkorny, A.D., Casey, J.F. and Katz, G. (1962). Drug therapy in depressions. Controlled evaluation of imipramine, isocarboxazid, dextroamphetamine—amobarbital and placebo. *Clinical Pharmacology and Therapeutics* **3,** 16–22.

Paxson, N.F. (1932). Obstetrical anesthesia and analgesia with sodium iso-amylethylbarbiturate and nitrous oxide-oxygen. *Current Researches in Anesthesia and Analgesia* **11,** 116–22.

Pocock, S.J. (1983). *Clinical trials, a practical approach*. John Wiley, Chichester.

Powell-Tuck, J., Macrae, K.D., Healy, M.J.R., Lennard-Jones, J.E., and Parkins, R.A. (1986). A defence of the small clinical trial: evaluation of three gastrointestinal studies. *British Medical Journal* **292,** 599–602.

Rickels, K., Lipman, R.S., Park, L.C., Covi, L., Uhlenhuth, E.H., and Mock, J.E. (1971). Drug, doctor warmth and clinic setting in the symptomatic response to minor tranquillisers. *Psychopharmacologia* **20,** 128–52.

Rogers, S.C., and Clay, P.M. (1975). A statistical review of controlled trials of imipramine and placebo in the treatment of depressive illnesses. *British Journal of Psychiatry* **127,** 599–603.

Rosenthal, R. (1967). Covert communication in the psychological experiment. *Psychological Bulletin* **67,** 357–67.

Salzman, C., Kochansky, G.E., Shader, R.I., Porrino, L.J., Harmatz, J.S., and Swett, C.P. (1974). Chlordiazepoxide-induced hostility in a small group setting. *Archives of General Psychiatry* **31,** 401–5.

Sarwer-Foner, G.J. (1960). The role of neuroleptic medication in psychotherapeutic interaction. *Comprehensive Psychiatry* **1,** 291–300.

Shader, R.I., Grinspoon, L., Harmatz, J.S., and Ewart, J.R. (1971). The therapist variable. *American Journal of Psychiatry* **127,** 49–52.

Shapiro, A.K. and Morris, L.A. (1978). The placebo effect in medical and psychological therapies. In: *Handbook of psychotherapy and behavior change*, 2nd edn (ed. S.L. Garfield & A.E. Bergin) John Wiley, New York.

Shepherd, M., Goodman, N., and Watt, D.C. (1961). Application of hospital statistics in the evaluation of pharmacotherapy in a psychiatric population. *Comprehensive Psychiatry* **2,** 11–19.

Skegg, D.C.G., Richards, S.M., and Doll, R. (1979). Minor tranquillisers and road accidents. *British Medical Journal* **i,** 917–9.

Smith, S.E. and Rawlins, M.D. (1973). *Variability in human drug response*. Butterworths, London.

Sneader, W. (1986). *Drug development from laboratory to clinic*. John Wiley, Chichester.

Speden, R.N. (1960). The effect of initial length on the noradrenaline-induced isometric contraction of arterial strips. *Journal of Physiology* (*London*) **154,** 15–25.

Spodick, D.H. (1982). Randomised controlled clinical trials. The behavioral case. *Journal of the American Medical Association* **247,** 2258–60.

Starkweather, J.A. (1959). Individual and situational influences on drug effects. In *A pharmacologic approach to the study of the mind* 3 (eds. R.M. Featherstone and A. Simon). Thomas, Springfield, Illinois.

Thoenen, H., Hurlimann, A., and Haefely, W. (1965). On the mode of action of chlorpromazine on peripheral adrenergic mechanisms. *International Journal of Neuropharmacolology* **4,** 79–89.

Tourney, G. (1967). A history of therapeutic fashions in psychiatry 1800–1966. *American Journal of Psychiatry* **124,** 784–96.

Urquhart, J. (1982). Rate-controlled drug dosage. *Drugs* **23,** 207–26.

Vaughn, C. and Leff, J.P. (1976). The influence of family and social factors on the course of psychiatric illness: a comparison of schizophrenic and depressed neurotic patients. *British Journal of Psychiatry* **129,** 125–37.

Venning, G.R. (1983). Identification of adverse reactions to new drugs. II. How were 18 important adverse reactions discovered and with what delays? *British Medical Journal* **286,** 289–92.

Vere, D.W. (1988). The ethics of adverse drug reactions. *Adverse Drug Reaction Bulletin* **128,** 480–3.

Whitehead, T.N. (1938). *The industrial worker: a statistical study of human relations in a group of manual workers*. Harvard University Press, Cambridge, Mass.

Wilder, J. (1958). Modern psychophysiology and the law of initial value. *American Journal of Psychotherapy* **12,** 199–221.

Wittenborn, J.R. (1980). Behavioral toxicity of psychotropic drugs. *Journal of Nervous and Mental Disease* **168,** 171–6.

Wolf, S. (1959). The pharmacology of placebos. *Pharmacology Review* **11,** 689–704.

Zito, J.M., Craig, T.J., Wanderling, J., and Siegel, C. (1987). Pharmacoepidemiology in 136 hospitalized schizophrenic patients. *American Journal of Psychiatry* **144,** 778–82.

7. The social aspects of prescribing

Treatment with psychotropic drugs is mostly initiated by family doctors. In considering the social function and consequences of this, some attention must be paid to what leads people to seek help from their doctor in the first place and what factors predispose to the inclusion of a prescription in the management package eventually offered, before attempting to assess the consequences, both good and bad, for society at large. The impact of specialist psychiatric opinion on the use of drugs in the treatment of nervous disorder, especially minor disorder, is not readily determined. However, any influence is presumably mainly through advice to general practitioners, at least in the United Kingdom where direct access to specialists is unusual. Psychiatrists themselves are, of course, exposed to similar psychosocial pressures as other doctors and the following analysis draws on evidence from several areas of medical practice.

Clinical skill is developed by the continuing interaction between an individual doctor and his patients. This has an immediacy and force which is not matched by knowledge gained by other means and can lead the clinician to have a rather myopic view of the nature of the problems which come to him and the efficacy of his management. It is important to recognize that both clinician and patient are subject to a variety of psychological forces which condition their encounter and which may be so powerful during the consultation itself that they have more effect than any specific treatments offered. As discussed in the previous chapter (Chapter 6), psychotropic drugs are not so potent that they consistently override these forces. Therefore, the responsible and effective use of these drugs requires an awareness of the broader scene within which the treatment process is carried out. The wisdom of the experienced clinician derives partly from an informal or 'amateurish' understanding of these matters which have become increasingly the subject of academic study. They are broadly discussed in this chapter.

Symptoms against which psychotropic drugs could be targeted are extremely common: fortunately perhaps, they remain amongst a mass of minor symptomatology unknown to doctors and aptly referred to by Hannay

(1980) as the 'symptom iceberg'. Minor symptoms are not unimportant because they absorb a great deal of medical time, they lead to the use of prescribed and non-prescribed medication, and they often cause distress in others which itself may require medical treatment.

The scale of the problem is illustrated by two community studies. Scambler *et al.* (1981) found in a study of health diaries kept for six weeks by women aged between 16 and 44 that symptoms were recorded one day in three, mostly minor and lasting 1–2 days; and a two week retrospective study of a random sample of 1000 adults living in London showed that only 46 had been symptom-free over this period (Wadsworth *et al.* 1971). The incidence or prevalence of psychiatric symptomatology of rather greater duration is much less although still substantial. Shepherd and his colleagues (1966) found that about 14 per cent of people consulted their doctors in primary care once in a twelve-month period for a condition diagnosed as largely or entirely psychiatric in nature: in about half of these patients the condition had been present for more than a year. Subsequent studies in Britain, Europe and the United States indicate that in the community at large about 15 per cent of people have a psychiatric disorder at any particular time, mostly minor affective disturbances, psychophysiological reactions or personality difficulties (Weissman *et al.* 1978 1981; Oliver and Simmons 1985; Marks 1986). In primary care settings about 25–30 per cent of new illness episodes carry a psychiatric diagnosis (Goldberg and Bridges 1987; Regier *et al.* 1985) although this often occurs in association with physical disease. These figures are influenced by the method of eliciting the symptoms and by the diagnostic criteria used, but, even when these are fairly testing, prevalence is quite substantial: for example, in a community study using Research Diagnostic Criteria the current prevalence for anxiety disorder was 4.3 per cent and depression was 5.7 per cent (Weissman *et al.* 1978). The severity of symptoms is substantially greater in patients attending psychiatric clinics the study of whom has provided, until recently, the basis of our current understanding of nosology and treatment response. Clearly, before reaching the psychiatric clinic the patient has passed through a series of formal and informal filters (Goldberg and Huxley 1980) so that studies in the community, in general practice, and in psychiatric clinics may give rather different results. Insufficient evidence exists at present to provide a consistent overall picture.

Given such a substantial prevalence of psychiatric symptoms it is not surprising that psychotropic drugs are widely prescribed and consumed. Surveys indicate that over any two-week period about 10 per cent of the adult population will consume such a drug on at least one occasion (Murray *et al.* 1981; Gabe and Williams 1986). Much of this use is short-term and about half of the patients who start treatment with a psychotropic drug will have stopped within a month. The remainder continue for much longer and there is evidence that the number of such patients is increasing (Williams 1983; Gabe and Williams 1986). Over the past twenty years the pattern of prescribing has steadily changed with the gradual elimination of older drugs such as barbiturates and the steady increase in non-barbiturate hypnotics, minor tranquillizers, and antidepressants. The rate of increase has lessened over the latter half of this period perhaps due in part to the use of non-psychotropic agents such as beta-adrenergic antagonists to manage psychiatric symptoms. The total volume of prescription for these disorders is probably not greatly changed over thirty years (Clare 1985).

It is perhaps fortunate that most people with psychiatric symptoms do not seek medical help: this is especially so for those minor or transient symptoms but quite disabled people also avoid such contact (e.g. Marks 1986). Many find their own solutions in non-prescribed medicines, alcohol, cigarettes, or comfort eating, or the use of medication as a 'resource' called upon when their favourite remedies and their family and social supports fail. For example, in one study (Dunnell and Cartwright 1972), 67 per cent of people interviewed had taken one or more non-prescribed medicines during the preceding two weeks, only one in ten of these were advised by the doctor, most being recommended by family, friends, or other lay sources. Indeed, evidence suggests that most people tolerate their symptoms for some time before they go to their doctors and that the symptoms themselves may not be sufficient to precipitate consultation.

Zola (1973) identified 5 types of trigger which lead the patient to present his symptoms to the doctor: interpersonal crises; pressure from others to consult; interference with vocational or physical activity or with personal and social relations; persistence of symptoms beyond a deadline considered by the patient to be safe or tolerable. Some patients resist consultation despite considerable discomfort and serious illness preferring their own nostrums or support systems (Anderson *et al.* 1977). Activities of this kind contain much illness, psychiatric or otherwise: 'It is the professional health services which should be seen as the stop-gaps, filling in when basic mutual self-help needs specific technical, organizational or expert assistance' (Robinson 1980). It is clear that even a small increase in the tendency to use medical services rather than other means of coping would have a major impact on these services and probably on the use of psychotropic drugs. Nevertheless, the number of people seeking medical help for what are mainly psychiatric problems is already considerable and the use of medicines to deal with them is on such a scale that up to 20 per cent of prescriptions are written for hypnotics, minor tranquillizers, and antidepressants (Skegg *et al.* 1981).

It would help to know what factors lead some people, but not others, to take prescribed psychotropic drugs and then to continue with them. In a questionnaire study of postal volunteers obtained through *Woman's Own*, most of whom had taken drugs for at least five years, Murray (1981) found that patients felt that their medication eased symptoms of tension, insomnia, and physical illness, and helped them to cope socially, with travel or with family problems. Many did not welcome their reliance on medication and many had tried to give it up. Many felt that doctors were too ready to write prescriptions and only one in five said that their doctors had tried to stop them. Women are more likely than men to use prescribed psychotropic drugs: family responsibilities and stress in family life being important causes of this difference between the sexes (Cafferata *et al.* 1983).

Factors leading doctors to prescribe psychotropic drugs have been less easily identified. Reviewing such evidence as exists, Hemminki (1975) concluded that 'No generalizations can be drawn from all these studies' which examined education, advertising, colleagues, regulation measures, patient demand, and doctors' characteristics. Presumably many complex factors constituting the 'sociocultural milieu' operate through doctor and patient, including advertising, drug company pressure, the changing climate of opinion concerning use of medication, the conditions of family and psychiatric practice, the existence of self-help groups and other supports, the patient's perception of the nature of drug action (Helman 1981), the level of social stress including unemployment and so on. There are therefore marked regional and national differences in the consumption of tranquillizers, Britain being near the top of the European league with about twice the per capita consumption of Italy (Balter *et al.* 1974). Similar factors presumably influence the consumption of alcohol and cigarettes. The path leading to the use of prescribed medicines is therefore highly complex and perhaps not too easily changed. For example, whilst the prescribing habits of doctors can be influenced by suitable educational programmes, the effect is short-lived (Harris *et al.* 1985).

Thus, by the time the doctor and patient have their first meeting a great many factors have exerted effects which continue during the consultation, the outcome of which is certainly not determined solely by the symptoms presented and the biomedical technology brought to bear upon them. The doctor–patient relationship is therefore a potent factor in the delivery of health care, including the use of psychotropic medication, and insight into the processes involved is an essential element of effective therapeutics.

The patient arrives at the consultation not altogether aware of the range of his symptoms or how he is to present it. He may have his own ideas as to the underlying cause and what ought to be done (e.g. he may disapprove of the use of drugs). He may be very apprehensive about whether the doctor will understand, give him time, respect his needs, cope with emotional display or recommend a course of management he would find difficult to accept. His motivation may arise partly from pressures in his family or working life of which he may only be dimly aware and exploration of which he would reflexly resist, initially at least. The doctor may conduct the consultation with an over-practised routine which is only dimly aimed at extracting what he considers to be relevant information within the allotted time in a manner which taxes him as little as possible: his interests and capabilities constrain the interaction between himself and the patient. The patient may therefore leave without having said all he intended, his questions remaining unanswered, his anxieties unrelieved, and he may have retained very little of the information and advice given him. The doctor may not have obtained a balanced view of the problem, may not have grasped the purpose of the consultation, may have been superficial or dismissive in his response, and may have spoiled the future relationship with the patient. The dynamics of these processes at the centre of medical practice have been extensively examined by Balint (1956), Fitton and Acheson (1979), Byrne and Long (1976), and Stimson and Webb (1975).

Of course, the doctor can only relate to patients through his own personality, and a professional manner must be built on this: to attempt otherwise is to risk appearing pompous, superficial, or insincere. His approach must be sufficiently flexible to adjust to the intelligence, age, and culture of the patient and it must change during a professional lifetime as social relationships in general and public sophistication on health matters develop. The doctor–patient relationship has changed considerably during the past 50 years, as can be seen in the comparison of the Goodenough (1944) and Todd (1968) reports on medical education: between these 'can be discerned a reformulation of the notion of clinical skills which involved a relative weakening of the importance of the clinical examination and the appearance of an inherently problematic doctor–patient relationship' (Armstrong 1982).

Nevertheless, studies of contemporary family and hospital practice indicate that only a minority of practitioners has made this change. In a study of 2 500 tape-recorded general practitioner consultations, Byrne and Long (1976) found 75 per cent to be 'doctor centred', involving a directive approach and tightly controlled interviewing aimed at getting the diagnosis as quickly as possible and providing little opportunity for patients to discuss their symptoms and worries. A similar situation was documented by Plaja and Cohen (1968) in hospital out-patient clinics where the most common style was 'bureaucratic, task-orientated', being marked by efficient questioning, limited sensitivity to the patient, and little variation from patient to patient. Few doctors were 'patient orientated' and therefore had no idea of the patient's own ideas about his illness or his anxieties and were therefore not in a position to understand and manage the cognitive and emotional factors associated with the illness. Yet there is considerable evidence that such awareness and understanding improves compliance and efficacy of treatment (Korsch *et al.* 1969; Davis 1968; Stewart 1984). Building a relationship with the patient ('personal doctoring') improves the patient's satisfaction with the care given, allows the patient to learn more about his illness, and to avoid undue anxiety and invalidism (Rudd *et al.* 1984) and permits effective training in the use of treatment methods including medication (Ettlinger and Freeman 1981; Norell 1979). For example, in Norell's study, in which an ingenious electronic monitor recorded when the cap of the medicine bottle was removed, the use and timing of pilocarpine eyedrops was greatly improved following a brief tape–slide presentation about the treatment recommended to the patient.

There is also clear evidence from various branches of medicine that the style of consultation influences efficacy. For example, Fitzpatrick and his co-workers (1983) interviewed patients at the time of their attendance at a neurological clinic for assessment of headache and again one year later. They found that patients whose initial reaction to clinic attendance was positive and who felt that the doctor had taken a personal interest in them and their anxieties reported more improvement after one year: specific medical treatment was unrelated to overall outcome. In anaesthetic practice the preoperative personal attention of the anaesthetist reduced post-operative pain, the need for narcotics and hospital stay (Egbert *et al.* 1964). Studies of psychiatric populations show that compliance with drug regimes and outcome are improved by 'promoting' therapists who take more interest and offer more reassurance and hope (Reynolds *et al.* 1965; Rickels 1968).

Personal doctoring brings other benefits to both doctor and patient. The doctor is more likely to be aware of important factors in the patient's life, particularly within the family, which have a fairly direct effect on the patient seeking treatment and his response to it. For example, in a retrospective study of drug use in 50 families attending a city practice, the children of the 10 mothers classed as high psychotropic drug users were seen twice as often with acute respiratory illness and received twice as many prescriptions for antibiotics as children of mothers who received no psychotropic drugs (Howie and Bigg 1980). The authors suggested that in many of these consultations the mother rather than the child should have been treated as the patient.

Compliance is poor among people who live alone and is improved where a relative or spouse is able to supervise treatment. Reducing the stress in key relatives by providing information and support can have a considerable effect on treatment response. This is particularly striking in acute situations. In a study of tonsillectomy, children were assigned randomly to either the hospital's usual procedure or to the care of a special nurse whose job was to provide the mother with information regarding the operation and its effects, on admission and at various times during the child's stay. Mothers given this support experienced less stress, as did the children who showed less disturbance of blood pressure and heart rate, vomited less and maintained a better fluid intake (Skipper and Leonard 1968).

Easing family distress for patients with psychiatric disorders probably also improves response to treatment. This has been studied mainly in relation to schizophrenic illnesses. The ability of maintenance medication to prevent relapse is much reduced in schizophrenic patients living in high stress households. Family therapy within the home of such patients has been shown to reduce the level of schizophrenic symptomatology, the number of acute exacerbations and the length of hospital stay if that proved necessary (Falloon *et al.* 1982).

The detection of such family and social factors requires a 'patient-centred' rather than 'doctor-centred' consultation, whether this be general practice or in specialist clinics, including psychiatric clinics. There is some evidence that this is happening (Cartwright and Anderson 1981). Patients are less happy to receive a prescription than they were, but the eagerness of doctors to prescribe has fallen less. This may be because a prescription helps doctors to cope with uncertainty by engaging in positive action, it allows a shorter consultation and may serve to communicate the doctor's concern to the patient. However, it also opens the door to repeat prescriptions, side-effects, and drug interactions, and may indicate to the patient that medical care is an appropriate way of dealing with his problem when this is not really the case.

Psychotropic drugs are therefore often used in situations which have been inadequately explored and where, as often as not, they do little good. How important is it that such drugs are used? Would there be serious consequences if they were used much less or only if there were clear and pressing indications? It is undoubtedly possible to overestimate the contribution of drugs,or any other treatment, to the outcome of illness especially where psychosocial factors are important as in the case for psychiatric disorders. Even in serious physical illness the value of specific remedies has probably been overdone (McKeown 1979). The reduced prevalence or severity of the infections, rheumatic fever, peptic ulcer, or schizophrenia may not be due, to a major degree at least, to the medical remedies employed over the past 40 years or so. The changing pattern of disease and the changing sociocultural environment makes these issues difficult to judge. It is certainly possible to effectively manage psychiatric conditions, in which drugs are commonly employed, without doing so. Catalan *et al.* (1984) were able to show that brief counselling was as effective as anxiolytic medication in treating minor illness over the course of 7 months without increased consumption of alcohol, tobacco, or non-prescribed drugs or increased demands on the doctor's time. Carpenter *et al.* (1977) reported that schizophrenic patients treated in a fairly intensive psychosocial programme with minimal medication did as well after one year as patients given antipsychotic drugs in the usual way. In the case of depressive illness it has been calculated that the use of antidepressant drugs produces a remission in only about 20 per cent more patients than if no drugs had been used (Paykel 1985).

Although psychotropic drugs may have a valuable role to play in the management of much psychiatric illness other factors are often as important. There is therefore no need to rush in with drug treatment in the vast majority of patients. It is important to be aware of pressures increasing the likelihood of prescribing and resisting them if they are not clearly in the interests of the patient rather than of the doctor. Premature and widespread use of psychotropics cannot be to the benefit of the individual patient or society at large and it only leads to increased exposure to harmful effects. The same can, of course, be said of other drugs which are commonly over-prescribed: beta-adrenergic blockers, diuretics, anti-inflammatory agents, H_2 antagonists. The hazards of long-term use can be minimized by initiating treatment only where there are clear indications, using minimal effective doses, evaluating the need for repeat prescriptions, and giving as much attention to terminating treatment as to initiating it.

Patients often protect themselves, wittingly or unwittingly, by not taking their treatment, but this in turn can lead to other problems because unused drugs are left about the house and may be accidently ingested, especially by children, used in suicidal bids, or consumed long after their shelf-life has expired, with possible toxic effects. The social cost of this misuse is considerable but perhaps rather modest compared to the cost of smoking and excessive alcohol consumption. The immediate dangers of drugs are usually easily recognised and, in principle at least, action can be taken to minimize them. Nevertheless, just as the dangers of smoking were not well recognized until the habit had been widespread for some decades, there must be concern over untoward effects of drugs which show themselves only after a considerable latency. Such effects may not be easily detected perhaps partly because of a reluctance to attribute them to drug exposure as in the case of antipsychotic drugs and tardive dyskinesia.

The long-term use of drugs, even where there are clear indications, must continue to cause anxiety to health workers. It is, for example, hard to believe that almost complete inhibition of monoamine oxidase for years will have no untoward long-term effect. Or again, whilst drug exposure *in utero* may be judged safe because it is not associated with defects of gross organogenesis, might it not affect the fine structure of neurones and hence intelligence and personality or be associated with pathology many years later as in the case of the vaginal carcinoma in girls exposed to the use of stilboestrol during their mother's pregnancy? The possibility, even if remote, of a pharmacological 'silent spring' should caution against the use of drugs to manage minor illness or personal problems and patients can undoubtedly be helped to manage much minor illness without medical supervision by providing them with a brief information booklet (Morrell *et al.*

1980). Such consideration should ensure that the benefits of psychotropic medication are maximized and the risks kept to the minimum.

Expenditure on health care is currently about 6 per cent of the gross national product in the United Kingdom and about 10 per cent in the United States, Sweden, and France. The economic activity of advanced nations is therefore inevitably influenced by it with a multiplicity of sociopolitical consequences. The pharmaceutical industry, contributing as it does so much to employment, the export trade, and scientific research has a powerful voice capable of influencing government on broad issues of policy or doctors on their attitudes to drug use. Doctors must therefore be aware of this influence on their clinical and scientific activities and be prepared to evaluate the consumption of resources which their work entails. Increasingly, cost-effectiveness of treatments is being discussed either in purely economic terms, as in comparing the cost of treatment with savings due to reduced hospital stay, or by comparing one treatment method with another, or by measuring the improvement in the quality of life obtained. The methods of measuring these are still being developed and have usually concerned serious physical illness and major interventions rather than psychiatric disorder. However, there is little doubt that in the future the allocation of health care resources will be guided by such analyses, so that what is technically possible will be purposely constrained by economic, social, and ethical considerations (Teeling-Smith 1985).

References

Anderson, J., Buck, C., Danaher, K., and Fry, J. (1977). Users and non-users of doctors: implications for self care. *Journal of the Royal College of General Practitioners* **27,** 155–9.

Armstrong, D. (1982). The doctor–patient relationship: 1930–1980. In *The problem of medical knowledge. Examining the social construction of medicine* (eds. P. Wright and A. Treacher). Edinburgh University Press, Edinburgh.

Balint, M. (1956). *The doctor, his patient and the illness.* Pitman, London.

Balter, M.B., Levine, J. and Manheimer, D.I. (1974). Cross-national study of the extent of anti-anxiety/sedative drug use. *New England Journal of Medicine* **290,** 769–74.

Byrne, P.S. and Long, B.L. (1976). *Doctors talking to patients.* HMSO, London.

Cafferata, G.L., Kasper, J. and Bernstein, A. (1983). Family roles, structure and stressors in relation to sex differences in obtaining psychotropic drugs. *Journal of Health and Social Behaviour* **24,** 132–43.

Carpenter, W.T., McGlashan, T.H., and Strauss, J.S. (1977). The treatment of acute schizophrenia without drugs: an investigation of some current assumptions. *American Journal of Psychiatry* 14–20.

Cartwright, A. and Anderson, R. (1981). *General practice revisited: A second study of patients and their doctors.* Tavistock Publications, London.

Catalan, J. Gath, D., Edmonds, G., Ennis, J., Bond, A., and Martin, P. (1984).

The effects of non-prescribing of anxiolytics in general practice. *British Journal of Psychiatry* **144,** 593–610.

Clare, A.W. (1985). Anxiolytics in society. In: *Psychopharmacology: Recent advances and future prospects.* (ed. S.D. Iversen). Oxford University Press, Oxford.

Davis, M. (1968). Variations in patients' compliance with doctor's advice: empirical analysis of patterns of communication. *American Journal of Public Health* **58,** 274–88.

Dunnell, K. and Cartwright, A. (1972). *Medicine takers, prescribers and hoarders.* Routledge & Kegan Paul, London.

Egbert, L., Battit, G., Welch, C., and Bartlett, M. (1964). Reduction of post-operative pain by encouragement and instruction of patients. *New England Journal of Medicine* **270,** 825–7.

Ettlinger, P.R.A. and Freeman, G.K. (1981). General practice compliance study: is it worth being a personal doctor? *British Medical Journal* **i,** 1192–4.

Falloon, I.R.H., Boyd, J.L., McGill, C.W., Razani, J., Moss, H.B., and Gilderman, A.M. (1982). Family management in the prevention of exacerbations of schizophrenia. A controlled study. *New England Journal of Medicine* **306,** 1437–40.

Fitton, F. and Acheson, H.W.K. (1979). *Doctor–patient relationship: A study in general practice.* HMSO, London.

Fitzpatrick, R., Hopkins, A., and Harvard-Watts, O. (1983). Social dimensions of healing: a longitudinal study of medical management of headaches. *Social Science and Medicine* **17,** 501–10.

Gabe, J. and Williams, P. (1986). Tranquilliser use: a historical perspective. In: *Tranquillisers. Social, psychological and clinical perspectives* (eds. J. Gabe and P. Williams). Tavistock Publications, London.

Goldberg, D. and Bridges, K. (1987). Screening for psychiatric illness in general practice: the general practitioner versus the screening questionnaire. *Journal of the Royal College of General Practitioners* **37,** 15–18.

Goldberg, D. and Huxley, P. (1980). *Mental illness in the community.* Tavistock Publications, London.

Hannay, D. (1980). The iceberg of illness and trivial consultations. *Journal of the Royal College of General Practitioners* **30,** 551–4.

Harris, C.M., Fry, J. Jarman, B., and Woodman, E. (1985). Prescribing—a case for prolonged treatment. *Journal of the Royal College of General Practitioners* **35,** 284–7.

Helman, C.G. (1981). 'Tonic', 'fuel' and 'food': social and symbolic aspects of longterm use of psychotropic drugs. *Social Science and Medicine* **15B,** 521–33.

Hemminki, E. (1975). Review of literature on the factors affecting drug prescribing. *Social Science and Medicine* **9,** 111–15.

Howie, J.G.R. and Bigg, A.R. (1980). Family trends in psychotropic and antibiotic prescribing in general practice. *British Medical Journal* **1,** 836–8.

Korsch, B., Gozzi, E., and Francis, V. (1969). Gaps in doctor–patient communication: patients' response to medical advice. *New England Journal of Medicine* **280,** 535–40.

McKeown, T. (1979). *The role of medicine: dream, mirage or nemesis?*, 2nd edn. Blackwell, Oxford.

Marks, I.M. (1986). Epidemiology of anxiety. *Social Psychiatry* **21,** 167–71.

Morrell, D.C., Avery, A.J. and Watkins, C.J. (1980). Management of minor illness. *British Medical Journal* **1,** 769–71.

Murray, J. (1981). Longterm psychotropic drug-taking and the process of withdrawal. *Psychological Medicine* **11,** 853–8.

Murray, J., Dunn, G., Williams, P. and Tarnopolsky, A. (1981). Factors affecting the consumption of psychotropic drugs. *Psychological Medicine* **11,** 551–60.

Norell, S.E. (1979). Improving medication compliance: a randomised clinical trial. *British Medical Journal* **2,** 1031–3.

Oliver, J.M. and Simmons, H.E. (1985). Affective disorders and depression as measured by the diagnostic interview schedule and the Beck Depression Inventory in an unselected adult population. *Journal of Clinical Psychology* **41,** 469–77.

Paykel, E.S. (1985). How effective are antidepressants? In: *Psychopharmacology: Recent advances and future prospects* (ed. S.D. Iversen). Oxford University Press, Oxford.

Plaja, A. and Cohen, S. (1968). Communication between physicians and patients in out-patient clinics: social and cultural factors. *Millbank Memorial Fund Quarterly* **46,** 161–213.

Regier, D.A., Burke, J.D., Manderscheid, R.W. and Burns, B.J. (1985). The chronically mentally ill in primary care. *Psychological Medicine* **15,** 265–73.

Reynolds, E., Joyce, C.R.B., Swift, J.L., Tooley, P.H., and Weatherall, M. (1965). Psychological and clinical investigation of the treatment of anxious outpatients with three barbiturates and placebo. *British Journal of Psychiatry* **111,** 84–95.

Rickels, K. (1968). *Non-specific factors in drug therapy.* Thomas, Springfield, Illinois.

Robinson, D. (1980). The self-help component in primary care. *Social Science and Medicine* **14A,** 415–21.

Rudd, P., Price, M., Graham, L., and Fortmann, S. (1984). More on labelling of hypertensive patients. *New England Journal of Medicine* **310,** 1126–8.

Scambler, A., Scambler, G., and Craig, D. (1981). Kinship and friendship networks and women's demand for primary care. *Journal of the Royal College of General Practitioners* **31,** 746–50.

Shepherd, M., Cooper, B., Brown, A.C. and Kalton, G. (1966). *Psychiatric illness in general practice.* Oxford University Press, London.

Skegg, D.G., Doll, R. and Perry, J. (1977). The use of medicines in general practice. *British Medical Journal* **i,** 1561–3.

Skipper, J. and Leonard, R. (1968). Children, stress and hospitalisation: a field experiment. *Journal of Health and Social Behaviour* **9,** 275–87.

Stewart, M. (1984). What is a successful doctor-patient interview? *Social Science and Medicine* **19,** 167–75.

Stimson, G. and Webb, B. (1975). *Going to see the doctor.* Routledge & Kegan Paul, London.

Teeling-Smith, G. (1985). *Measurement of health.* Office of Health Economics, London.

Wadsworth, M., Butterworth, W., and Blaney, R. (1971). *Health and sickness: The choice of treatment.* Tavistock Publications, London.

Weissman, M.M. and Myers, J.K. (1978). Affective disorders in a US urban community. The use of Research Diagnostic Criteria in an epidemiological survey. *Archives of General Psychiatry* **35,** 1304–11.

Weissman, M.M., Myers, J.K. and Harding, P.S. (1978). Psychiatric disorders in a US urban community. *American Journal of Psychiatry* **135,** 459–62.

Weissman, M.M., Myers, J.K., and Thompson, W.D. (1981). Depression and its treatment in a US urban community—1975–1976. *Archives of General Psychiatry* **38,** 417–21.

Williams, P. (1983). Patterns of psychotropic drug use. *Social Science and Medicine* **17,** 845–51.

Zola, I. (1973). Pathways to the doctor: from person to patient. *Social Science and Medicine* **7,** 677–89.

8. Pharmacokinetics

Introduction

Pharmacokinetics is the study of the body's effects on drugs and determines whether the drug gets to its site of action and in what concentrations. As both a theoretical and practical topic it has become increasingly important in recent years. An excellent detailed account is given by Grahame-Smith and Aronson (1984).

The pharmacokinetic approach, already established in the treatment of infectious diseases and epilepsy, was first used in psychopharmacology with the introduction of lithium salts. Much information is now available about pharmacokinetic properties of other psychotropic drugs and a basic understanding in this field has become increasingly relevant to psychiatrists over the past few years. For example, when confronted with such different sleep disorders as initial insomnia, repeated awakenings or early morning waking, it would be difficult to prescribe rationally a hypnotic drug without knowing its half-life and the time to its peak plasma concentration.

Because of the mass of factual material, it is unrealistic to expect the clinician to know the pharmacokinetic details of every psychotropic agent, its absorption characteristics, distribution, liver metabolism, kidney excretion, drug interactions, and so on. The important pharmacokinetic variables are covered in the chapters on the individual drugs. This chapter is intended to introduce some basic principles and to emphasize how important these principles are to the rational use of psychotropic agents. It follows the traditional headings of absorption, distribution, metabolism, and excretion. First, however, some basic definitions are described.

Definitions and basic principles in pharmacokinetics

Pharmacokinetics aims to provide a mathematical model for the description and prediction of the time-course of drugs in the body. This is achieved by measuring the drug concentrations in plasma and sometimes other body fluids, e.g. urine, saliva, or cerebrospinal fluid (CSF), over a period of time following administration. The pharmacokinetic variables obtained from these data are essential factors for rational therapy. For each drug they give important information about:

(1) the optimal dosage intervals;

(2) the time-lag and duration of action of a single dose;

(3) the delay of maximal effect of repeated doses;

(4) the influence of physiological (e.g. sex, pregnancy, age) as well as pathological states upon the usage of the drug;

(5) the likelihood of drug interactions.

However, these variables represent mean values for populations of normal adults and can vary widely for the same drug between individuals and, to a lesser extent, within the same person on different occasions. Thus, if such variation is suspected, the dosage regimen needs adjustment for some people according to their own pharmacokinetic capabilities. This may be pertinent in those who fail to respond to treatment or develop severe side effects during usual dosage regimens.

Several parameters are important:

1. The biological half-life (T) is the time required for the plasma drug concentration to decrease by half. It is constant for a given individual if the rate at which the drug is eliminated is proportional to its plasma concentration (known as first-order kinetics). The half-life can be calculated graphically or by the formula

$$T = \frac{0.693}{K}$$

where T is expressed in hours and K is the elimination constant measured as units per hour. K is the slope of the linear curve obtained from graphically plotting the logarithm of the plasma concentration against time. T will be large for drugs which are eliminated slowly and small for drugs eliminated quickly. The biological half-life is an important parameter to determine the dosage interval of a drug and the delay necessary to achieve steady-state on repeated administration or complete elimination after the drug has been stopped. In both cases this delay is roughly equal to five times T. In some instances T can help to understand the duration of action of a drug after acute administration.

2. The apparent volume of distribution (V_d) is a purely theoretical ratio (expressed in litres per kilogram), without any physiological meaning, between the amount of drug present in the body (mg per kg) and its plasma concentration (milligrams per litre). It is usually calculated by dividing the intravenous dose (D) by the plasma concentration at the start of the injec-

tion—a purely fictional value obtained by extrapolating the graph of the plasma concentration against time to zero time (C_0).

$$V_d \text{ (litres per kg)} = \frac{D \text{ (mg per kg)}}{C_0 \text{ (mg per litre)}}$$

For most psychotropic drugs V_d is large because of their distribution throughout the body fluids and their significant uptake by the tissues due to their lipophilic properties. A V_d of about 10 litres per kilogram will mean that the average drug concentration in tissues is ten times higher than in plasma, indicating important binding to tissue proteins.

3. The total body clearance (*Cl*) is the fraction of the apparent volume of distribution which is completely cleared from drug per unit time. Thus, *Cl* is a general index of all the elimination mechanisms leading to the disappearance of the drug from the central compartment. These mechanisms are mainly contributed by hepatic metabolism and renal elimination.

$$Cl \text{ (ml per min per kg)} = V_d \text{ (ml per kg)} \times K \text{ (per min)}.$$

The total body clearance is directly proportional to the elimination constant and thus is commonly used to quantify drug elimination. Of course, the processes of absorption, distribution, metabolism and excretion are complex and interactive. Simple models do considerable violence to the truth but they may be of practical value. More complex models can correspond more closely to physiological systems and the mathematical description and analysis of them is inevitably rather forbidding. These matters can be explored more fully in texts of pharmacokinetics.

Absorption

Most drugs are distributed in the body in the water phase of the plasma. Hence, drugs must first enter the bloodstream by crossing lipoprotein cell membranes. The rate at which a drug reaches its site of action, such as the brain, is thus dependent on (a) the blood flow through the organ, and (b) the speed with which the drug can pass across lipoprotein membranes.

A drug enters the circulation either by being placed there directly or by absorption from depots, or 'sumps', such as the gastrointestinal tract, the muscles, or subcutaneous tissue. The latter two sites represent the parenteral mode, and the gut represents the enteral mode.

Intravenous injection

An obvious advantage of the intravenous method of drug administration is the minimal delay before the drug enters the circulation (Fig. 8.1). Moreover, intravenous administration is easy to control, especially with an

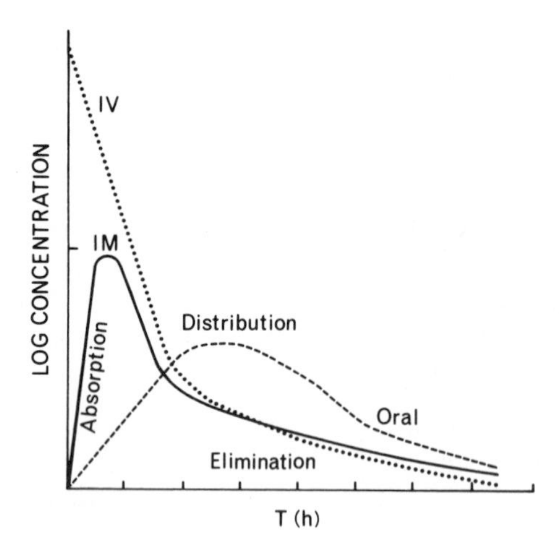

Fig. 8.1. Blood concentrations after intravenous (IV), intramuscular (IM), and oral administration of a drug.

infusion rather than a bolus injection. An example of controlled injection is the use of intravenously infused drug to induce an abreaction. Intravenous infusions are a useful way of building up body concentrations as has been advocated in the acute use of clomipramine. The disadvantage of intravenous injection is that dangerously high concentrations may be attained during the bolus injection. Furthermore, once injected the drug cannot be removed except by metabolism and excretion, whereas an emetic or stomach lavage can remove an oral overdose.

Intramuscular injection

Intramuscular injections of antipsychotic drugs are commonly used by psychiatrists to quieten the disturbed patient. Blood flow through resting muscles is about 0.02 to 0.07 ml/min/g tissue and may increase tenfold during emotional excitement. Thus, the agitated or frenzied, disturbed patient should rapidly absorb antipsychotic injections. However, for some drugs such as diazepam or chlordiazepoxide, absorption is erratic after intramuscular injection. Long-acting depot injections comprise highly lipid-soluble formulations of drugs, such as fluphenazine decanoate in oil, which are absorbed very slowly from their depot in the muscle, probably because they dissolve in the fatty tissues of the muscle.

Oral administration

Drugs are traditionally given by mouth, absorption being possible along the whole length of the gastrointestinal tract from buccal mucosa to rectum (Fig.

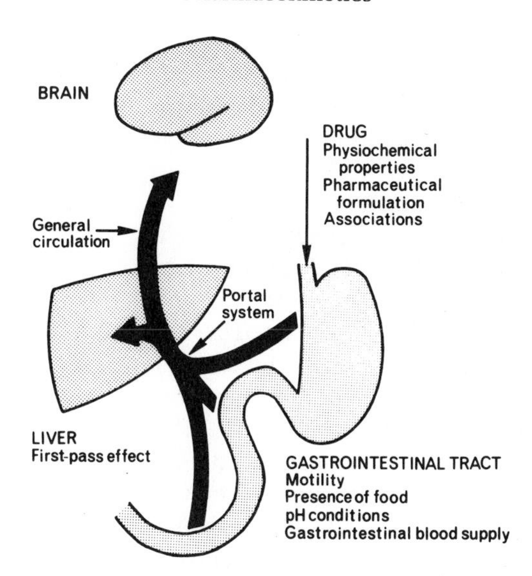

Fig. 8.2. Factors influencing availability of a drug after oral administration.

8.2). The absorption in the stomach and jejunum is the most important, but the site of most rapid absorption depends on the chemical properties of the drug. Gastric absorption is favoured by an empty stomach, the drug coming into unimpeded contact with the mucosal walls. A full stomach can also postpone absorption of drugs from the intestine by causing delayed gastric emptying. Thus, if rapid action is required, drugs (except for gastric irritants such as aspirin) should be given on an empty stomach. For a smoother, delayed absorption, the drug should be taken after meals. In some instances, however, the extent of drug absorption is increased by food intake (propranolol, phenytoin, carbamazepine). In some patients, an increase in gastrointestinal motility due to anxiety can lead to a quicker absorption of drugs like diazepam.

Some drugs such as iron, methyldopa, and several amino acids are actively absorbed by specific carrier mechanisms. Most, however, diffuse passively into the body. To do so the molecule must be either very small or non-ionized and lipid-soluble. Gastric juice is acid (pH about 1), and intestinal contents are neutral or slightly alkaline. Many drugs are weak acids or bases; most psychotropic drugs are weak bases that exist in two forms—the non-dissociated (or non-ionized) form, and the dissociated (or ionized) form, e.g.:

$$\underset{\text{(non-ionized)}}{\text{Drug base} + \text{HCl}} \rightleftharpoons \underset{\text{(ionized)}}{\text{Drug base}.\ H^+} + Cl^-$$

The degree of dissociation depends on the pH of the medium. The drug is half-ionized at the pH of the solution indicated by its pK_a (negative logarithm of the dissociation constant). In practice, weak bases are absorbed better in the higher pH conditions of the jejunum, where their ionization is largely suppressed.

Absorption also depends critically on the lipid solubility (better termed 'lipophilicity') of the undissociated drug. Thus, barbitone and quinalbarbitone have almost the same pK_a, yet the latter is more rapidly absorbed because of its higher lipophilicity.

Some drugs for oral use are formulated as sustained-release preparations: the tablet slowly dissolves or the drug leaches out of an inert matrix. If release is too slow and the rate of movement through the gut too rapid, the drug will be incompletely absorbed.

Other substances can affect gastrointestinal absorption of psychotropic drugs. A modification of gastric pH by antacids can modify the degree of dissociation (ionization) of drugs like diazepam or chlordiazepoxide and delay their absorption. With clorazepate, antacids decrease the hydrolysis of the drug to nordiazepam which takes place in the stomach and can reduce the sedative effects of single doses. Anticholinergic drugs like tricyclic antidepressants, and some antipsychotics, can decrease the motility and delay the emptying of the stomach. Thus, the extent of absorption can be increased for drugs absorbed in the stomach and decreased for those absorbed in the intestine.

Bioavailability

Bioavailability strictly speaking means the relative amount of an administered drug which reaches the general circulation, but is sometimes used to mean the rate at which it occurs. Bioavailability is commonly referred to as a fraction of the drug dosage and is calculated by comparing the area under the curve (AUC) of the given formulation with the AUC obtained after IV administration.

$$\text{Bioavailability (per cent)} = \frac{\text{AUC after oral or IM dose}}{\text{AUC after IV dose}} \times 100$$

The rate of absorption is estimated as the delay to the peak plasma concentration and its value, i.e. the quicker a drug is absorbed the higher and sooner will be its peak plasma concentration.

In Fig. 8.3 are depicted three curves representing the theoretical plasma concentrations following the oral administration of three different preparations of the same dose of a drug. It can be seen that A is too rapid, with the peak occurring early (t_{max} less than 30 min) and with a high and potentially toxic peak concentration. Conversely, C is too slow and prolonged and

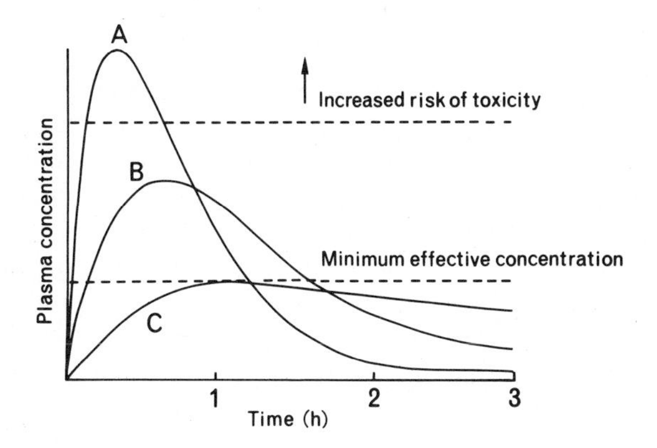

Fig. 8.3. Theoretical plasma concentrations following oral administration of three different formulations of same dose of a drug. (Modified from Grahame-Smith and Aronson 1984, with permission.)

effective concentrations are not attained, at least in single dosage. Preparation B lies between the two giving 1.5 h of effectiveness without toxicity. Note that the bioavailability—the area under the curve (AUC)—is the same in each.

All the factors influencing absorption can modify the bioavailability of a drug. Differences in the product formulation is another factor which can lead to important modifications in the rate and extent of absorption of a drug. This has been clearly documented for drugs like phenytoin, digoxin, aspirin, and to a lesser extent for some psychotropic drugs like chlorpromazine, dextroamphetamine, chlordiazepoxide, methaqualone, and amitriptyline.

Furthermore, the amount of hepatic metabolism of the drug during its passage from the portal system to the general circulation can influence the bioavailability of drugs. As shown later, this hepatic 'first-pass' effect is especially important for some psychotropic drugs.

Distribution

Protein binding and distribution

Most drugs are distributed throughout the body fluids in the water phase of plasma. From there, they reach their sites of action at a rate depending on the blood flow through the organ and on the ease with which the drug can pass across lipoprotein membranes. Only drug which is not bound to plasma protein (i.e. the unbound or 'free' drug) is able to cross the membranes and reach the site of action. Thus, plasma protein binding is another crucial factor governing drug distribution within the body.

Plasma protein binding

Tricyclic antidepressants, phenothiazines and benzodiazepines are highly and strongly bound to plasma proteins. The amount of free drug is usually less than 10 per cent of the plasma drug concentration, and remains constant for a wide range of concentrations. However, binding varies among individuals and the free fraction varies about twofold across most subjects. The characteristics of protein binding depend strongly on the chemical structure of the drug. While acidic drugs bind mainly to albumin, basic drugs, as are most psychotropic drugs, can also be bound to lipoproteins, alpha$_1$-glycoproteins and globulins. In the case of imipramine and chlorpromazine the binding to lipoprotein is actually as high as that to albumin. The extent of binding for some common psychotropic drugs is shown in Table 8.1.

The binding is reversible and can be modified by different factors:

1. The plasma drug concentration. Usually the percentage of binding increases linearly with the plasma drug concentration until it reaches a plateau and then remains constant. Thus, the percentage of drug binding is a meaningless value unless the drug concentration is specified.

2. The plasma protein concentration. While variations in plasma albumin concentrations are narrow and usually in the direction of decreasing concentrations, large fluctuations in both directions are possible for other proteins. Thus a decrease, or sometimes an increase, in protein binding of psychotropic drugs can be observed in pathological conditions. These conditions are detailed in Table 8.2. Furthermore a decrease of plasma albumin concentration can be observed in different physiological conditions, e.g. ageing or pregnancy.

3. The presence of other substances which can compete with the drug for binding sites or modify their affinity by inducing structural changes in the tertiary conformation of the protein. This can be due to other drugs

Table 8.1. Values of percentage protein binding for some common psychotropic drugs

95–99% bound	90–95% bound	50–90% bound	50% bound
Amitriptyline	Phenytoin	Carbamazepine	Alcohol
Chlorpromazine	Propranolol		Phenobarbitone
Diazepam	Valproate		Trichloroethanol
Imipramine			(chloral metabolite)

From Grahame-Smith and Aronson (1984), with permission.

Table 8.2. Pathological conditions affecting plasma concentrations of different proteins

Change in plasma protein concentration	Pathological conditions
Hypoalbuminaemia	Hepatic diseases, nephrotic syndrome, malnutrition, cancer, surgery, renal failure, cardiac failure, burns, inflammatory diseases
Hypo alpha$_1$-glycoproteinaemia	Nephrotic syndrome, hepatic diseases, malnutrition
Hyper-alpha$_1$-glycoproteinaemia	Inflammatory diseases, Crohn's disease, rheumatoid arthritis
Hyperlipoproteinaemia	Hyperlipoproteinaemia of various types

administered concomitantly or to changes in concentration of physiological substances, e.g. bilirubin, free fatty acids or urea.

For psychotropic drugs that are highly bound, a small decrease in binding can cause a large increase in the free fraction. As the free fraction is the only part susceptible to diffusion, glomerular filtration and hepatic metabolism, its increase will lead to an increase of these processes. Thus, the increase of the free drug concentration in plasma will usually be transient due to the large volume of distribution of these drugs. After a variable period of transition the original drug concentration at its sites of action is re-established.

Important clinical consequences are unlikely to occur with psychotropic drugs as a result of modifications of their binding, given their wide apparent therapeutic concentration range. However, adverse reactions to phenytoin, diazepam, and flunitrazepam have been reported to be more common in hypoalbuminaemic patients.

Ideally the free concentration of a drug should be measured when studying the relationships with therapeutic effects. However, even in physiological conditions with human proteins, binding studies are difficult, poorly reproducible and not fully predictive of the extent of binding *in vivo*. Consequently, other methods have been developed to estimate the concentration of free drug at its sites of action, e.g. measuring the drug concentration in saliva or cerebrospinal fluid (CSF). These methods are based on the assumption that only the free drug diffuses into the given fluid without intervention of any active process. Good correlations with plasma free drug have been described for CSF concentrations of diazepam, phenytoin, and nortriptyline and for salivary concentrations of phenytoin, carbamazepine, diazepam, and caffeine.

Passage of drugs into brain

A drug may enter the brain directly from the circulation or indirectly from the cerebrospinal fluid. Areas of brain vary in vascularity, the cortex having a richer blood supply than white matter. The brain has the best blood supply of all organs; it comprises only 2 per cent of the body weight but receives 15 per cent of cardiac output. Thus, drugs should equilibrate rapidly between brain and blood. However, the histological organization of capillaries in the brain is that of a continuous layer of vascular endothelial cells, which has given rise to the concept of the 'blood–brain barrier'. Nevertheless, there is no such absolute barrier, and the rate of diffusion from blood to brain depends on a number of factors:

1. *Protein binding.* Highly bound drugs will diffuse into the brain slowly because unbound drug concentrations, which determine the rate of diffusion, are low. After equilibration, the concentration in the CSF is usually close to the free plasma water concentration because the fluid is virtually protein-free. Brain tissues, by contrast, can strongly bind many psychotropic drugs, forming a central pool.

2. *Ionization.* As with absorption from the gut, the drug diffuses into the brain in its non-ionized form. Thus, at the plasma pH of 7.4, or the slightly lower pH values of extracellular fluid, knowledge of the pK_a of the drug allows one to calculate the nonionized proportion.

3. *Lipophilicity.* The brain is a highly lipid tissue, and the lipid solubility of a drug gives a good indication of how rapidly the drug will enter the brain. This factor is the most important of the three. Most psychotropic drugs are quite lipophilic and enter the brain rapidly (see Table 8.3).

Because they are highly ionized, quaternary ammonium compounds such as neostigmine are not taken into the brain. Dopamine and serotonin have low lipophilicity and also fail to diffuse into the brain. Finally, simple cations or anions such as lithium and bromide diffuse readily because the molecules are small.

Table 8.3. Penetration time of barbiturates to the brain depends on degree of protein binding and pK_a but especially on lipid solubility

	Per cent bound	pK_a	Per cent non-ionized at pH 7.4	× Lipid solubility	= Effective partition coefficient	Penetration half-time (minutes)
Thiopentone	75	7.6	61	× 3.3	= 200	1.4
Pentobarbitone	8.1	8.1	83	× 0.05	= 0.42	4.0
Barbitone	2	7.5	56	× 0.002	= 0.001	27.0

Metabolism

Some drugs, mainly those that are relatively lipid-insoluble or ionized, or elemental, are excreted unchanged by the kidney; barbitone, lithium and bromides are examples. However, most highly lipophilic drugs diffuse readily across body membranes and are reabsorbed by diffusion from the glomerular filtrate in the kidney. Such substances have a very low renal clearance rate and persist in the body. To be eliminated, drugs of this type must be metabolized to derivatives that are more polar, i.e. more soluble in water and less in lipids. This process is not equivalent to 'detoxification', since the metabolite may be more active than its parent.

Drug metabolism takes place mainly in the liver and is by four main processes:

1. Oxidation is the most common form of drug metabolism. Liver microsomal enzymes catalyse a variety of reactions, including hydroxylation, *N*-dealkylation, *O*-dealkylation, and sulphoxide formation. Examples of such reactions are shown with chlorpromazine, and also with the metabolic pathways of the biogenic amines.

   Some drug oxidations are not catalysed by the typical liver microsomal enzymes. Examples are the alcohol and aldehyde dehydrogenases, which oxidize ethanol to acetaldehyde and then to acetic acid. The monoamine oxidases, another example, are widely distributed mitochondrial enzymes that oxidatively deaminate a whole range of substances.

2. Reduction, as by the aldehyde reductases, is not common.

3. Hydrolysis is also uncommon, metabolism by cholinesterases being an example.

4. Conjugation consists in the coupling of molecules such as glucuronic acid, acetyl radicals, and sulphate to form less lipid-soluble and hence easily excretable metabolites. The molecular weight of the complex is increased so that active transport excretion can also take place.

Psychotropic drugs are extensively metabolized, often through several pathways. As a result of this, several metabolites may appear in the plasma, and most of the time almost no drug is excreted unchanged. The metabolites may be pharmacologically inactive, or active with the same or different properties than the parent drug.

Another aspect of the metabolism of psychotropic drugs is the wide inter-individual variability. The differences in the rate of metabolism are probably the major source of variability among individuals in the pharmacological action of a given drug.

Some other practical aspects of the drug hepatic metabolism need further discussion.

First-pass metabolism

After oral absorption a drug must pass through the liver before it reaches the general circulation. The rate of metabolism occurring in the liver is referred to as the hepatic 'first-pass' effect. The effect can be quantitatively very important. For example, more than 90 per cent of orally administered fluphenazine is oxidized in the liver after absorption before even reaching the systemic circulation and some individuals metabolize phenothiazines almost entirely. These patients in particular may benefit from a switch to depot administration of antipsychotic drugs, which obviates first-pass metabolism.

For antidepressants the interindividual variability of the first-pass effect is wide: from 20 to 70 per cent for imipramine and nortriptyline. Consequently, the bioavailability of the drug will vary in the same proportions between subjects. The clinical consequences of such differences depend on whether or not the metabolism creates active metabolites, and on the pharmacological profile of those metabolites.

Inhibition of drug metabolism

In multiple drug therapy different drugs may compete for a common enzymatic site of metabolism. This can lead to an inhibition of the biotransformation of one of the drugs and to its accumulation. For example, dicoumarol inhibits the metabolism of phenytoin and tolbutamide and consequently may induce severe adverse effects due to the high bodily concentration of these drugs.

Disulfiram may have the same effect on the metabolism of phenytoin, tolbutamide, chlordiazepoxide, and diazepam. Furthermore, disulfiram inhibits aldehyde dehydrogenase thus causing the accumulation of acetaldehyde after the ingestion of ethanol. Acetaldehyde accumulation is believed to produce the unpleasant flushing, throbbing, nausea, and vomiting of the 'disulfiram reaction'.

Phenothiazines and haloperidol inhibit the metabolism of tricyclic antidepressants, leading to an increase in their steady-state concentration. The clinical consequences of this concentration increase are unknown but probably limited.

The MAO inhibitors are another example. The inhibition is irreversible (except for some compounds currently under development) and the effects of the drug wear off only when new enzyme has been synthesized. The MAO inhibitors thus potentiate the action of amines that are broken down primarily by MAO. The prime example is tyramine, a constituent of fermented foods such as cheese. On ingestion, tyramine is not metabolized by the inhibited MAO, but instead reaches the circulation and releases noradrenalin from the noradrenergic nerve endings. Thus, a potentially fatal hypertensive crisis may ensue from the combination of an MAO inhibitor and a tyramine-containing food.

Hepatic diseases are another factor in drug metabolism, oxidation usually being more impaired than conjugation. The total clearance of drugs such as barbiturates, narcotic analgesics, chlordiazepoxide, and diazepam can be reduced in patients with hepatic function impairment. Thus, patients with liver disease are unduly sensitive to these drugs, which means that the dose should be reduced.

Stimulation of drug metabolism

Some drugs administered over a few days may induce an increase in concentrations of microsomal metabolizing enzymes due both to an increased synthesis and a decreased destruction. The induction leads to a stimulation of the metabolism of the drug and may produce an apparent condition of drug tolerance. Furthermore, due to the low-specificity of these enzymes, which can deal with a wide variety of substrates, the metabolism of other drugs can be accelerated. Consequently, enzyme induction is a major potential mechanism of drug interaction.

Barbiturates are a well-known example of inducing drugs. Patients treated chronically with barbiturates metabolize the drugs more rapidly than do non-exposed persons. Many drugs are inducers in animals, but species differences are important and each drug must be assessed in man. For example, benzodiazepines are good inducers in rats, but induction is of little or no clinical importance in man. Among other psychotropic drugs known to induce their own metabolism are glutethimide, chloral hydrate, meprobamate, chlorpromazine, and the anticonvulsants, carbamazepine and primidone.

Caffeine, cigarette smoking, adrenal steroids, sex hormones, dicoumarol, and phenylbutazone are also capable of induction. This probably explains why the incidence of drowsiness during chlorpromazine or diazepam treatment is lower in smokers than in non-smokers.

Induction usually occurs within a few days of administration and wears off a week or so after the drug is discontinued. The phenomenon can be quite marked, resulting in a 50 per cent reduction in plasma concentration of the drugs. Response to enzyme inducers is partly genetically controlled. Another example of genetically determined differences in drug metabolism is acetylation. Isoniazid and probably phenelzine are metabolized mainly by acetylation: about half the population acetylate rapidly, the other half slowly. Higher concentrations of unmetabolized drug are maintained in the slow metabolizers, with greater chance of side effects, but clinical response seems less influenced.

Some physiological conditions can affect hepatic metabolism. The microsomal enzymes that metabolize drugs are not fully active until about eight weeks after birth. Hence, neonates metabolize most drugs slowly. Conjugation to form glucuronides is less deficient. Adults and children metabolize drugs similarly, but smaller doses must be used in children, especially prepubertal children, because of their smaller size. During pregnancy, the rate of hepatic metabolism of drugs like phenytoin and barbiturates can be increased and thus the clinical effects of the drug may be diminished.

Excretion

Each day 190 litres of plasma water are filtered through the glomeruli, all but 1.5 litres being reabsorbed. Only drug dissolved in free (i.e. unbound) plasma water can be filtered, and lipid-soluble non-ionized drugs will be reabsorbed because they diffuse back into the tubules.

This reabsorption cannot occur with lipid-insoluble (water-soluble) drugs, which, along with their metabolites, are therefore cleared from the plasma. The pH of the urine is an important factor influencing the rate of drug excretion. Thus, it is the non-ionized form of the drug that tends to diffuse back across the tubule cells and out of the urine. Weak acids tend to be excreted in alkaline urine because they form ions, whereas weak bases remain in acidic urine. For example, amphetamine, a weak base, is excreted rapidly in urine of low pH but slowly and erratically in alkaline urine. Acidification of the urine with ammonium chloride therefore hastens the excretion of amphetamine in cases of overdose. Conversely, barbiturates, being weak acids, are excreted more rapidly if the urine is made alkaline by administering bicarbonate.

Lithium is a prime example of a drug for which renal excretion is quantitatively important. A decrease in clearance due to renal impairment may cause an increase in plasma lithium concentrations and lead to severe side-effects. Conversely, the increase in renal clearance observed at the end of pregnancy may induce a decrease of both plasma concentration and the therapeutic effect of lithium salts.

Drugs can also be excreted by the liver cells into the bile, where they can then be reabsorbed from the intestine, a process that forms the entero-hepatic cycle. Other ways of excretion are the expired air, the saliva, the sweat, and the intestine. Some basic drugs can be excreted into the stomach after intravenous administration. Furthermore, the lactating mother is likely to secrete lipophilic drugs into the milk. This is known to occur with diazepam, which has been reported to have appreciable effects on the baby. Milk excretion may also occur with other benzodiazepines, lithium, meprobamate, barbiturates, imipramine, phenytoin, and phenothiazines which thus should be avoided during lactation.

Pharmacokinetics and pharmacological effect

Variability in response to a given drug varies widely in psychopharmacology. On the basis of the fundamental pharmacological relationship $E = f(C \times S)$ where the clinical effect (E) is described as a function of the concentration of the drug at the site of action (C) and of the sensitivity of that site of action (S), the variability of drug response can be examined as follows:

1. The function relating the effect to the concentration $\times$ sensitivity combination. This function is not always linear and one example of complex relationship concerns nortriptyline. In this case there is believed to be a parabolic relationship between clinical response and plasma concentration, both low and high concentrations being associated with a lack of response.

2. The receptors' sensitivity, i.e. the responsiveness of tissues. This factor is probably critical, but attempts to assess receptor sensitivity have until now only been indirect. Examples of such attempts are the measurement of inhibitory constants for MAOIs, the prolactin response to antipsychotics, or the growth hormone response to clonidine. In practice, there is no way by which the sensitivity of the receptor response in man to any psychotropic drug can be estimated directly. This reflects the lack of knowledge of the precise biological mechanisms of action underlying the clinical properties of psychotropic drugs as well as the inaccessibility of human brain response systems.

3. The concentration of drug at its site of action. This factor cannot be measured directly for the same reasons as indicated above. But, because the therapeutic response to drugs usually correlates better with the plasma concentration than with the drug dosage, it is assumed that the former is a better indicator of the drug concentration at its site of action than the latter. However, such estimations are only an approximation of receptor site concentrations because of complicating factors such as plasma binding, active metabolites, penetration and binding in the brain. Consequently, it is not usually possible to define for a given drug an optimal concentration but only a therapeutic range wherein the majority of patients will experience maximal therapeutic effects for minimal toxicity and side-effects. Two different situations have to be considered in the attempt to correlate plasma drug concentrations and clinical effects (Fig. 8.4).

Acute dosage

In psychopharmacology, drugs administered on an acute basis are mainly hypnotics and anti-anxiety agents. For both types of drugs, when groups of patients are compared, no precise correlation is found between the plasma concentration and the clinical effects but higher concentrations usually correspond to greater effects in the patients. The correlation is not increased when drugs without active metabolites are used, e.g. lorazepam, or when

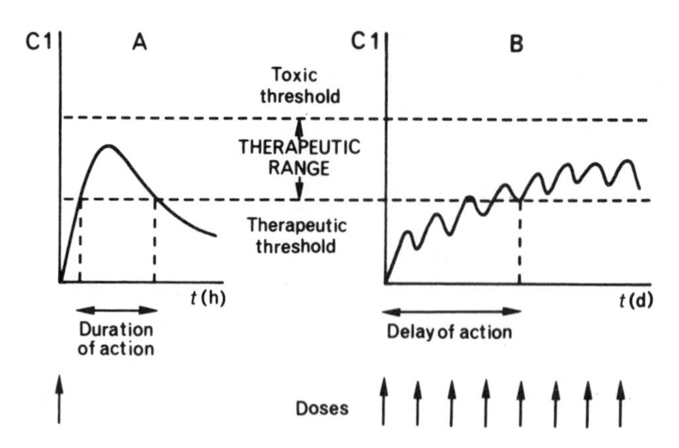

Fig. 8.4. Theoretical curves describing blood concentrations following single and repeated doses of a drug.

these metabolites are taken into account, e.g. *N*-desmethyldiazepam for diazepam.

However, if the comparison is made within the same subject, there is usually a good correlation between dose, plasma peak concentration and clinical effect. Thus, when using hypnotics, one should begin to administer small doses to test the patient's sensitivity, then progressively increase the doses until the therapeutic effect is achieved.

Other pharmacokinetic properties like elimination half-life or the delay of the peak plasma concentration are important guides for acute administration of drugs. These two variables are not related and oxazepam is a good example of a drug with an intermediate half-life but some delay of peak plasma concentration, e.g. 2–3h.

Repeated dosage

In patients receiving medications for a long period of time blood concentrations cannot be continuously monitored. Blood must be drawn at a given time regularly during treatment. This time is usually between 8 a.m. and 10 a.m., before the patient has received the morning dosage. Therefore, the sample is taken after a delay corresponding to the maximum dosage interval and the concentration is likely to reflect the lowest of the day.

Correlation of plasma drug concentrations and clinical effects should only be sought when the steady state is reached because the drug effects should then be maximal. The steady-state plasma concentrations (C_{ss}) vary considerably between individuals: after repeated administration of the same dose the variability in C_{ss} is about tenfold to twenty-fold for the majority of

Table 8.4. Main factors of variability in steady-state concentration (C_{ss}) of a given drug

	Drug dosage
Pharmacological	Drug physico-chemical properties Pharmaceutical formulation Route of administration Duration of treatment (if induction) Co-prescription of other drugs
Individual	Age Weight Genetic factors influencing metabolism Pathological factors Pregnancy
Others	Compliance Diet Time of administration of the drug Cigarettes Alcohol

psychotropic drugs. The main factors involved in the variability of C_{ss} are summarized in Table 8.4.

The free drug concentration, which is more likely to reflect concentrations at the receptor site, has been proposed to be more relevant in correlation studies with clinical effects. However, this measure is of little value in practice for several reasons:

(1) the technical difficulty of measuring binding accurately;

(2) the small interindividual variability in binding (twofold) compared to the variability in steady-state concentrations (at least tenfold);

(3) for each individual, the percentage of drug bound is a constant.

Except for lithium, only a few positive results have emerged from attempts to correlate steady-state plasma concentrations and clinical effects of psychotropic drugs (Lascelles 1981). The best documented examples of positive correlations are those related to adverse effects, e.g. the sedative and hypotensive effects of chlorpromazine, the extrapyramidal effects of haloperidol, and the cardiotoxicity of tricyclic antidepressants. In most of the cases, attempts to correlate C_{ss} with therapeutic results remain controversial, e.g. for tricyclic antidepressants. Several reasons may explain this absence of correlation:

1. Some drugs have an irreversible action which is maintained despite the disappearance of the drug from plasma. This is the case of drugs qualified as 'hit-and-run' like MAOIs and reserpine.

2. Receptor sensitivity may be modified so drug concentrations bear no constant relation to receptor effects. With benzodiazepines such modifications may explain the tolerance developing over time for sedative effects and the increased sensitivity of elderly people to the same effects because of slower tolerance.

3. The presence of active metabolites, with different pharmacokinetic properties and sometimes a different mode of action. This is the case with most psychotropic drugs except a few like haloperidol, lorazepam, and oxazepam.

4. The inability to confirm in man that plasma concentration reflects the concentration at receptor sites. When the drug has an active transport mechanism, the plasma concentration will clearly not reflect that at the receptor site.

5. The selection of patients, their diagnosis and subtyping, or the choice of outcome criteria may be irrelevant. Furthermore, the measures available, e.g. the rating scales, may lack precision. The absence of data about the rate of spontaneous remissions is another factor which can make the interpretation of such studies difficult.

In practice, lithium is the only psychotropic drug whose plasma concentrations are routinely monitored because a correlation exists between plasma concentrations and clinical responses. Furthermore, there is a narrow range between therapeutic and toxic levels of the drug. For other psychotropic drugs the measurement of plasma concentrations will only be helpful in some particular situations, summarized in Table 8.5.

The young, the old, and the physically ill

The lactating mother is likely to secrete lipophilic drugs into the milk. This is known to occur with diazepam, which has been reported to have appreciable

Table 8.5. Main reasons for the monitoring of psychotropic drugs

Doubts about compliance.
Therapeutic failure at usual dosages.
Adverse drug reaction at usual dosages.
Drugs whose clinical efficacy is related to a minimum steady-state concentration.
Drugs with a narrow therapeutic range.
Diagnosis of drug intoxications.
Drugs likely to induce their own metabolism.
Consequences of drug interactions.
Consequences of diseases.
Necessity to mimimize plasma concentrations (children, pregnancy, coexisting disease, elderly patients).

effects on the baby. Similarly, lipophilic drugs would be expected to reach the fetus *in utero*.

Neonates metabolize most drugs slowly. Furthermore, especially in the premature infant, the blood–brain barrier is immature so that centrally acting drugs penetrate the brain readily and have enhanced effects. Finally, renal excretion mechanisms may be impaired. Thus, babies in the first weeks of life, especially the newborn, are usually very sensitive to psychotropic drugs.

The elderly, like the newborn, are particularly sensitive to psychotropic drugs. The effects of the patient's age on pharmacokinetic mechanisms are many, and they vary from drug to drug. In some cases, the drug distribution is altered; in others, hepatic metabolism is slowed; and with other drugs, renal clearance seems impaired. Differences from effects in young persons can be substantial. For example, the plasma half-life of diazepam in hours is on average about the same as the age of the patient in years.

Patients with liver disease are unduly sensitive to most psychotropic drugs. However, hydroxylation is more impaired than conjugation. Protein binding may also be affected because of hypoalbuminemia. Renal disease may impair excretion, especially of lithium.

Drug interactions

Drug interactions can occur at the metabolic level (pharmacokinetic interaction) or at the site of action (pharmacodynamic interaction). The former includes competition for plasma albumin binding sites, but no important example concerning psychotropic drugs is known. Enzyme induction interactions are very important. The concurrent administration of phenobarbitone with chlorpromazine or nortriptyline produces liver enzyme induction, more rapid metabolism of the psychotropic drugs, and a drop in plasma concentrations. Other barbiturates also induce enzymes and counteract other psychotropic drugs. Antiparkinsonian drugs such as orphenadrine are powerful liver inducers and should not be given routinely with antipsychotic medication. Enzyme induction by alcohol partly explains the tolerance that alcoholics have to alcohol and the cross-tolerance they have to barbiturates; cellular changes are also an important factor. Phenytoin is also a powerful enzyme inducer and can interact with other drugs.

Relatively weak inducing agents may compete for the metabolizing enzymes more than they induce those enzymes. Thus, chlorpromazine and amitriptyline given together result in plasma concentrations of each that are higher than those attained by the individual drugs given alone. Similarly, cimetidine and diazepam may interact to increase concentrations of diazepam.

References

Grahame-Smith, D.G. and Aronson, J.K. (1984). *Oxford textbook of clinical pharmacology and drug therapy*. Oxford University Press, Oxford.

Lascelles, P.T. (1981). Drug assays in neuropsychiatry. *Psychological Medicine* **11,** 661–7.

9. Depression and antidepressants

Of the three main groups of psychotropic drugs, the antipsychotics are useful in treating all forms of psychosis and the antianxiety compounds are really antiarousal or antiemotion compounds and therefore less specific than their names would imply. Only the antidepressants appear to exert a specific or selective action on a recognizable psychiatric entity. For this reason an outline of the features of depression is presented, including some of the problems of classifying this condition.

Depression

Introduction

The term 'depression' can apply to a transient mood, a sustained change in affect, a symptom, a syndrome, or a psychiatric illness. It can be normal as an understandable reaction to adverse circumstances or loss; or abnormal when it is inappropriate in severity, persistence, or precipitating circumstances, or contains features of psychosis. Abnormal depression can be secondary to a physical illness such as influenza or carcinoma (Kathol and Petty 1981), to another psychiatric condition such as schizophrenia (Johnson 1981*a*), or to drug therapy, particularly some antihypertensive agents and steroids (Lewis and Smith 1983). Its relationship to anxiety is complex (Stavrakaki and Vargo 1986).

Most commonly, however, depression is a primary illness with a wide range of symptoms. Some are primarily physical, some essentially psychological, but definite symptom clusters can be identified.

Psychological symptoms

Even in the mildest depressive illness, there is a prevailing sadness with lowering of mood. Patients are downcast, miserable, despairing, despondent, and jaded. In the early stages they may forget their sadness when with others or at work, but later the depression is persistent. Uncontrollable weeping is common, giving relief initially, but more ill patients still feel depressed after 'a good cry'. Even more deeply depressed patients are anguished beyond any normal human experience, the mood having an ineffably painful quality. But at the greatest levels of severity patients become incapable of any emotion and describe a complete emptiness of emotional experience.

Patients feel guilty and worthless, mulling over the past and reproaching themselves for imagined wrong behaviour. They believe that they have failed themselves and their families. They ruminate over peccadillos, exaggerating them to heinous sins. These deficiencies are confessed to the family and self-imposed penances may be performed. Depressed patients become unsociable and shun the company of others, even old friends. As the depression deepens, the patient's preoccupation with the waste of his life, the futile nature of his present existence, the enormity of his neglect and abuse of his family and friends reaches psychotic intensity with delusions of guilt.

Many patients develop paranoid states becoming secretive, suspicious, and blaming others for their predicament. This may become delusional in intensity, with beliefs that neighbours are puffing poison gas through the letter box or that everyone around is a foreign agent.

Lack of energy is a common complaint, every routine task becoming a major chore. Women find their housework exhausting and meals become perfunctory exercises in opening cans. At work, patients no longer innovate or carry out their duties with zest. Tasks are postponed or avoided and this procrastination is accompanied by indecisiveness, self-depreciation, and lack of confidence. Loss of interest is seen as inability to concentrate or to take a job through to a successful conclusion. Patients complain of loss of attention and concentration or of depressive thoughts intruding. Self-neglect is quickly noticeable, the dapper man becoming slovenly, the bandbox-dressed woman slouching around in old jeans. Make-up is absent or carelessly applied. More severely depressed patients become apathetic, self-neglect endangers hygiene and even survival, and patients are totally incapable of work.

Closely related to these symptoms is a loss of the patient's ability to enjoy himself. This 'anhedonia' is particularly upsetting to patients of aesthetic disposition. Patients' families no longer inspire them with tender feelings, their hobbies become boring. Favourite music loses its appeal, scenery becomes insipid, interest in sports wanes. Everyday sights and sounds become dulled. Many describe the slowness of passage of time—everything drags on, an hour seems a day, a day an eternity.

Suicidal thoughts, preoccupations, and tendencies increase roughly in parallel with the depth of the depression. First, the future seems grey to patients, then black. Next, no future at all can be envisaged, with patients living from day-to-day. They wish they had never been born and that they could fall asleep and not wake up. Existence is bleak or agonizing and it seems logical to end it all. Such thoughts occur infrequently at first and are firmly resisted. Later, suicidal thoughts become more frequent, intense, and insistent. Ways of committing suicide begin to suggest themselves and plans may be laid. Tablets are stored up or a connector between car exhaust and hose pipe obtained. Impulses to commit suicide become more frequent and the patient may carry out a 'dummy-run'. However, the lack of energy, interest, and initiative may become so strong that patients are incapable of carrying out their intentions.

Symptoms of anxiety are very common (Leckman *et al.* 1983), especially in the mildly ill. The patients are anxious, tense, jumpy, irritable, and apprehensive, worrying about trivial matters and agonizing over decisions. Agitation is a prominent feature of many of the severely depressed.

Physical symptoms

Sleep disturbances are very common in depressive disorders and patients often complain miserably of their insomnia. Typically, sleep is lighter throughout the night, with less deep sleep. Dreaming is not altered in duration, but the content becomes gloomy or frightening. Sleep is restless and fitful, culminating in early wakening. Patients then lie awake in the depths of despair, unable to return to sleep. Patients usually fall asleep quite rapidly, being exhausted by the early wakening and the strains of the day. Some with anxiety, however, have difficulty getting off to sleep. About 10 per cent of depressives, mainly the young, sleep longer than usual during their depressive episodes.

Loss of appetite starts as lack of enjoyment of food and can progress to almost total anorexia. The weight loss which follows is a good index of the depth of depression. In more severe cases, weight loss seems more than would be expected from the loss of appetite, and may reflect increased energy requirements because of agitation. Some depressives, especially the young, overeat.

Sexual disturbances

Disturbances of sexual function are early symptoms of depression and include frigidity in women and impotence in men. In severely depressed patients, delusions and hallucinations often have a sexual content. Oligomenorrhoea and amenorrhoea are frequent in women; menorrhagia occurs occasionally.

Retardation and agitation

Retardation comprises a general slowing down of bodily functions. Patients sit motionless, but not stiff, and the usual small movements are infrequent or absent. The facial expression is fixed in careworn lines with deep furrows in the forehead and beside the mouth. Walking is slow and an immense effort. In particular, the patient's voice is monotonous, lifeless, empty of cadences and inflexions. Replies are delayed, but speech is not slowed (Greden and Carroll 1981). Patients complain of jumbled thoughts, or, in more severe cases, that their minds are empty and no spontaneous thoughts occur. Finally, retardation can be so marked that the patient sits inertly, responds in monosyllables, and needs dressing and feeding. Rarely, a retarded stupor supervenes.

Agitation is a motor disorder with overactivity of the extremities. It is closely related to anxiety and anguish. Patients clasp and unclasp their hands, twiddle rings on their fingers, pace up and down, and importune attendants seeking reassurance that they will eventually recover. Milder degrees of agitation are subjective, the patient describing his emotional turmoil.

Some degree of retardation is common in all but the mildest depressive, but it can be masked by agitation. Retardation and agitation are good indicators of the depth of the depression.

Somatic symptoms

These take two main forms, the emergence of new physical symptoms and the exacerbation of existing ones (Davies 1973). Elderly patients are particularly likely to be affected. Constipation, indigestion, and dry mouth reflect slowing of bowel and glandular function. Anxious depressives may complain of palpitations, tremor, sweating, urgency of micturition, feelings of tightness in the chest and breathlessness. Pain is a very common complaint and can affect almost any part of the body: headache, low backache, and vague rheumaticky pains are the commonest. Atypical facial pain or 'neuralgia' can be agonizing in intensity. Analgesics are of limited effectiveness and patients can become demoralized by the pain. The preoccupation with the pain becomes hypochondriacal, the patient fears cancer or some incurable disease and fails to be reassured by physical investigations.

If the depressive already suffers from chronic pain, symptoms become worse. Headaches become more frequent and often more diffuse in distribution, joint pains become more chronic, and so on. The close relationship between depression and pain has led some observers to regard depression as a 'psychic pain'.

Types of depression

The classification of types of depression has given rise to much controversy and this problem has led in turn to difficulties in deriving clinical factors predictive of drug response (Paykel 1979). Some typologies relate to the symptom patterns, some to the history of the condition, and some to the prognosis with treatment. The most researched division is into 'endogenous' and 'reactive'. Endogenous implies that the illness arises out of factors in the patient rather than from external circumstances as in the reactive cases. There are also clinical distinctions, endogenous features including retardation, self-blame, weight loss, and early morning wakening (Nelson and Charney 1981), reactive depressions showing signs of anxiety, self-pity, restless sleep and projection of blame. Many studies, using a wide range of statistical techniques of varying sophistication and justification, have examined the hypothesis that endogenous and reactive cases form two separate entities. In general, this has not been supported: although primarily endogenous and primarily reactive cases can be identified (Nelson and Charney 1980), most patients show mixed features clinically and the aetiology is also mixed, reactive external factors interacting with the endogenous depressive diathesis of the individual. Thus, an umbra of endogenous cases exist surrounded by a penumbra of cases in which reactive factors are increasingly important.

Another division which has found increasing favour in the last decade or so is into the bipolar manic-depressive illnesses and the unipolar recurrent depressions. The differentiating criterion is usually that of an identifiable manic episode. Family history, sex incidence, clinical features and course and treatment response differ between the two types. Manic-depressive patients tend to be more retarded in type with more physical changes. Antidepressant therapy is liable to swing them over into hypomania. Recurrence is more likely and at a shorter interval than with the unipolar depressives.

Another distinction of therapeutic relevance is that of agitated/retarded. However, patients can show mixed features or swing from one clinical picture to the other during the course of an episode.

Many subgroups of depression have been proposed, both on clinical grounds and following statistical manipulations of the data from groups of patients. As well as the endogenous–reactive groups mentioned earlier, the following have been suggested on clinical evidence:

1. Psychotic depression. This implies hallucinations and delusions with loss of insight in distinction to so-called neurotic depression. It is essentially a grouping of the severest form of depressive illnesses.

2. Anxious depression is not well-defined, but can refer to any depressive illness in which anxiety is a prominent feature. Mildly anxious and depressed patients are common in general practice, but do not form a separate entity.

3. Involutional melancholia is a syndrome of late onset, prone to occur in

obsessional people, and characterized by agitation and hypochondriacal preoccupations. It is very doubtful whether it is a separate entity.

4. Atypical depressives are anxious, phobic, obsessional, or hypochondriacal without the full panoply of depressive symptoms. Others are of a previously histrionic personality so that the affective changes appear shallow. These patients are claimed to respond well to the monoamine oxidase inhibitors.

Numerical taxonomy techniques have been applied to the classification of depression. Their use is not without its hazards, both with respect to the initial selection of patients and the historical and clinical data used. Paykel (1971) described four overlapping groups: severely ill 'psychotics', less ill 'neurotics', 'hostile' depressives, and mildly depressed patients with personality disorders. Personality attributes of depressive patients were evaluated by Matussek and Feil (1983). In depression-free intervals, depressives were more 'autodestructive–neurotic' than controls. The non-endogenous patients were overautonomous and aggressive, the endogenous unipolar patients lacked autonomy and the bipolar patients were anarchistic, aggressive, and striving for success and achievement.

Severity in a dimensional rather than a categorical sense is the most useful approach from the point of view of therapy (Ashcroft 1975). The number of points in the dimension of severity is arbitrary. Perhaps mild, moderate, and severe is sufficient. Symptoms tend to vary with severity so a moderately depressed patient would be expected to have some bodily upsets, feelings of guilt, failure to see a future, and so on.

Antidepressant drugs

Debates about the clinical features and course and the typologies of depression have also taken account of developments in experimental pharmacology and of the introduction of effective antidepressants. The amphetamines were introduced in the 1930s as psychological stimulants but were found to be of very limited usefulness in the treatment of depression; a very real risk of inducing dependence was appreciated later. Then reserpine was found to trigger retardation and depressive reactions and to induce a state in animals which appeared to reproduce some, but by no means all, of the physical features of depression in humans. Two groups of antidepressant drugs were discovered, the tricyclic compounds and the monoamine oxidase inhibitors (MAOIs). Hypotheses concerning the biochemical mode of action of reserpine and the antidepressants led to various amine hypotheses of depression, the indoleamine and the catecholamine neurotransmitters being the focus of attention (van Praag 1981*b*). It was generally held that depression

was associated with a state of insufficient activity in neuronal systems using either indoleamine or catecholamine neurotransmitters, or both. Antidepressant drugs were believed to correct this insufficiency.
So influential did these hypotheses become that the ability to increase amine neurotransmitters became a criterion for antidepressant activity, despite accumulating evidence that some drugs with putative therapeutic efficacy in depression had other actions. Though many psychotropic agents can induce some elevation of depressed mood, the tricyclics and the MAOIs have been the centre of interest.

The drugs used to alleviate depressive illnesses are generally termed 'antidepressants'. This implies an action against 'depressant' drugs which, though true in the case of reserpine does not apply to either the antipsychotics or the tranquillizers. Some authors favour the term 'antidepressive', which is more correct but still not an entirely felicitous choice. Other terms include 'thymoleptics' and 'mood elevators'. We will use the term 'antidepressant' simply because it is the most widely accepted.

Even more problems surround the nomenclature of the first main class of antidepressants. 'Tricyclic' refers to the chemical structure, so it is non-specific; phenothiazines are also tricyclic. Also, some newer drugs of this type are tetracyclic or have only one or two rings. The term 'monoamine re-uptake inhibitors' has been proposed to parallel the other main group, the monoamine oxidase inhibitors. However, some of the newer drugs have little effect in blocking re-uptake. For want of a better term we have chosen 'tricyclic-type antidepressants'.

Tricyclic-type antidepressants

History

The first of these compounds, imipramine, is an iminodibenzyl compound. In the later 1940s, iminidobenzyl derivatives were investigated as possible antihistaminic and antiparkinsonian agents (Fig. 9.1). They were found to be relatively ineffective until the introduction of chlorpromazine rekindled interest in them. Again, they were disappointing, but Kuhn used imipramine, the analogue of promazine, in depressed patients as well as schizophrenics, and discovered its antidepressant properties. In an early account of his open clinical observations he described the clinical characteristics of those who benefited, the dosage regimens required, the two-week delay before improvement becomes noticeable, the failure of some patients to respond, and the numerous unwanted effects (Kuhn 1958).

Imipramine was introduced in 1959 and gradually became an important drug in the treatment of depression. Other tricyclic compounds were synthesized, evaluated, and introduced. Amitriptyline, a dibenzocyclo-

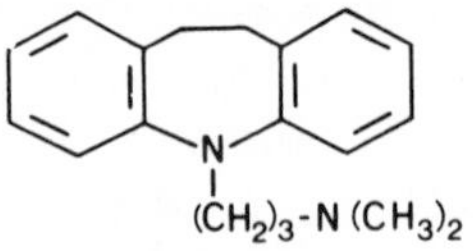

$(CH_2)_3-N(CH_3)_2$
IMIPRAMINE

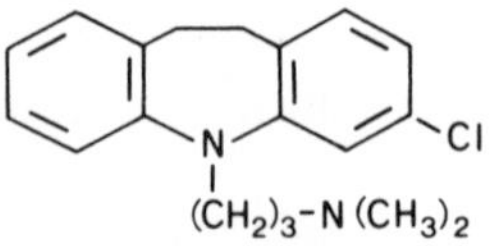

$(CH_2)_3-N(CH_3)_2$
Cl
CHLORIMIPRAMINE

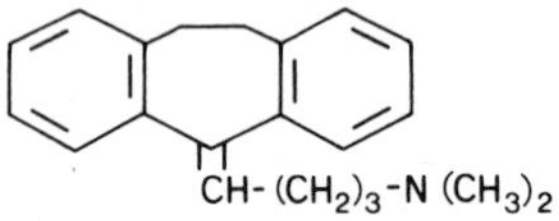

$CH-(CH_2)_3-N(CH_3)_2$
AMITRIPTYLINE

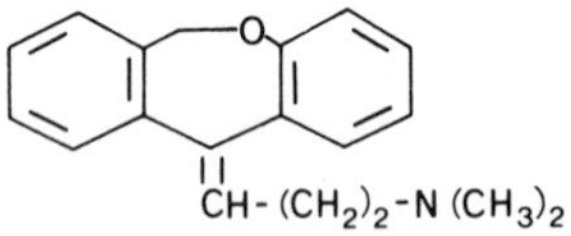

O
$CH-(CH_2)_2-N(CH_3)_2$
DOXEPIN

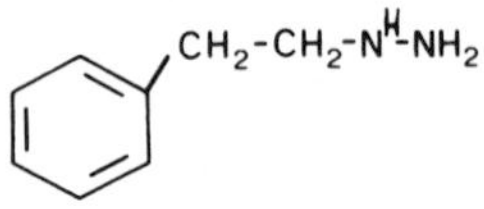

$CH_2-CH_2-NH-NH_2$
PHENELZINE

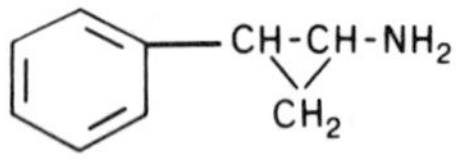

$CH-CH-NH_2$
CH_2
TRANYLCYPROMINE

Fig 9.1. Chemical formulae of some antidepressants.

heptadiene, has in addition some of the properties of a sedative antipsychotic, and in many countries is still the most popular tricyclic antidepressant, despite its pronounced side-effects. Many other compounds have been marketed, most of which have few if any advantages over imipramine and amitriptyline. In the last years, however, antidepressants with untypical clinical profiles and anomalous biochemical pharmacology have been introduced. Viloxazine and mianserin are instances. Unfortunately, some of these compounds have had to be withdrawn because of untoward effects.

Almost all these compounds are characterized by a complex ring structure, dihydrobenzapine, dibenzycycloheptadiene and -triene being the commonest examples. Instead of these rings lying flat as with the phenothiazines, the molecule is three-dimensional. Within each series, variation in pharmacology and clinical profile is achieved by alterations in the side chain and by substitution in the structure (Baldessarini 1989). Over the years, other indications have been explored and include bulimia, chronic pain, and migraine (Orsulak and Waller 1989).

Imipramine

Pharmacokinetics

Imipramine is rapidly absorbed, being detectable in the plasma a few minutes after oral administration. Absorption is slower after intramuscular injection. Distribution is rapid, imipramine readily crossing the blood–brain barrier. Concentrations are highest in the liver, adrenals, lungs, brain, and heart muscle. Brain concentrations are maximal 45 min after oral administration in the rat. As with many psychotropic drugs, imipramine is extensively bound to plasma albumin and in the tissues.

Imipramine is extensively metabolized in the body, a number of pathways having been identified. Four routes are important in man:

1. *N*-desmethylation in the side-chain producing the active compound desipramine.
2. *N*-oxidation of the side-chain.
3. Hydroxyl substitution in the ring structure.
4. Glucuronide conjugation of the resulting hydroxylated compound with subsequent excretion via the kidneys.

The liver is, of course, the main organ of metabolism, the liver microsomal oxidizing enzymes being involved. Between a quarter and three-quarters of orally administered imipramine is metabolized 'first-pass' in the liver (Gram and Christiansen 1975).

Imipramine and its metabolite has an effective half-life in the plasma of a little under 24 h, so it takes about a week for steady-state levels to be attained (Gram *et al.* 1977) (Table 9.1). In depressed patients on the same oral dose of imipramine, wide variations are found from patient to patient with respect to the levels attained. The ratio of imipramine to desipramine also varies from subject to subject, but does not usually differ much from unity.

Table 9.1. Half-lives of various tricyclic antidepressants

Tricyclic	Half-life (hours)	
Antidepressant	Mean	Range
Amitriptyline	15	10–26
Desipramine	17	13–26
Desmethyldoxepin	51	33–81
Doxepin	17	8–25
Imipramine	8	4–18
Nortriptyline	27	13–47
Protriptyline	78	55–125

Basic pharmacology (Green and Costain 1979; Kopin 1981; Stahl and Palazidou 1986)

Imipramine has an extensive range of pharmacological actions, interacting with several neurotransmitters including 5-hydroxytryptamine, noradrenalin, and acetylcholine. Since the early demonstration that imipramine potentiates the action of noradrenalin on the cat nictitating membrane, it has become apparent that its sympathomimetic effects are due to its ability to inhibit the re-uptake of noradrenalin from the synaptic cleft into the presynaptic neurone (Axelrod 1971). It does this by blocking the active uptake transport system. A similar effect is seen on 5-HT uptake. *In vivo*, in the blockade of uptake of 5-HT, imipramine is more potent than desipramine. Conversely, desipramine is several times more potent than imipramine in blocking noradrenalin uptake. Thus, on chronic administration uptake of both amines is blocked. Dopamine is weakly affected. In high doses, imipramine loses its amine-potentiating effects because it blocks postsynaptic receptors at supratherapeutic levels. Another complication is that adaptive processes occur within the neurone and in receptors to overcome the amine re-uptake blockade (Stahl and Palazidou 1986) (see Fig. 9.2). The synthesis of the neurotransmitters is reduced as is the consequent turnover. The effects on brain amines are therefore complex (Iversen and Mackay 1979).

Imipramine interacts with several other groups of drugs. It can prevent and partly reverse the depressant effects of reserpine and tetrabenazine by preventing depletion of amines. It potentiates amphetamine and other central stimulants. It prevents the uptake of indirectly acting sympathomimetic amines such as tyramine. Some antihypertensive agents such as guanethidine and debrisoquine also have to be taken into presynaptic noradrenergic nerve endings in order to exert their effects. Imipramine blocks this uptake and attenuates or negates the therapeutic actions of these drugs.

Imipramine has anticholinergic properties similar to those of atropine: it

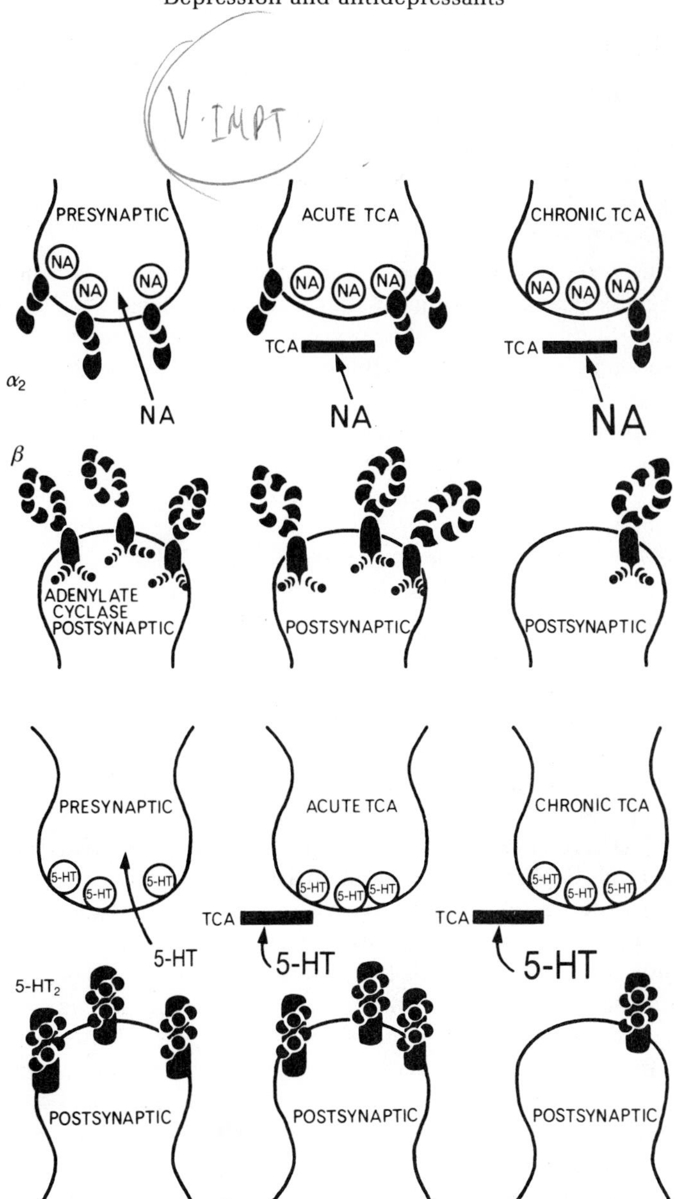

Fig 9.2. Down-regulation of beta-adrenergic receptors (above) and (5-HT_2) receptors (below) by chronic tricyclic antidepressants (TCAs) is shown. Monoamine re-uptake (left panels) is inhibited acutely by TCAs (middle panels), but no clinical response or receptor downregulation is evident. After chronic treatment with TCAs (right panels) receptors are down-regulated and clinical antidepressant effects are seen. (From Stahl and Palazidou 1986, with permission.)

inhibits acetycholine-induced spasm of the guinea-pig ileum and physostigmine-induced arousal of the cat's EEG. Antihistaminic effects are weak.

Normal animals are little affected by imipramine, some mild sedation being the usual effect. Many behavioural tests fail to distinguish between tricyclic-type antidepressants and antipsychotic drugs.

Clinical pharmacology

Imipramine produces slow-wave (theta) activity in the EEG of man with generalized desynchronization. It may activate epilepsy. REM sleep is suppressed. Studies of cognitive, psychomotor, and affective changes in normal subjects have revealed definite impairment (Seppala and Linnoila 1983). Memory is particularly affected. Mood changes can only be demonstrated in groups of normal subjects selected for their high scores on ratings of depressive affect; thus, these subjects are essentially a sub-clinical group.

Of other effects of imipramine, the anticholinergic actions are the most easily demonstrable. Potentiation of noradrenalin can also be shown. The blockade of amine uptake is demonstrable by giving bolus injections of intravenous tyramine: after imipramine, acutely or chronically, more tyramine is needed to provide a standard increase in blood pressure.

Clinical uses

Kuhn (1958), in his original account of the clinical effects of imipramine in over 500 patients with various types of depressive illness, concluded that: 'The main indication is without doubt a simple endogenous depression', and that 'every complication of the depression impairs the chances of success of the treatment'. These statements are still generally true. Nevertheless, many cases of reactive depression do respond to tricyclic-type antidepressants as do some cases of depression associated with early dementia (Raskin and Crook 1976). Depressed schizophrenics and depressive reactions in the context of personality disorders are much less amenable to treatment. In one early controlled trial, 48 depressed out-patients were given either imipramine in the high dosage of 250 mg daily, or placebo for 4 weeks. Among those suffering from the endogenous type of depression, three-quarters improved on imipramine as compared with less than a quarter receiving placebo; the improvement rate for reactive depressives was 60 and 20 per cent respectively (Ball and Kiloh 1959).

Accumulated data from many controlled clinical trials have shown imipramine to be consistently superior to placebo. Overall, two-thirds of depressed patients on imipramine improve compared with one-third on placebo. However, a few trials have suggested that imipramine is not so effective in the severely depressed, where any improvement is partly attributable to admission to hospital and other non specific effects. In these patients, imipramine is less effective than electroconvulsive therapy.

One major study examined the efficacy of imipramine as compared with placebo in mildly depressed out-patients. Patients with the less mild degrees of depression improved significantly whereas those who only just exceeded the criterion for inclusion did not (Stewart *et al* 1983).

Some studies have attempted to safeguard double-blind procedures by using an 'active' placebo; that is, a compound which mimics the side-effects of imipramine. Atropine, 0.3–1.0 mg, is generally used. Again, imipramine has proved consistently superior to atropine.

The symptoms which improved significantly with anti-depressant treatment have been selected by Nelson and his colleagues (1984*b*) and collated with those found in two previous studies (Montgomery and Asberg 1979; Bech *et al.* 1981). These symptoms are set out in Table 9.2; a fair degree of concordance is apparent. Symptoms susceptible to improvement, common to all three studies are depressed mood (sadness), guilt and worthlessness and decreased involvement in work and interests.

The time course of response has received some attention. Improvement in somatic symptoms is often the first feature to be noted. For example, patients remark that they sleep better and longer, feeling less tired when they awaken. General activation also improves, the patient becoming more

Table 9.2. Comparison of symptoms useful for measuring change in severity of depression

Nelson *et al* (1984*b*)	Montgomery and Asberg (1979)	Bech *et al* (1981)
Depressed mood (includes apparent and reported sadness) Hopelessness	Apparent sadness Reported sadness (includes hopelessness)	Depressed mood (includes apparent and reported sadness and hopelessness
Guilt Worthlessness	Pessimistic thoughts (includes guilt and worthlessness	Guilt (includes worthlessness)
Early morning awakening	Reduced sleep	———
Decreased interest in work and activities	Lassitude (difficulty initiating and performing work)	Decrease in work and interests
Decreased appetite	Reduced appetite	———
Loss of energy	———	Somatic symptoms: general (includes loss of energy)
Anhedonia	Inability to feel	———
Somatic anxiety	———	———
———	Inner tension	Psychic anxiety
———	Concentration difficulties	———
———	Suicidal thoughts	———
———	———	Retardation

alert, able to attend and concentrate, and retardation becomes less marked. Later, the depressive affect begins to lift, but may be delayed for up to four weeks from the initiation of drug therapy. In anxious depressives, anxiety may be slow to respond or refractory to treatment (Lader *et al.* 1987). In bipolar patients a hypomanic swing may be evident with drug treatment.

A major multicentre study of the effects of imipramine and other antidepressant treatments and placebo was carried out under the aegis of the Medical Research Council (1965) in the UK. The effects of imipramine, phenelzine, and placebo were compared with those of ECT in 250 depressed in-patients. In the short term (4 weeks), ECT was the most effective treatment, but over a longer period of 12 weeks, both ECT and imipramine improved about two-thirds of patients. The improvement rates for phenelzine and placebo were only a half of this. Imipramine particularly benefited male patients.

Other studies have attempted to characterize those patients particularly likely to respond to drug therapy. Findings have not been entirely consistent, but age and educational background seem not to affect outcome. Patients with neurotic, hypochondriacal, and histrionic personality traits respond poorly. A favourable outcome is associated with a few previous episodes, insidious onset, brief duration, and lack of precipitating causes. Patients with anorexia, weight loss, early wakening, and psychomotor slowing usually do best, whereas deluded patients may fail to respond (Joyce and Paykel 1989).

In schizophrenic patients, imipramine may increase hostility, belligerence, agitation, delusions, and thought disorder. Its effect on the depressive symptoms is usually disappointing. The combination with an antipsychotic drug is popular, but fixed-formulation combinations of tricyclic-type antidepressants and antipsychotics have little to commend them.

Imipramine has also proved efficacious in some patients with anxiety and phobias. It is also used to suppress nocturnal enuresis temporarily; its mode of action here is obscure.

Amitriptyline

Amitriptyline resembles imipramine in its pharmacology and clinical effects, but is more sedative, with somewhat more pronounced anticholinergic effects. In animal studies it more closely resembles chlorpromazine than does imipramine; for example, in high dosage it has neuroleptic effects.

Like imipramine, amitriptyline is mainly metabolized by demethylation (to nortriptyline) and by hydroxylation and glucuronide formation. It also has a fairly long plasma half-life.

Many controlled trials have established its effectiveness in depression, especially when anxiety or agitation coexist. It is now generally established as the archetypal tricyclic antidepressant with which newly developed putative antidepressants are compared. Overall, about 70–80 per cent of depressed in-patients, and 60–70 per cent of depressed out-patients, achieve substantial symptomatic relief with amitriptyline.

Nortriptyline

This is the most extensively studied antidepressant from the pharmacokinetic point of view because it happened to be the first compound for which adequate methods were developed for estimation. Treatment with standard dosage results in an up to thirtyfold variation in steady-state concentrations. Twin and family studies suggest that genetic factors strongly influence metabolism. Plasma binding is high. Plasma concentrations correlate with biological effects, such as inhibition of noradrenalin uptake into rat iris, or cerebral cortex, or as shown by the reduced pressor effects of intravenous tyramine. Side effects increase with plasma concentrations as judged by subjective complaints or by measurements of visual accommodation. The relationship of clinical response to plasma concentrations is discussed later.

Clinically, nortriptyline is about as effective as amitriptyline, but is less sedative and rather less useful in agitated and anxious patients.

Other tricyclic antidepressants

As mentioned earlier, more than 20 such compounds have been introduced throughout the world, and it is often difficult to distinguish any special characteristics of many of them. Uptake inhibition of brain amines varies greatly among these and related drugs (Table 9.3) (Rudorfer and Potter 1989). *Desipramine* was introduced in the belief that it was the active principle of imipramine and would therefore have a quicker onset of action. This has not proven the case. Desipramine is slightly stimulant rather than sedative. *Clomipramine*, the dihydrobenzazepine analogue of chlorpromazine, is strongly sedative. It is a powerful inhibitor of 5-HT uptake, but on repeated administration its metabolite, desmethylclomipramine, accumulates and preferentially blocks noradrenalin uptake. Claims that it is rapidly therapeutic following intravenous administration have not been adequately tested. It has also been promoted as the treatment of choice in patients with obsessional and phobic neuroses. Its usefulness in these conditions has been shown to depend on its primary antidepressant action but some evidence suggests that it is distinctly better in this respect than the other tricyclic-type antidepressants (Ananth *et al.* 1979). *Trimipramine* (Settle and Ayd 1980) with a branched side chain, is strongly sedative and is favoured by those few clinicians who advocate combined therapy with MAOIs.

Lofepramine is a tricyclic compound which resembles imipramine except that it has a more complex substitution in the terminal nitrogen atom of the

Table 9.3. The relative inhibitory potencies of antidepressant and related drugs on the uptake of NA, 5-HT, and DA in the rat brain *in vitro* (synaptosomes), *in vivo* (various techniques), and 5-HT uptake in human platelets under clinical conditions.

	RAT BRAIN						HUMAN PLATELETS
	In vitro			*In vivo*			
Drug	NA	5-HT	DA	NA	5-HT	DA	5-HT
Alaproclate	−	+(+)	−	−	++	−	+
Amitriptyline	++	++	−	+	(+)	−	+(+)
Citalopram	−	+++	−	−	+++	−	++
Clomipramine	++	+++	−	++	+(+)	−	+++
Desipramine	+++	(+)	−	+++	(+)	−	+
Doxepin	+	+	−	+	+	−	+
Femoxetine	+	++	−	+	++	−	++
Fluoxetine	+	++	−	−	++	−	++
Fluvoxamine	−	++	−	−	+	−	
Imipramine	++	+(+)	−	+++	+	−	++
Iprindole	−	−	−	−	−	−	−
Lofepramine	+++	(+)	−	+++	(+)	−	+
Maprotiline	++	−	−	++	−	−	−
Mianserin	+	−	−	−	−	−	
Nomifensine	++	−	+	++	−	+	
Nortriptyline	++	(+)	−	++	(+)	−	
Viloxazine	+	−	−	(+)	−	−	
Zimeldine	(+)	++	−	(+)	++	−	++

The data are compiled from numerous reports. Very high potency +++, high potency ++, moderate potency +, low potency −. Brackets denote possible effects.

side chain. It binds poorly to cholinergic receptors and has less anticholinergic actions in clinical use while retaining the efficacy of imipramine (Feighner *et al.* 1982, Rickels *et al.* 1982). Despite being partly metabolized to desipramine it has less cardiotoxicity and seems safer in overdosage than typical tricyclic antidepressants (Lancaster and Gonzalez 1989).

Butriptyline has the same side chain as trimipramine and is also sedative. By contrast, *protriptyline* is strongly stimulant and may produce restlessness and insomnia if taken during the late afternoon or evening.

Iprindole is a puzzling compound in that it does not inhibit amine uptake, has weak anticholinergic and antihistaminic effects and does not block the effects of indirectly acting amines. A number of comparisons with imipramine suggest that it is an effective antidepressant (despite doubts expressed in some quarters), but has fewer unwanted effects. *Dothiepin* is similar to amitriptyline whereas *doxepin* may have fewer unwanted effects. Both drugs are sedative antidepressants and have been advocated in the treatment of anxious depressives and patients with anxiety states uncomplicated by depression. *Dibenzepine* is not sedative but slightly stimulant. It is less potent than most other tricyclic antidepressants. *Maprotiline* is chemically a tricyclic compound with a bridge structure. It closely resembles the tricyclic compounds in its pharmacology but does not block 5-HT uptake. It is similar to imipramine or amitriptyline in its efficacy, speed of onset of action, and type and frequency of side effects.

Other tricylic-type antidepressants (Blackwell and Simon 1986)

Viloxazine is an oxazine derivative, chemically related to propranolol but unrelated to any other psychotropic drug. It has some properties in common with tricyclics such as the ability to block the re-uptake of noradrenalin, reversal of reserpine effects, and potentiation of catecholamines. It hardly antagonizes acetylcholine or histamine. It has a shorter half-life than most tricyclics. It has few side effects but nausea and vomiting may be troublesome.

Mianserin is a most interesting newer antidepressant. Chemically it is a true tetracyclic and was discovered in 1969. Its pharmacological actions are generally dissimilar to those of the standard tricyclic agents. Thus, it does not potentiate amphetamine and only weakly antagonizes reserpine, and it has no central anticholinergic actions. It is only moderately active as an inhibitor of noradrenalin and 5-HT uptake and it is a 5-HT receptor antagonist. It is believed that its major pharmacological property is to block presynaptic noradrenergic synapses ($alpha_2$), thereby increasing noradrenalin turnover in the brain. This action offers an alternate method to amine re-uptake blockade for increasing noradrenalin availability in synapses. In view of this novel pharmacological profile, it is not surprising that the potential value of mianserin as an antidepressant was not uncovered in routine animal tests. However, its EEG effects resemble those of the conventional tricyclics and this action in man provided the clue to its therapeutic action. In man it is devoid of significant peripheral anticholinergic actions, its main side effect being drowsiness early in treatment. Clinical trials have suggested that it is about as efficacious as imipramine and amitriptyline.

Trazodone is another unusual compound. It is chemically unrelated to other antidepressants and its mechanism of action is unclear (Brogden *et al.* 1981; Cazzullo and Silvestrini 1989). Its efficacy compares with those of imipramine and amitriptyline, but it has fewer anticholinergic side effects. It is also quite an effective anti-anxiety medication. It appears to be well-tolerated by the elderly and seldom exacerbates psychotic symptoms.

Amoxapine is available in the USA and many other countries. It is chemically related to the antipsychotic compound, loxapine (Jue *et al.* 1982). It appears fairly similar in efficacy to the standard tricyclic antidepressants with a similar profile of unwanted effects.

Currently, great interest revolves around the so-called selective 5-HT inhibitors. Although clomipramine is highly potent and selective, its metabolite, desmethylclomipramine is not. *Zimeldine* was the first compound which maintained most of its selectivity *in vivo* (Heel *et al.* 1982). It was withdrawn because of toxicity. *Fluvoxamine* is a recently introduced selective 5-HT uptake inhibitor whose clinical properties closely resemble those of zimeldine, without the toxicity (Benfield and Ward 1986). It causes fewer anticholinergic side effects than standard tricyclics, but is associated with more nausea and vomiting. *Fluoxetine* is another selective 5-HT uptake inhibitor, with a broadly similar profile (Sommi *et al.* 1987).

Plasma concentrations and clinical response

This is a complex and highly controversial subject about which few conclusions can be drawn. Nevertheless, some discussion of this topic is necessary because of the potential usefulness of plasma concentration measures in optimizing clinical dosage (Preskorn 1986).

In essence, the major question is whether a range of plasma concentrations can be established, within which a clinical response is to be expected (Risch *et al.* 1979*a*,*b*). It will be remembered that the very earliest accounts of the therapeutic effects of the tricyclic antidepressants noted that 20–30 per cent of depressed patients fail to respond adequately. Some of these patients are not taking their medication as prescribed or are prescribed insufficient quantities because they metabolize the drug rapidly. Thus, the establishing of a lower therapeutic level would be in line with other classes of drug and with basic pharmacological principles. Even so, studies vary as to the lower limit of effectiveness.

Nortriptyline has been the most widely studied tricyclic antidepressant in this respect. In an early study it was claimed that a curvilinear relationship existed between clinical response after two weeks' treatment with nortriptyline and its plasma concentration. Patients with plasma concentration in the 50–139 ng/ml range stood the best chance of improvement (Asberg *et al.* 1971). In a subsequent study, the upper limit was about 170 ng/ml. Patients above this level who had their dosage decreased showed a rapid resolution of their depressive symptoms (Kragh-Sorensen *et al.* 1976). However, in the largest series of patients studied, there was no discernible relationship between plasma nortriptyline levels and clinical response (Burrows *et al.* 1972).

Routine monitoring of nortriptyline plasma concentrations is not justified (Risch *et al.* 1981). In non-responders, however, sufficient studies have shown enough of a relationship to make it worthwhile taking a standardized plasma sample (i.e. just before the morning dose) and adjusting the dosage of nortriptyline if the plasma drug concentration seems excessively high or inadequately low (between 50–200 ng/ml). Clinical response follows reduction in dosage fairly rapidly.

There is a rationale for this presumed curvilinear relationship. High doses of tricyclics block postsynaptic receptors and consequently prevent the action of the increased intrasynaptic amine neurotransmitter.

The situation concerning plasma amitriptyline concentrations and clinical response is even more complex. First, both amitriptyline and its active metabolite, nortriptyline, have to be taken into account, and it is by no means self-evident that simple addition of the two concentrations is warranted. Secondly, the studies which have been carried out are even more contradictory than those with nortriptyline (Robinson *et al.* 1979). One large-scale study concluded that patients with plasma concentrations of amitriptyline plus nortriptyline above 120 ng/ml responded well whereas those patients below these concentrations responded poorly (Braithwaite *et al.* 1972). There was no indication of an upper limit as with nortriptyline alone. Unfortunately, in another large scale study carried out under the auspices of the World Health Organization, no such correlation was apparent (Coppen *et al.* 1978). Again, it is difficult to discern any guidelines through the obscurity but it is unlikely that the amitriptyline plus nortriptyline level has a relationship to response totally dissimilar to that of nortriptyline alone. Accordingly, it is sensible to lower dosage if the levels of the two together exceed 250 ng/ml or if that of nortriptyline exceeds 150 ng/ml (Vandel *et al.* 1978). Adverse effects begin to appear at levels above 350 ng/ml (Preskorn 1986).

One other relationship seems to hold up: patients with the most severe subjective side effects have the poorest clinical outcome, although no relationship to plasma concentration is evident. This might be because patients with severe side-effects tend to stop taking their medications or because the side effects reflect excessively high concentrations on normal dosage. The safest course is to change the medication to a drug with fewer side-effects.

The data from studies with imipramine are perhaps the clearest (Task Force 1985). When the combined levels of imipramine and desipramine exceed 200 ng/ml, clinical response is better than in patients with lower levels. Higher levels (over 250 ng/ml) are associated with no better clinical response than 200–250 ng/ml but side effects are increased. Studies of clomipramine yield essentially similar data, the threshold value for satisfactory antidepressant effect being combined clomipramine and desmethylclomipramine concentrations of 160–200 ng/ml (Faravelli *et al.* 1984).

With other drugs, studies have been too few to permit any definite conclusions (Amsterdam *et al.* 1980). The practical implication, that decrease in dosage may as well effect an improvement as increase in dosage, is explored further in the section on management of refractory depression.

Unwanted effects

The unwanted effects of the tricyclic antidepressants are often more than a minor or a transient nuisance (Blackwell 1981*a*,*b*). They may be so unpleasant for the patient as to preclude his attaining an adequate therapeutic dose level or they may lead the patient to fail to take his drugs as prescribed. Many systems of the body are involved. As depressives have many subjective complaints anyway, it is often difficult to disentangle drug effects (Nelson *et al.* 1984*a*).

Central nervous system

A common side effect of many of the antidepressants is drowsiness and torpor. This comes on quickly, is maximal in the first few days and then lessens over the ensuing week or two. Amitriptyline, doxepin, prothiadin, trimipramine, clomipramine, and mianserin are the most sedative; imipramine, nortriptyline, desipramine, and dibenzepine have much less effect, and protriptyline is definitely stimulant. As well as drowsiness, the patient often feels light-headed, almost to the point of psychological detachment and depersonalization. Thinking, attention, concentration, and especially memory are impaired with high doses. However, these functions are typically impaired anyway in depressives and antidepressants may improve cognitive performance as a harbinger of clinical improvement (Glass *et al.* 1981; Thompson and Trimble 1982).

In the elderly, a persistent tremor may be induced. At high doses, especially of amitriptyline, extrapyramidal reactions have been recorded and one or two cases of syndromes resembling tardive dyskinesia have been reported. Rare neurotoxic reactions have also been documented, comprising ataxia, nystagmus, dysarthria, agitation, tremor, and hyperreflexia.

Almost all tricyclic/tetracyclic drugs lower the convulsive threshold. Epileptic patients may have an increase in fit frequency or an apparently normal subject may convulse for the first time (Burley *et al.* 1978). Maprotiline is particularly likely to induce fits (Edwards *et al.* 1986).

As with all antidepressant therapy, the patient may swing into hypomania when treated with tricyclic drugs. Patients with bipolar illnesses and with a pronounced diurnal variation are most at risk.

Confusional reactions of the atropine-type may occur, especially in the elderly. The initial symptom is heightened visual awareness progressing to visual illusions such as shimmering and moiré effects, flashes of colour, and eventually visual hallucinations, usually of a fairly unformed type. Rarely, a full-blown delirium is induced, with fully organized hallucinations. Confusional reactions, as with other anticholinergic reactions, are more likely when the tricyclic antidepressant is combined with an anticholinergic antipsychotic drug.

The abrupt withdrawal of tricyclic antidepressants is occasionally followed by an akathisia-like syndrome with acute anxiety and restlessness, malaise, muscular aches, nausea, vomiting and dizziness (Disalver and Greden 1984, 1987; Disalver 1989). The drug should be resumed and withdrawn more gradually. Alternatively, atropine can be given to combat the cholinergic overactivity (Disalver *et al.* 1983).

Cardiovascular

Postural hypotension is particularly common in the very young, the very old and the physically debilitated. The tachycardia noted in many patients on tricyclics is a reflex mechanism to compensate for the hypotension. The effect is most pronounced during the first few weeks of medication but it may persist. It is less of a problem if the dose is gradually increased at the onset of treatment.

The changes in cardiac conduction in patients on tricyclic antidepressants resemble those seen with phenothiazines (Taylor and Braithwaite 1978). Repolarization is prolonged as shown by a lengthened Q–T interval, flattened or inverted T-waves and prominent U-waves in the ECG. In addition, tricyclics have a quinidine-like effect with prolongation of A–V conduction and even A–V block. More serious conduction defects include bundle branch and complete heart block. Bradycardia or tachycardia, ventricular extrasystoles and atrial and ventricular arrhythmias may occur. The pharmacological mechanisms are complex and include cholinergic blockade of the vagus, a direct toxic effect on the myocardium and a heightened sensitivity of the heart to circulating catecholamines.

The cardiac arrhythmias are suspected of accounting for an excess of sudden deaths in depressed patients with a history of cardiac disease treated with tricyclic antidepressants. However, the evidence implicating tricyclic drugs is inconsistent. Amitriptyline seems most suspect but this may reflect its extent of usage. Nevertheless, it is wise to avoid its use in cardiac patients and to give any tricyclic drug in divided doses rather than as one large dose at night in the elderly. Congestive cardiac failure may be precipitated or aggravated by tricyclics in patients with recent myocardial infarctions.

Some of the tricyclics and particularly the newer antidepressants seem less cardiotoxic. Lofepramine is one of these. Of the newer drugs, mianserin and trazodone appear so far to be almost devoid of cardiotoxicity, even in overdose. If these initial impressions are maintained, one of these drugs would be the treatment of choice in the depressed patient with cardiovascular pathology. Orme (1984) concluded that one should be very careful about the use of tricyclic antidepressants in patients with severe heart disease and placed in that category patients suffering from heart failure, those with bundle branch block or heart block in their ECGs, and patients with a recent myocardial infarction.

Gastrointestinal

Anticholinergic effects comprise reduced gut motility with constipation which may become severe or even culminate in paralytic ileus. Achalasia of the oesophagus and relaxation of the oesophageal sphincter may produce a hiatus hernia or exacerbate a pre-existing one. The best treatment is to lower the dose rather than to administer cholinomimetic drugs such as neostigmine or bethanecol.

Acid formation in the stomach is diminished by tricyclic drugs which are therefore particularly helpful in depressed patients with peptic ulcer.

Genitourinary

Increased bladder sphincter tonus results from the cholinergic blockade of the tricyclic drugs. Some degree of urinary retention may ensue but this is usually only of clinical significance in patients with pre-existing pathology such as prostatic enlargement. Therefore, elderly males should be asked about difficult micturition before being prescribed tricyclic antidepressants.

Another drug effect is delayed orgasm with slow ejaculation, a property sometimes made use of therapeutically in patients with premature ejaculation. Erectile dysfunctions and changes in libido may also occur (Mitchell and Popkin 1983; Segraves 1989).

Trazodone has marked alpha-adrenergic antagonistic properties and this underlies the rare but serious complication of priapism which has been reported. Treatment is by local irrigation with adrenalin.

Metabolic-endocrine

Weight gain is often marked in patients treated with tricyclic antidepressants, many women in particular finding it both upsetting and costly because of the need for new clothes. Part of the weight gain is reversal of the weight loss earlier in the illness. Many patients report a craving for carbohydrates, and tricyclics are known to have complex effects on blood glucose levels.

Effects on the pituitary–gonadal axis result in menstrual irregularities, breast enlargement, and galactorrhea in women, impotence, gynaecomastia, and testicular swelling in men. Libido may be increased or decreased but such changes are difficult to interpret because of alterations in sexual function associated with the depressive illness itself.

Miscellaneous

Anticholinergic effects include pupillary dilatation and loss of accommodation with blurring of vision. Intraocular pressure rises, so these drugs should be given with the utmost care in patients with narrow angle glaucoma. It is probably wisest to choose one of the newer antidepressants with few anticholinergic actions. Paradoxically, hyperhidrosis has been described, especially with imipramine, and was claimed to be a sign of good therapeutic response; the mechanism is unclear.

Minor symptoms include headache, fatigue, nausea, anorexia, stomatitis, peculiar taste sensations, and nightmares. Liver function tests may show minor impairment, but usually return to normal even though the drug is continued. Occasionally, mild cholestatic jaundice develops. Allergic reactions include rashes, urticaria and oedema (Warnock and Knesevich 1988). Agranulocytosis, thrombocytopenia, and eosinophilia are on record.

A rare syndrome of nephrogenic diabetes insipidus, unresponsive to vasopressin, has been described. Plasma sodium concentrations are low and polyuria is present.

Teratogenicity

Imipramine has been implicated in teratogenic effects in animals but reports of congenital limb deformities in babies born of mothers who had taken this drug during pregnancy have not been confirmed. Unless there is a compelling need to use these drugs in pregnant women, they should be avoided, especially in the first trimester. If a depressed woman on a tricyclic antidepressant becomes pregnant, the possibility of recommending a therapeutic abortion should be considered.

Overdoses

Tricyclic antidepressants are a major problem in overdose (Proudfoot 1986). They are prescribed for depression, a major feature of which can be suicidal tendencies or intentions, and most of these drugs are dangerous in overdose, causing a complex clinical picture which is difficult to treat. For this reason, prescriptions should be for conservative amounts, but even a week's supply of an antidepressant at full dosage can be lethal. Also, the determined patient can hoard his supplies. Entrusting antidepressants to a trustworthy relative or friend is a wise precaution. The problem of accidental overdosage among children is also worrying, even 250 mg proving fatal on occasion. The toddler may take a parent's antidepressants or those prescribed to an elder sibling for enuresis.

The standard tricyclic drugs of the imipramine and amitriptyline family are all dangerous in overdose, any dose above 600 mg likely to produce serious effects in adults. Doses over 2.5 g, that is one hundred 25 mg tablets, are likely to prove fatal. Some of the newer tricyclics may be a little less toxic. Experience so far suggests that the later compounds, mianserin and trazodone, may be significantly less toxic and bear considering when prescribing for a patient who is socially isolated and whom one suspects of harbouring suicidal intent. Lofepramine also appears to be safer (Dorman 1985).

Symptoms usually appear within 4 h (Crome 1982). Features commonly include dry mouth, blurred vision, dilated pupils, sinus tachycardia, extra-pyramidal signs, and either drowsiness or excitement.

The cardiovascular effects of overdosage are the most life-threatening and range from sinus tachycardia to major arrhythmias. The serious arrhythmias are more likely in the elderly, those with pre-existing problems and in patients with respiratory difficulties. The ECG may show prolongation of the QRS complex and ST segment. T-waves are often abnormal. The ECG changes may resemble ventricular or supraventricular tachycardia or bundle branch block. Atrioventricular block and bradycardia sometimes occur. The more serious effects probably stem from a quinidine-like myocardial depressant action of the tricyclic compounds. All patients with overdoses of tricyclic drugs need ECG monitoring until they have fully recovered.

Central effects comprise excitement, or coma with shock. The latter state suggests that a sedative drug such as a barbiturate may have been taken as well. Metabolic acidosis is sometimes present. Convulsions may occur, especially in children. Respiratory depression may develop, with sudden apnea. Other effects recorded include hypotension, agitation or delirium, hyperreflexia, myoclonus and chorea, and bowel and bladder paralysis. Total recovery is still possible despite a flat EEG and dilated non-reactive pupils.

As the anticholinergic actions of the drug may delay gastric emptying, it is worth washing out the stomach within the first 12 h. Activated charcoal may also help reduce absorption. Because of the high tissue and plasma binding, forced diuresis, haemodialysis and haemoperfusion are useless.

Respiration must be rendered adequate and electrolyte and blood gas disturbances rectified. The correction of the metabolic acidosis by intravenous infusion of bicarbonate may of itself lessen the cardiac abnormalities. Intravenous physostigmine salicylate 2 mg over 5 min may reverse both peripheral and central anticholinergic effects but it tends to cause convulsions, and on balance, is best avoided. Diazepam 10 mg may be needed to combat any fits which develop although some centres prefer intravenous phenytoin as it has an antiarrhythmic effect as well. Otherwise, treatment is generally supportive, bodily temperature and vital functions being monitored and maintained.

Drug interactions

CNS drugs. The sedative actions of many tricyclic/tetracyclic antidepressants are potentiated by central depressants such as alcohol, barbiturates, and benzodiazepines. Thus, patients on antidepressant medication must be warned about drinking and enjoined never to drink and drive. The interaction with barbiturates is especially complicated. As well as the initial central potentiation, the barbiturates accelerate the metabolism in the liver of the tricyclic drug. This results in the attenuation of antidepressant effects. Benzodiazepines lack any significant inducing effect in man so mild potentiation of central sedation is the only action.

The stimulant effects of amphetamine, as with other sympathomimetics, are potentiated.

Potentiation of phenothiazines is only a problem at high doses. Anticholinergic effects include confusion, constipation, dry mouth and urinary retention. Toxic effects on the heart may develop. The potentiation is both at the receptor level and in the liver where drugs compete for the microsomal liver enzymes.

Cardiovascular drugs. Tricyclic antidepressants prevent some antihypertensive agents—guanethidine, bethanidine, debrisoquine, and perhaps methyldopa—from being taken up by the amine pump to their site of action in the presynaptic noradrenergic neurone (Cocco and Ague 1977). Consequently, if a tricyclic drug is used to treat a depressed hypertensive patient maintained on one of these antihypertensive agents, control of the blood-pressure may be lost. The rise in blood-pressure is sometimes marked and difficult to control.

Clonidine is more complex. It also is transported by the noradrenalin pump, but it acts as well as a presynaptic noradrenergic agonist, the stimulation of these receptors producing a feedback inhibition of noradrenalin synthesis. These receptors are blocked by mianserin which is thus to be expected to antagonize the actions of clonidine but not of the other antihypertensive drugs.

The practical management of the depressed hypertensive patient is first to review whether specific antihypertensive therapy is necessary or whether salt restriction and a diuretic might suffice. If drugs are judged necessary, a beta-adrenoceptor antagonist should be used. Otherwise, mianserin could be tried as the antidepressant, except when clonidine is being administered.

Tricyclic/tetracyclic drugs markedly potentiate some directly acting sympathomimetic amines, especially noradrenalin. Attacks of severe hypertension may be caused. Patients receiving injections of local anesthetics formulated with adrenalin are at risk, so dentists and others using such injections should inquire of their patients whether they are taking antidepressants.

Tricyclics may potentiate antiarrhythmics such as quinidine and cardiac drugs of the digoxin type. Coumarin anticoagulants are occasionally potentiated by tricyclic drugs. Thyroid hormones are also mildly potentiated.

Monoamine-oxidase inhibitors

These compounds are much less popular than the tricyclic-type antidepressants, comprising less than 10 per cent of antidepressant prescriptions in the U K and even less in the U S A. However, some revival of interest has recently occurred (Zisook 1985). Their biochemical pharmacology has been extensively researched, although the relationship of M A O inhibition to clinical response is still not clear. The following account of the M A O Is reflects their clinical importance and is thus less detailed than that of the tricyclics.

Only two M A O Is are available in the U S A, phenelzine and tranylcypromine, five in the U K. As phenelzine and tranylcypromine are the most widely used, by choice in the U K, by necessity in the U S A, their pharmacology will be emphasized.

History

In the late 1940s isoniazid and iproniazid were introduced for the treatment of tuberculosis. Both drugs, iproniazid in particular, were noted to induce euphoria and overactivity. Iproniazid was tried in schizophrenic patients and was found to bring about a small, and by no means entirely beneficial, increase in activity. In other studies on schizophrenics, effects were less noticeable and interest in iproniazid waned.

Meanwhile, Zeller and Barsky (1952) had discovered that iproniazid (but not isoniazid) was a powerful inhibitor of the enzyme monoamine oxidase. They speculated that the general mental stimulation and mood elevation in patients with iproniazid was related to an inhibition of M A O with a subsequent increase in brain amines. This hypothesis fired the imagination of many clinicians who then carried out a series of studies, mostly uncontrolled, which showed useful antidepressant properties for iproniazid.

Unfortunately, the drug, a hydrazine derivative, produced a significant number of cases of liver toxicity. New M A O Is were developed in an attempt to obviate this problem. The first of these were also hydrazine derivatives and still produced some adverse effects. Non-hydrazine derivatives were therefore produced and introduced into clinical practice. Some were found to produce other untoward effects and were later withdrawn.

Pharmacodynamic adverse effects, such as the 'cheese reaction' were described and their mechanism elucidated. The realization of the difficulties this entailed for clinical usage, together with a disillusionment with the therapeutic efficacy of the M A O Is led to a marked decrease in their prescription. Occasionally, it seems that the drugs are going to be revived but they are still used in a very limited way. Although they still have their enthusiastic advocates, these are far outnumbered by practitioners who regard the M A O Is as too toxic and too inefficacious for any but the most occasional use.

Pharmacokinetics

The pharmacokinetic properties of the MAOIs can be construed as of little importance. This is because these drugs are irreversible, non-competitive inhibitors of MAO so that the kinetics of drug action are primarily dependent on the properties of MAO rather than those of the MAOI. Thus, iproniazid is no longer detectable in the brain 24 h after administration; however, MAO activity remains low for several days until new enzymes are synthesized.

Iproniazid is changed to an active metabolite, probably isopropylhydrazine, which is a more potent MAOI than iproniazid itself, and has a longer half-life in the tissues. Isocarboxazid, nialamide, and phenelzine are also rapidly absorbed and metabolized. The routes of metabolism of phenelzine include acetylation by hepatic acetyl transferase. The rate of acetylation is genetically determined. It is possible that slow acetylators have more unwanted effects and a better clinical response than do rapid acetylators but this is still controversial (Rose 1982). Determination of acetylator status is not of much use in clinical practice (Marshall *et al.* 1978). Tranylcypromine is closely related to amphetamine and is rapidly absorbed and excreted.

Basic pharmacology

Monoamine oxidase is an enzyme which is widely distributed throughout most tissues. It is localized within the cell in the outer mitochondrial membrane where a major function is to inactivate by oxidative deamination aromatic amines including noradrenalin, dopamine, and 5-hydroxytryptamine. In humans, neuronal MAO is not directly accessible so resort has been made to peripheral tissues such as blood platelets. The activity of MAO is influenced by many factors including age, hormonal status, and several diseased states. Evidence of altered activity in depression is not consistent. Monoamine oxidase may exist in a variety of forms (isoenzymes) which vary from tissue to tissue and have different effects on different substrates. For example, type A breaks down noradrenalin and 5-HT, but not phenylethylamine; type B acts in the reverse way: both types deaminate tyramine. Most MAO inhibitors are active against all forms, but some research compounds have a more specific action (Pare 1985). Clorgyline inhibits type A preferentially and selegiline (deprenyl) type B. The latter has been introduced for the treatment of parkinsonism, but seems to have few if any antidepressant properties.

Monoamine-oxidase inhibition leads to the accumulation in the tissues, including the brain, of several aromatic amines usually present in only minute amounts, including several neurotransmitters. Monoamines from exogenous sources also build up. Secondary pathways of metabolism may become important, leading to the formation of unusual amines. For example, tyramine may be metabolized by hydroxylation to octopamine, the monohydroxy analogue of noradrenalin. Deaminated products of metabolism such as 5-hydroxyindoleacetic acid (5-HIAA) are decreased in concentration. Since an excess of MAO exists in cells, very high levels of inhibition are needed before amine changes can be detected in the brain.

Monoamine oxidase inhibitors raise amine levels widely especially after the prior administration of precursors such as tryptophan and L-dopa. Thus, MAO inhibition enhances amine effects such as tryptamine-induced convulsions and tyramine-induced elevations in blood-pressure. Changes in urinary excretion patterns have been demonstrated in man and include increased tryptamine, and free and methylated catecholamines.

A single dose of a MAO inhibitor such as iproniazid produces little physiological or behavioural effect. Repeated doses cause overactivity and sympathomimetic effects including mydriasis and vasoconstriction. In very large doses, the EEG shows an alert pattern. MAO inhibitors can prevent the effects of reserpine but cannot reverse them once they have occurred. Monoamine-oxidase inhibitors are relatively non-selective in that they can inhibit a range of other enzymes such as amino acid decarboxylases and transaminases.

Tranylcypromine has a somewhat different spectrum of effects. Its inhibitory effect is more rapid in onset than that of the hydrazine MAO inhibitors and it is more effective against type B MAO. It is structurally similar to amphetamine and has some effects in common. However, these stimulant effects are usually present only in dose levels above those necessary for MAO inhibition and are weaker than those of amphetamine itself. Like amphetamine, tranylcypromine releases noradrenalin from nerve terminals and inhibits its re-uptake into the nerve terminals. In man, tranylcypromine produces marked increases in urinary tryptamine and can activate the EEG.

Some doubts have been cast on the idea that clinical response is a direct consequence of MAO inhibition and elevation of brain amines. It has been suggested that the hypotensive properties of MAO inhibitors are due to the formation of octopamine from tyramine and its cumulation in nerve endings where it displaces noradrenalin, and acts as a 'pseudotransmitter'. The hypothesis explains the delay in action, as the octopamine builds up, but predicts a decrease in noradrenergic activity on chronic administration of a MAO inhibitor. If this model also applies to the brain, then depression would have to be associated with elevated rather than diminished brain amine levels.

Clinical pharmacology (McDaniel 1986)

Early clinical studies were uncontrolled and generated a great deal of uncritical enthusiasm. Improvement of depressive symptoms were often delayed for two or three weeks, but dramatic improvements were then claimed. Controlled trials showed much less effect (Quitkin *et al.* 1979). One early study (Cole *et al.* 1959) failed to find a difference between iproniazid, placebo and psychotherapy in a group of patients with depression as a prime symptom. Rees and Benaim (1960) in a cross-over trial against placebo reported that restlessness and depressive speech content were reduced, and Wittenborn *et al.* (1961) showed increased verbal and motor activity and shorter reaction times even though the change in mood was unimpressive.

Phenelzine is fairly effective (Robinson *et al.* 1978) and has become the main hydrazine MAO inhibitor since iproniazid fell into disuse. Most comparative trials find it better than placebo but less effective than the standard tricyclic drugs, imipramine and amitriptyline. Isocarboxazid and nialamide have proved even more disappointing in comparative clinical trials. Tranylcypromine, by contrast, is undoubtedly effective in treating depressed patients, being superior to placebo in 3 out of 4 controlled studies and equal to imipramine in 3 (Morris and Beck 1974). Although tranylcypromine might be suspected to particularly affect noradrenalin and dopamine disposition, 5-HT also seems important.

Some trials have suggested that larger doses of an MAO inhibitor are associated with better clinical response than the usual recommended clinical doses (Robinson *et al.* 1978; Pare 1985). For example, in one study, phenelzine 60 mg, but not 30 mg, relieved anxiety and depression more than placebo. In another study, patients were allocated randomly to receive either 45 or 90 mg daily. The latter group improved significantly more with a more rapid rate of improvement. Acetylator status did not influence clinical response (Tyrer *et al.* 1980). Also, treatment must be continued for at least 6 weeks. Patients with inhibition of platelet MAO greater than 90 per cent are more likely to improve than those with lower levels of inhibition but the relationship is not simple and prediction of response is not accurate.

Clinical uses (Tyrer 1979)

While it is generally accepted that overall the MAO inhibitors are less efficacious than the tricyclic antidepressants, many attempts have been made to delineate their clinical uses by attempting to define the clinical characteristics of the patients who respond. In a retrospective study of 58 patients who responded to iproniazid, West and Dally (1959) found responders tended to suffer from 'anxiety hysteria with secondary atypical depression', to have phobias, and to have responded poorly to ECT. Similar findings apply to phenelzine which has been found valuable in cases of 'atypical depression' in which irritability, somatic anxiety, hypochondriasis and phobic symptoms are prominent (Tyrer 1976). Such a clinical picture merges into that of anxiety states, and phenelzine has been shown to be effective in phobic anxiety states (Tyrer *et al.* 1973). Phenelzine is less effective against classical endogenous depression especially in its more severe forms. However, no differential predictive indicators of response were found in a controlled trial of MAOIs versus tricyclic antidepressants in unselected outpatient depressives (Young *et al.* 1979).

Thus, MAO inhibitors are most often indicated in patients with atypical depression characterized by phobic anxiety, irritability, and hypochondriasis, often with a histrionic element to the illness (Nies and Robinson 1982; Tollefson 1983) (Table 9.4). However, the predictive value of such features is not so high as to identify a group of patients for which MAO inhibitors are drugs of first choice, nor a group in which response is totally unlikely. Monoamine-oxidase inhibitors have been tried in depressed schizophrenics but benefits are scanty and psychotic phenomena may be activated.

Unwanted effects

Orthostatic hypotension is a common and troublesome side effect and often limits the dose which can be attained. Tolerance does not develop for it. It is dose-related and tends to build up in the days or weeks after initiation of treatment or an increase in dose. Severe hypotension can be dealt with by recumbency but pressor amines should be avoided in patients on MAO inhibitors.

An unexplained adverse effect is oedema of the legs, often quite gross, bilateral or unilateral. The effect is usually dose-dependent but may persist until the MAO inhibitor is totally discontinued.

Restlessness and hyperactivity are extensions of the central stimulating properties of the MAO inhibitors, particularly tranylcypromine. Patients

Table 9.4. Typical symptom profile of MAOI-responsive patients.

Psychopathological symptoms	*Vegetative symptoms*
mood reactivity retained	initial insomnia
irritability	hypersomnia
panic episodes	weight gain
agoraphobia	hyperphagia
social fears	craving sweets
hypochondriasis	lethargy and fatigue
obsessive preoccupations	tremulousness
Interpersonal reactions	*Historical features*
self-pity/blaming others	personal loss before intensification
communicative suicidal actions	poor ECT response
rejection sensitive	liking amphetamines
vanity/applause seeking	dysphoric tricyclic responses
histrionic personality	alcohol/sedative abuse

From Nies and Robinson (1982), with permission.

with retarded depression may become agitated. Schizophrenic patients may show activation of symptoms or become paranoid. As with other antidepressants, patients may swing over into hypomania.

Paraesthesias of the fingers or toes may be noticed by the patient; very rarely, peripheral neuropathy ensues. Muscle twitches in the limbs may occur especially after waking up, often in conjunction with hyperreflexia.

Iproniazid, the first MAO inhibitor to be marketed, has been implicated in hepatocellular damage, often fatal. The other hydrazine derivatives, phenelzine, isocarboxazid, and nialamide, have also been associated with such reports. The clinical syndrome resembles that of viral hepatitis with jaundice, diffuse cellular damage, elevated serum liver enzymes, and bile stasis. However, the condition is rare and may incorporate some element of drug sensitivity. Hydrazine MAO inhibitors should not be given to patients with a history of liver disease. The drug should be stopped immediately if jaundice supervenes in any patient.

Autonomic side effects include dry mouth and skin, constipation, hesitancy of micturition and dysuria, and blurring of vision. Changes in libido and inhibition of ejaculation are also documented. Patients with angina may note an anti-anginal effect. Uncommonly, allergic skin reactions and leucopenia may occur.

Drug interactions

The dangers of taking certain foodstuffs while on MAO inhibitors is well known. The MAO inhibition prevents the breakdown of exogenous amines in the gut wall and liver and also increases noradrenalin stores throughout the body. The amines, mainly tyramine, reach the systemic circulation and thence noradrenergic nerve endings where they release noradrenalin resulting in vasoconstriction and hypertension. Symptoms comprise severe headache, and death from intracranial haemorrhage may ensue. The treatment of hypertensive crisis is to administer phentolamine 5–10 mg intravenously or chlorpromazine 50 mg intramuscularly, thereby blocking alpha adrenergic receptors.

The list of foods implicated is fairly small. Many foodstuffs have been excluded on dubious grounds (Folks 1983; Sullivan and Shulman 1984). McCabe and Tsuang (1982) after an exhaustive review of the literature listed foods which must be avoided (see Table 9.5). The food interactions are unpredictable and some patients break the rules with apparent impunity. Nevertheless, having eaten cheese uneventfully on one occasion does not mean that it is safe to ignore warnings in the future.

Interactions with sympathomimetic amines are more dangerous and more predictable (Davidson *et al.* 1984) (Table 9.6). Indirectly acting amines which release noradrenalin include ephedrine, phenylethylamine, phenylpropanolamine, and other compounds available in pharmacies as nasal

Table 9.5. MAOI dietary restrictions

High tyramine content—not permitted
Unpasteurized cheeses (aromatic): Cheddar, Camembert, Stilton, Bleu, etc.
Meat extracts: 'Bovril', 'Marmite', etc.
Smoked/pickled protein: herring, sausage
Aged/putrifying protein: chopped chicken liver, tuna, etc.
Red wines: chianti, burgundy, sherry, etc.
Italian broad bean (fava) pods
Limited tyramine—limited amount allowed
Meat extract: bouillon, consommé
Pasteurized light and pale beers
White wines: champagne
Ripe avocado, ripe banana
Sour cream, yoghurt
Low tyramine—permissible
Distilled spirits (in moderation)
Pasteurized cheeses: cream, cottage
Chocolate
Yeast breads
Fruits: figs, grapes, raisins
Soy sauce, meat tenderizer
Caffeine containing beverages

From McCabe and Tsuang (1982), with permission.

Table 9.6. Monoamine-oxidase inhibitor drug incompatibilities

Contraindication
Stimulants: amphetamines, cocaine, anorectic drugs
Decongestants: sinus, hay fever, cold tablets
Antihypertensives: methyldopa, guanethidine, reserpine
Antidepressants: imipramine, desipramine, clomipramine, trimipramine
MAOIs: tranylcypromine after other MAOIs
Relatively contraindicated (marked potentiation)
Narcotics: pethidine
Sympathomimetics: adrenalin, noradrenalin, dopamine, isoprenaline
General anaesthetics
Amine precursors: L-dopa
Potentiation
Narcotics: morphine, codeine, etc.
Sedatives: alcohol, barbiturates, benzodiazepines
Local anaesthetics: containing vasoconstrictors
Hypoglycaemic agents: insulin, tolbutamide, chlorpropamide
Insufficient knowledge
Antidepressants: maprotiline, amoxapine, trazodone

decongestants. Dangerous hypertensive crises can be induced. Patients taking MAO inhibitors should be issued with a standard card warning of dietary and drug interactions (Table 9.7). Levodopa is markedly potentiated as its product dopamine is a good substrate for MAO. Amphetamines may also interact dangerously. Directly acting amines such as adrenalin and noradrenalin are not potentiated.

Narcotic analgesics and anticonvulsants such as pethidine, meperidine and dextromethorphan can be dangerously potentiated by MAO inhibitors. The interaction can take two forms: excitatory with restlessness, muscular rigidity, hyperpyrexia, and hyperreflexia; and a depressive type with respiratory depression, hypotension, and coma (Brown and Linter 1987). The mechanism of these interactions is complex, but is not just an increase in narcotic action.

Antihypertensive agents may be potentiated because MAO inhibitors produce hypotension themselves. Beta-adrenoceptor antagonists do not seem to interact with MAO inhibitors.

Dangerous interactions can occur with tricyclic antidepressants. The typical syndrome comprises restlessness, excitement, pupillary dilatation, sweating, muscular rigidity or twitching, hyperpyrexia, and coma, all features of aminergic overactivity. Deaths have been reported especially when a tricyclic drug has been given to a patient already on an MAO inhibitor or within two weeks of cessation of an MAO inhibitor. The tricyclics vary in the hazard they pose. Clomipramine and imipramine seem most

Table 9.7. Instructions to patients taking MAOI's

While taking this drug and for 10 days after your treatment finishes, you must observe the following simple instructions:

1. On no account take any other MEDICINES (including tablets, capsules, nose drops, inhalants, or suppositories) whether purchased by you from a chemist or previously prescribed by your doctor, *without first consulting him*.
   NB Cough and cold cures
Pain relievers
Tonics
Laxatives } ARE MEDICINES
2. Avoid CHEESE, BOVRIL, OXO, MARMITE, BROAD BEAN PODS and PICKLED HERRINGS.
3. Drink ALCOHOL only in moderation and avoid CHIANTI WINE completely.

Keep a careful note of ANY FOOD OR DRINK THAT DISAGREES with you, avoid it and tell your doctor.

Report any unusual or severe symptoms to your doctor.

dangerous, trimipramine and amitriptyline safer. Tranylcypromine in combination is more dangerous than phenelzine or isocarboxazid. The pharmacology of antidepressant interactions in man is complex (Pare *et al.* 1982).

Overdose

Twelve hours or more may elapse after an overdose of an MAO inhibitor before effects are noticed. Headache, chest pain, and hyperactivity progress to confusion, hallucinations, and delirium (Crome 1982). Other signs include nausea, vomiting, photophobia, hyperpyrexia, and dilated pupils. Attacks of paroxysmal hypertension may culminate in intracranial haemorrhage, pulmonary oedema, or acute circulatory collapse. Hyperreflexia may be seen, together with trismus, laryngeal stridor, muscle spasms, and convulsions. Finally, profound hypotension and death may supervene.

Treatment is symptomatic and supportive. Difficult pharmacological problems are often presented because of the complex clinical picture and the dangers of interactions with any drugs given symptomatically.

Other antidepressants

Antipsychotic drugs

Since the introduction of the antipsychotic drugs there have been many reports (including those of controlled trials) that they possess useful antidepressant properties (Robertson and Trimble 1982). Some of the earlier studies were concerned with psychotic patients with marked paranoid features and both chlorpromazine and thioridazine were found to be as effective as imipramine. More recently, claims have been made concerning thiothixene and flupenthixol in moderately depressed out-patients. Controlled studies have confirmed uncontrolled observations that these thioxanthene derivatives are as effective as amitriptyline (Johnson 1979). The dosage used in establishing the antidepressant effect is low, say flupenthixol 1.5–3 mg a day. Higher doses are not usually effective, although occasionally high doses can produce a gratifying response in very refractory patients. Response, if it occurs, usually happens quickly, with full recovery. Partial response is usually followed by relapse in a month or two so these drugs are not useful as maintenance therapy.

In view of the low dosage, extrapyramidal effects are uncommon, and tardive dyskinesia is rare although not unknown. Nevertheless, this use of the thioxanthene drugs is still experimental; the results of further trials are awaited.

Benzodiazepines

Many studies have evaluated benzodiazepines in the treatment of depressed patients. One problem is that many of the patients involved in these studies are anxious as well as depressed, most rating scales of depression contain items relating to anxiety, and consequently spurious antidepressant properties may be ascribed to pure anxiolytics. However, some useful therapeutic effects of anxiolytics can be discerned in depressives. For example, in one large-scale trial 425 outpatients were randomly assigned to double-blind treatment with imipramine, chlordiazepoxide or placebo (Lipman *et al.* 1986). Chlordiazepoxide treatment produced early improvement but by 4 weeks imipramine produced more improvement than either the benzodiazepine or the placebo. By 6 and 8 weeks, imipramine was definitely the most effective on measures of depression, anxiety, anger-hostility, interpersonal involvement, and global improvement. Chlordiazepoxide-treated patients did best on sleep difficulty.

One benzodiazepine which has been extensively evaluated for antidepressant properties is the triazolobenzodiazepine, alprazolam, given at dosage levels higher than those used for anxiety effects. Several trials have suggested definite antidepressant effects (Feighner *et al.* 1983). Side-effects were least with alprazolam. However, because of the high dose and the duration of treatment, the risk of dependence seems appreciable. Currently, further trials are awaited.

Amine precursors

The idea that affective disorders are associated with reduced cerebral utilization of neurotransmitter amines led logically to attempts to treat depressive illnesses by administering drugs which increase the synthesis of these brain amines (van Praag 1981*a*). The transmitters themselves, dopamine, noradrenalin and 5-hydroxytryptamine, cannot be given because they do not penetrate the brain and have major peripheral effects. Precursors can be given providing that they pass the blood–brain barrier and that the synthesis of transmitter depends on the concentration of precursor. Thus, L-dopa is effective in parkinsonism because it is a constituent in the chain of dopamine synthesis beyond the rate-limiting enzyme, tyrosine hydroxylase. Even so, the biochemical consequences of loading with precursors are complex, and changes in brain chemistry can occur in systems other than the one directly involved.

L-tryptophan

L-tryptophan is an essential amino acid, a constituent of the normal diet, the daily requirement being 0.5 g. A very small percentage is involved as the precursor of 5-HT, most being incorporated into proteins or metabolized to kynurenine derivatives. L-tryptophan is the only amino acid which is bound to plasma albumin, which thus complicates its pharmacokinetics. For example, stressful procedures mobilize unesterified fatty acids, which displace tryptophan from its binding sites on plasma albumin. The concentration of unbound tryptophan determines its biological activity. It is taken up into the brain by complex carrier-mediated mechanisms which are shared by other aromatic amino acids such as tyrosine, phenylalanine, and histidine. Excess of tryptophan will competitively inhibit the uptake of the other amino acids.

In man, tryptophan is rapidly absorbed from the gut, plasma concentrations being maximal 1 to 2 h after ingestion. Distribution to brain and tissues is rapid, EEG changes being apparent within 30 min. Within 5-HT neurones, tryptophan is hydroxylated by tryptophan 5-hydroxylase to 5-hydroxytryptophan. However, the availability of this enzyme is the rate-limiting step in synthesis, so administering tryptophan may have less effect in elevating 5-HT levels than expected. The next step is decarboxylation, the enzyme involved being L-aromatic amino acid decarboxylase. Administration of a tryptophan-free diet to animals lowers brain 5-HT levels which recover when tryptophan is added to the diet. In man, giving large doses of tryptophan results in an increase in 5-HT metabolites in the CSF, although it is doubtful whether 5-HT at the nerve endings actually increases. In animals, tryptophan alone produces little change in behaviour; pretreatment with an MAO inhibitor, which prevents breakdown of the extra 5-HT formed, does result in behavioural changes.

The breakdown of tryptophan to kynurenine derivatives involves the enzyme tryptophan pyrrolase which cleaves the indole ring, Factors such as adrenocortical steroids, oestrogens and stress can increase the activity of this enzyme and thus direct tryptophan away from 5-HT synthesis. Tryptophan metabolism shows diurnal variation, pyrrolase activity being maximal at 6 a.m. and minimal at 8 p.m. In man, plasma tryptophan levels are highest at 8 p.m. and it might be predicted that more of a dose of tryptophan would be available at that time.

A number of cofactors are involved in the metabolism of tryptophan, further complicating the issue. Ascorbic acid is a cofactor in the hydroxylation step, pyridoxal-5-phosphate in decarboxylation and later steps in breakdown. Many trials have used both these substances added to the tryptophan, but the evidence that they are needed in patients on normal diets is unconvincing.

In normal men, large doses have little effect. In one study, intravenous doses of L-tryptophan which increased free plasma levels fortyfold merely produced a little drowsiness, but no objective impairment of psychological function. Effects reported in other studies include euphoria, disinhibition, and increased libido.

L-tryptophan in doses of 1–3 g has been advocated as a natural hypnotic, but the evidence is conflicting. It is supposed not to affect REM sleep, nor slow-wave-sleep, and to have no rebound effects on withdrawal but other studies have suggested that lack of effect extends to its hypnotic properties also.

Clinically, tryptophan has been assessed as an empirical treatment without much reference to possible 5-HT deficits in depressed patients and their rectification by the amine precursor. Depressed patients appear to absorb tryptophan normally and metabolize it normally, although some studies suggest free tryptophan may be low in some patients. In the initial clinical trials, L-tryptophan was used in conjunction with MAO inhibitors and found to be more effective in alleviating depression than the MAO inhibitors alone. Later, the claim was made that D, L-tryptophan, 5–7 g daily, was as effective as ECT; this claim has not been sustained, nor does it potentiate ECT (d'Elia *et al.* 1977). However, in a number of controlled studies, L-tryptophan alone has proved as effective as imipramine and amitriptyline. In one large trial in general practice (Thomson *et al.* 1982), tryptophan was superior to placebo, but it is not certain that the therapeutic response to tryptophan is sustained over long periods. Enzyme induction or the accumulation of kynurenine metabolites may underlie this fading of antidepressant effect in some patients.

L-tryptophan has also been used in conjunction with tricyclic antidepressants, particularly those such as amitriptyline and clomipramine which affect 5-HT disposition (Walinder *et al.* 1976). Some potentiation of effect has been claimed. L-tryptophan has also been tried in mania with some apparent success (Chambers and Naylor 1978; Chouinard *et al.* 1985).

To summarize, the therapeutic properties of L-tryptophan are by no means firmly established (Boman 1988). It has few side effects, only nausea, anorexia, and epigastric fullness for an hour or so following each dose. It is safe in overdosage. Animal studies suggested that prolonged usage in high dosage might result in neoplasms in the bladder, because of the carcinogenic properties of some kynurenine derivatives; no human cases have been reported. Thus, L-tryptophan might be useful in patients intolerant of the side effects of other antidepressants. The elderly may benefit especially.

L-tryptophan has very recently been implicated in an eosinophilia–myalgia syndrome in the USA. The cause is believed to be an as yet unidentified contaminant in some batches. The compound has been withdrawn from health food stores in the USA and UK but is still available on prescription in the UK.

5-hydroxytryptophan

L-tryptophan's 5-hydroxy derivative is still at the research stage (Byerley *et al.* 1987). Administration of this compound should result in greatly increased 5-HT concentrations. However, it is taken up into other monoaminergic neurones and there decarboxylated. Its effects are difficult to interpret (d'Elia *et al*. 1978).

Levodopa

This has been given to depressed patients without a great deal of useful effect. In some retarded patients it appeared therapeutic and mania was precipitated in some bipolar patients. In other patients, anger, hostility and increased psychotic phenomena resulted without alleviation of depression.

Management of depressive illnesses

Conceptual models

Depression is a complex condition ranging from sustained unhappiness to severe and life-threatening stupor. Many schemata have been proposed within which to set patients presenting with the prime complaint of depression. The following is suggested (Fig .9.3) as one which is based on clinical observation rather than theoretical or statistical abstractions. It has the advantage that it leads to the logical use of physical treatments.

The model comprises three interactive elements, namely, personality, external circumstances, and biological changes. The personality factor relates to the usual mood state of the individual. Every person has some

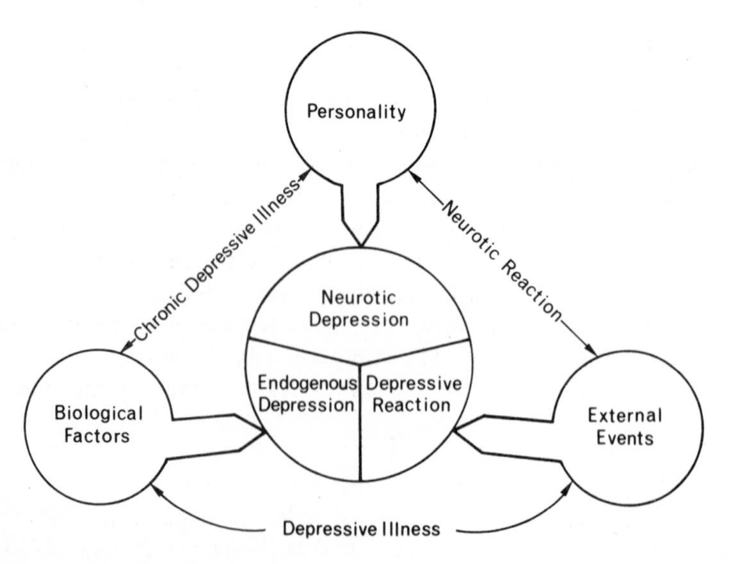

Fig 9.3. A model of depression.

depressive element in his make-up. Some cheery, happy-go-lucky, 'hyperphoric' individuals have very few depressive constituents in their temperament, but others are pessimistic and lugubrious, looking on the dark side of things, 'every silver lining has its cloud'. When this pessimism and blackness of outlook becomes excessive, the patient suffers from an abnormally depressive personality and may seek treatment. The depressive outlook is neurotic and excessive. 'Pure' forms of this type of depression are uncommon and are typically seen in younger individuals, often with a flavour of hostility about the condition. This type of depression is termed 'characterological' in the USA.

The second factor constitutes the circumstances of the individual. Life events such as bereavement, loss of employment, loss of self-esteem, or threat to family happiness may precipitate a reactive depression. Usually, this is within the limits of normal, or follows a defined pattern, the best example being the mourning process after bereavement. The depth of the depression is entirely consistent with the life stresses borne by the individual. The life events can be internal as well as external, for example, the very common depressions which accompany physical illnesses, especially those of an incapacitating or terminal nature.

The third factor, the biological one, is manifested as a wide range of physical changes. Loss of appetite and weight, poor sleep, loss of libido, amenorrhea, retardation, and autonomic dysfunction are the commonest examples. The cause of such changes is unknown. The 'pure' form of this type of depression is endogenous depression, which implies that no external circumstances are operating. Such depressive illnesses are uncommon but are sometimes seen in the cyclic manic-depressive where the depressive episodes occur regularly without the intervention of external influences.

These three uncomplicated forms are greatly outnumbered by the depressive illnesses compounded of two of the factors. The interaction of the neurotic depressive personality and external events results in the neurotic depressive reaction. The abnormal grief reaction is one example, the hypochondriacal depressive reaction to a physical illness is another. Because the depressive reaction is bound up with the personality it tends to become chronic.

The second interaction is that between external circumstances and endogenous factors, and this is probably the commonest mechanism in the aetiology of depression. Two types of interaction can be postulated and both can be discerned in different patients. In the first type, the depressive illness starts off as a depressive reaction to life events. However, the biological predisposition of the person is then activated and somatic features become increasingly pronounced. In the second case, a 'spontaneous' change in biological vulnerability takes place. Response to pharmacological treatment does not seem to be influenced by any history of a stressful environmental event (Garvey *et al.* 1984). The individual is a little out-of-sorts, somewhat labile emotionally, with minor symptoms such as occasional bouts of insomnia. This episode lasts a few months to a few years. If life-circumstances remain favourable, no overt illness develops. However, if life events, particularly of loss, impinge on the person, a depressive illness, apparently 'reactive' in aetiology but with obvious 'endogenous' features, supervenes. Recurrent illnesses are likely until the phase of biological vulnerability remits.

Thirdly, personality and endogenous elements may interact producing a depression with biological features and an exaggeration of hostile, hypochondriacal, histrionic, and impulsive traits. The condition, being personality-bound, tends to be chronic. Alcoholism may develop as a complication although other types of depression may also lead to secondary alcoholism. The biological features may become very intractable with severe insomnia; or chronic inadequacy and indecision may exacerbate the personality problems. Finally, a three-way interaction can be postulated, with life events deepening the chronic depression engendered by personality and endogenous elements.

To anticipate later sections, the three elements of depression have three types of management most appropriate to them: personality – psychotherapy; life circumstances – social manipulation; biological factors – physical treatments.

History and examination

With the above simple scheme in mind, history-taking can be made purposeful in evaluating the three factors. The previous personality should be assessed both from the patient's account and from that of a reliable informant. The general and typical affective tone should be carefully elicited. The reactive element needs to be assessed for the possibility of life events, physical illness, etc. Events of loss seem particularly relevant. Major bereavements in early life may also be important. Biological elements are judged from the symptoms and signs of the present illness and also from the history of affective illnesses previously in the patient and also in his family. The presence of definite or possible hypomanic elements should be carefully sought.

The depressive episode should be evaluated both in terms of present state and also in longitudinal historical terms. Any prodromata such as anxiety or physical symptoms should be enquired for and the nexus between personality, external circumstances, and bodily changes should be evaluated. A drug history is important, since depression can follow drugs such as antihypertensive agents and steroids. Secondary problems such as insomnia or sexual difficulties should be listed as these may require separate symptomatic treatment.

Non-pharmacological measures

The above schema simply equates biological factors to drug therapy, personality features to psychotherapy, and external circumstances to pragmatic counselling and social manipulation. Of course, in practice, the management of a patient with depression is much more complex and many more aspects need to be considered—in particular, the risk of suicide. The different modes of management intermesh and indeed, there are few patients for whom a multidimensional therapeutic approach is inappropriate.

Admission to hospital is necessary if the patient is deemed actively suicidal; that is, states his intention openly, admits to specific plans, and so on. It is also advisable if any doubts concerning the patient's intentions are raised. In general, suicidal intent parallels the severity of the depression so any patient with a depressive illness of more than moderate intensity should be admitted unless he or she can be strictly supervised by a responsible relative or friend.

Supportive psychotherapy is a long term commitment but specific goals can be set in the short term (Winokur and Rickels 1981). One of these is increasing the patient's adherence to any medication which might be prescribed. The patient's co-operation is essential in ensuring the success of any drug therapy. Too often the patient is unprepared for medication, suspicious of medical interventions, and resentful of the unpleasant side-effects of most antidepressant drugs. The first step is to explore the patient's attitudes towards his illness and towards drugs. Many patients regard their miserable condition as just retribution for their previous (grossly exaggerated) sins and oppose any attempts to alleviate their anguish.

Medicines may be regarded as inappropriate because the patient refuses to acknowledge that he is ill. Less ill patients may be reluctant to take medication because, although agreeing they are not well, they are determined to overcome their difficulties on their own, without 'chemical crutches'. Thus, each patient must be carefully prepared for his relevant drug treatment with sympathetic reassurance combined with gently repeated insistence that drug therapy is essential. Even in patients in whom medication is not immediately indicated, the possibility of resorting to it may be usefully raised at quite an early stage. If drugs do eventually prove necessary, the ground will have been prepared.

Doctors should warn the patient of the possible unwanted effects, state their belief that these effects will prove transient, and offer help and advice about any effects which eventuate. Commoner side-effects such as drowsiness and dry mouth should be enumerated in the presence of a caring relative or friend. Even better, a printed list of instructions should be provided, and in the case of the MAO inhibitors, this should include drug and dietary precautions (see Table 9.7).

Environmental manipulation and counselling about the reality situation is an important part of the management of the depressed patient. It must be borne in mind that depressives are indecisive, but that if they do make a decision, it is likely to be coloured by their morbid outlook on the world. Thus, important decisions such as resigning a job, or suing for divorce should be delayed. Deliberate prevarication is essential to prevent the patients doing irrevocable things that they will regret later.

Depressed patients often focus on just one of their difficulties and magnify it to the status of sole cause of their depression. For example, a woman with noisy neighbours may complain bitterly of them and attribute her depression to this annoyance. Yet often, rehousing will effect only a temporary amelioration of symptoms and it becomes apparent that the illness is not primarily reactive at all. It is useful to try and test the situation, for example, by seeing if symptoms remit during a holiday.

Many other facets of management are important but space precludes a more detailed discussion.

Drug therapy

In this section, the indications for drug therapy are discussed in terms of severity and type of depressive illness (Quality Assurance Project 1983). The main decision is whether or not to use drugs and then which of the two main groups to use (Stern *et al.* 1980).

Meta-analyses were carried out with respect to the efficacy of various antidepressant therapies in the treatment of endogenous depression and neurotic depression (Quality Assurance Project 1983). By this means, the average of the total improvements during treatment with a variety of therapies was calculated and expressed in terms of standard deviations of the initial severity level ('effect size'). It can be seen from Fig. 9.4 that MAOI therapy in endogenous depressives is generally less effective than placebo whereas both ECT and antidepressant therapies more than double the placebo effect. In neurotic depressives, the placebo response is greater, psychotherapies and drug treatment have somewhat more effect but not more than sedatives or neuroleptics (Fig. 9.5).

The first decision depends on the severity of the depressive illness, patients with either severe or mild illnesses responding less well than those with moderate illnesses. At the severe end of the spectrum, the treatment of choice remains electroconvulsive therapy (Avery and Winokur 1977). The detailed indications are set out in Chapter 19. ECT and tricyclic antidepressants neither potentiate nor negate each other. Some patients, particularly the elderly, tend to relapse despite an initial encouraging response to ECT. The addition of antidepressant therapy is then most useful to prevent relapse. Other patients respond only partially to ECT and the prescription

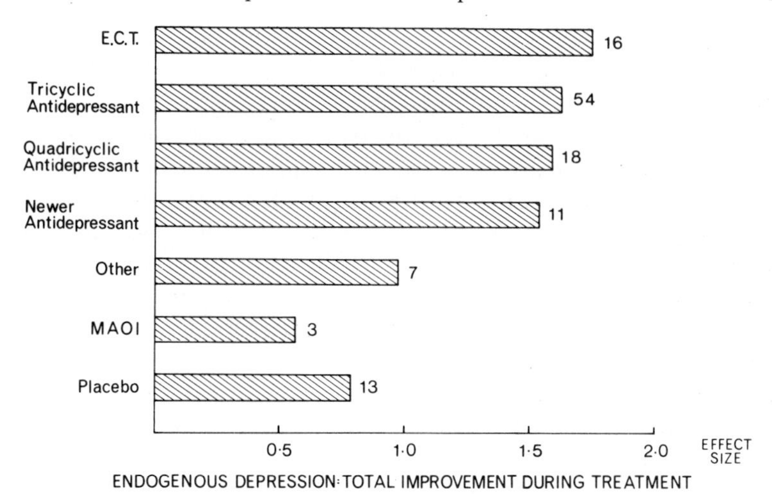

Fig 9.4. A pooled estimate of the improvement with various treatments in endogenous depression expressed as a proportion of the initial standard deviation of the severity ratings ('effect size'). The number to the left of each histogram is the number of clinical trials of that treatment included in the meta-analysis (redrawn from Quality Assurance Project 1983, with permission.)

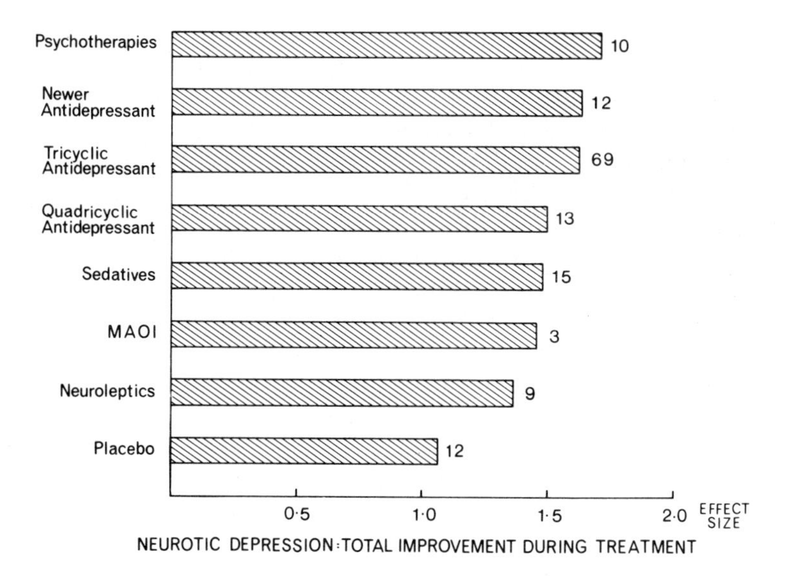

Fig 9.5. A pooled estimate of the improvement with various treatments in neurotic depression expressed as a proportion of the initial standard deviation of the severity ratings ('effect size'). The number to the left of each histogram is the number of clinical trials of that treatment included in the meta-analysis. (Redrawn from Quality Assurance Project 1983, with permission.)

of a tricyclic antidepressant may produce a worthwhile further improvement.

Milder cases of depression often show little response to tricyclic antidepressants (Paykel *et al.* 1988). This type of illness is usually reactive in nature and, as outlined above, social manipulation to alter circumstances is more likely to be successful. However, the clinician must be aware that mildness does not necessarily equate with reactivity of depression. A common error is to fail to recognize mild endogenous type depressions. The patient feels out of sorts, loses his zest for life, sleeps poorly, lacks confidence about the future and complains of odd aches and pains. All these symptoms are mild expressions of features which are unmistakable in their full-blown form in endogenous depression. However, the patient may not admit to being really depressed, and the other features, such as loss of interest, poor attention and concentration, and in particular failure to feel gratification, are more prominent. Careful history taking is needed to elicit all these features. The administration of antidepressant medication is usually followed by prompt and complete relief of symptoms.

The use of MAO inhibitors remains controversial. Their advocates regard them as the treatment of first choice in a wide range of patients but mainly those untypical in being phobic, hypochondriacal, or histrionic in their symptoms. These claims have, however, not been evaluated systematically: although some studies do confirm that such patients respond to MAO inhibitors, it is not certain that distinct advantages exist over the tricyclic group of antidepressants. Consequently, and in view of the dietary and drug interactions of the MAO inhibitors, most clinicians relegate them to drugs of second choice. Their place in therapy will be discussed in the section on refractory depression.

Some psychiatrists still advocate the occasional use of stimulants in judiciously chosen patients (Chiarello and Cole 1987).

Choice of tricyclic and related antidepressants

The strong clinical impression exists that amitriptyline is marginally more effective than any other tricyclic. Despite its troublesome side-effects, it is the most widely prescribed antidepressant in many countries. Objective evidence for the belief in its superiority is very difficult to come by. Most of the hundreds of clinical trials using it as the comparison antidepressant find no differences between it and the test drug. A few trials report it as inferior and, of course, it will appear superior in other trials, It must be regarded as the standard drug against which to assess the others.

Amitriptyline is a highly sedative compound and is usually regarded as appropriate treatment for anxious or agitated or depressed patients. Accordingly, the use of amitriptyline is more related to whether sedation is wanted or unwanted in that particular patient. Someone driving a car, operating complex machinery, or carrying out intellectual tasks for their livelihood, might be incapacitated during the first week or two of treatment. By contrast, an agitated patient in hospital would benefit even if sedation was quite marked.

Amitriptyline, trimipramine, clomipramine, prothiaden, and doxepin are all definitely sedative, and patients will often complain of the heaviness and drowsiness produced by them. Imipramine, desipramine and nortriptyline are much less sedative. Dibenzepine and iprindole have no sedative properties and protriptyline is definitely stimulant. Of the newer antidepressants, mianserin, trazodone, and maprotiline are sedative, viloxazine not so.

Attempts have been made to relate these secondary psychotropic effects to the biochemical effects of the drugs (Cowdry and Goodwin 1981). Thus, it has been suggested that sedative antidepressants are those that primarily affect 5-HT, stimulating ones those that affect noradrenalin. The basis of this is not firmly established, but it might conceivably explain the waning of sedative effects over the first two weeks or so as follows: the tertiary, sedative, 5-HT uptake blocking drugs are metabolized to secondary, non-sedative noradrenalin blocking drugs; as the latter accumulate, the sedative actions are counteracted. Another possible mechanism concerns the antihistaminic properties of the drugs. Whatever the basis of the 'tolerance', the lessening of unpleasant sedative actions is usually noticeable and patients can be reassured that this will happen.

Tricyclic and related antidepressants also vary with respect to their anticholinergic actions. The older tricyclics such as amitriptyline and imipramine have marked atropine-like activity. Newer and non-tricyclic drugs such as iprindole, viloxazine and mianserin have few if any such effects.

Cardiotoxicity also varies, as outlined earlier. Consequently, patients with pre-existing cardiac pathology should not be prescribed amitriptyline; one of the newer compounds such as mianserin or trazodone is preferable. Patients on antihypertensive therapy also need special consideration. Beta-adrenoceptor antagonists, e.g. propranolol, pose no problems with interactions but the antiadrenergic drugs such as guanethidine and bethanidine attenuate the actions of many tricyclics. As these obsolescent antihypertensive drugs are not very effective and might conceivably be contributing to the depression, they are best discontinued and the antihypertensive medication reviewed.

A particular problem is encountered in the management of depressed patients with epilepsy because almost all the tricyclic antidepressants lower the convulsive threshold (Robertson and Trimble 1983). Maprotiline should be avoided. A second complication concerns possible interactions between anticonvulsive medication and antidepressants. Careful monitoring of plasma drug concentrations is essential.

Apart from these special indications for particular antidepressants, the choice of tricyclic-type antidepressants reflects the secondary actions—sedation and anticholinergic effects—rather than real differences in efficacy (Nystrom and Hallstrom 1985). Compliance is likely to be higher with the new drugs as they have fewer-side effects. On the other hand, most practitioners are well-practised with the older drugs such as amitriptyline. Patients known to be intolerant of the sedation and anticholinergic effects should be started on a newer drug, as they will be greatly incommoded by amitriptyline or imipramine.

Another consideration is the suspected suicidal patient who cannot be persuaded to enter hospital and yet is not certifiable. So far, the newer drugs, mianserin, lofepramine, and trazodone, seem much less toxic in overdose than older drugs, and their prescription could just prove life-saving in the occasional patient.

Of the several antidepressants available, the practitioner should be familiar with one sedative and one non-sedative older drug. Together with the use and evaluation of one or two of the newer drugs with fewer side effects, this should prove sufficient to treat almost all depressed patients in which tricyclic and similar drugs are indicated.

Dosage (Table 9.8)

Ever since the introduction of the tricyclic antidepressants over 20 years ago, it has been customary to initiate dosage at about half the therapeutic dose. Thus, 25 mg three times daily of amitriptyline or imipramine is typical for an adult, not elderly, in good, physical health. This dosage is maintained for at least a week, except in the more severely ill in-patient where the dose may be pushed up after 4 days or so. Increase in dose is usually necessary, but if the patient shows an improvement in the first few days it is worth delaying a little in case further remission occurs. It is also impossible to increase the dose if the side-effects (mainly sedation, dry mouth and constipation) are not tolerated by the patient.

Table 9.8. Daily Dosage Ranges of some Antidepressants

Drug	Out-patients	In-patients
Tricyclic		
Imipramine	75–150	75–225
Amitriptyline	75–150	75–225
Doxepin	75–150	100–300
Tetracyclic		
Mianserin	30–90	60–120
MAO Inhibitors		
Phenelzine	15–45	30–75

Typically, after a week the dosage is increased to 50 mg three times per day. In the more severely ill, or in those who show neither therapeutic effects nor side effects, a further increase at the end of the next week to 75 mg three times per day should be considered. It is doubtful if doses above this will effect any further improvement, and doses totalling 300 mg per day carry some hazard of major anticholinergic effects, a toxic confusional state, or rarely extrapyramidal reactions. If no side effects are seen at high dosage, the patient is probably not adhering to treatment.

A variant of dosage regimen which is popular is to give the drug as one dose at night. Only sedative tricyclics are appropriate and will act as hypnotics obviating the need for an additional hypnotic. In view of the possible cardiotoxicity of some tricyclics, particularly amitriptyline, care should be taken in elderly patients not to overdo this single dosage but rather to give the bulk of the dose at night with smaller amounts during the day.

Stimulant antidepressants must be given in divided dosage, the last dose being in the afternoon; otherwise insomnia will occur. Other antidepressants such as viloxazine have short plasma half-lives so once nightly dosage is not appropriate. Not all tricyclic antidepressants are effective in the 75–150 mg dosage range and reference should be made to the detailed literature on each compound. Dosages in the USA tend to be higher than in the UK (Quitkin 1985) but have been claimed to be safe (Schuckit and Feighner 1972).

The elderly vary more than younger patients with respect to interindividual dosage requirements. As a consequence, it is necessary to start at very low dosage levels—a quarter normal for the very old and frail and half normal for the less old. The dosage should be very carefully increased according to the clinical response and tolerance of the individual. Some quite old patients need and can tolerate full clinical doses providing the dosage increase is gradual.

It is generally found that clinical response is delayed for 2–4 weeks (Quitkin *et al.* 1984*b*). Part of this is due to the traditional dosage schedules, so that adequate levels are unlikely for at least 10 days. Nevertheless, the observant clinician may often remark an improvement within a few days of initiation of therapy (Lapierre 1985). One early sign is an amelioration in the severe insomnia so that patients sleep longer and feel a little refreshed when they awake. Weight loss may be halted and the appetite may perk up. A little later, psychomotor slowing starts to remit, so the patient becomes more active and is able to attend and concentrate on matters. Finally—and this may certainly be delayed for 2–4 weeks—the depressed mood starts to lift. The patient is always the last to acknowledge that improvement has occurred. In the more severely depressed, this is a dangerous time because the patient can still see no future yet is more active and more able to execute any plans for suicide.

In general practice depressed patients, outcome at 20-week follow-up could be predicted by the degree of improvement in the first few weeks, even as early as the sixth day (Parker *et al.* 1986). Factors predictive of good outcome included a history of recurrent episodes, a more severe illness, lower social class, break up of an intimate relationship as a precipitant and family support. Similar data and predictive factors were found in 43 patients with non-endogenous depressive disorders referred to psychiatrists (Parker *et al.* 1985).

In more severely ill in-patients, response to tricyclic antidepressants was related to Newcastle Scale scores in a complex way (Abou-Saleh and Coppen 1983). The Newcastle Scale arrays each patient along a continuum of reactive–endogenous. Patients with scores in the middle range (4–8) showed significantly higher percentage improvement than those with low (neurotic type) and high (endogenous—psychotic) types of depression.

Patients with previously abnormal personalities, especially of an obsessional type, respond worse than those with previously normal personalities (Shawcross and Tyrer 1985).

The dexamethasone suppression test (DST) has been extensively evaluated as a predictor of response to biological treatments. However, in only 6 out of 16 published studies reviewed by Gitlin and Gerner (1986) did DST predict response. No simple explanation was adduced for this discrepancy. Only 2 out of 7 studies examining the relationship between DST suppression and response to 'transmitter-specific' antidepressants were positive. Accordingly, the DST does not add anything useful to the usual clinical criteria in predicting clinical response (Stokes 1987; Joyce and Paykel 1989).

Duration of therapy

If treatment with antidepressants is discontinued soon after apparent remission of symptoms, relapse is quite likely, suggesting that the clinical action of these drugs is to suppress manifestations of the illness until natural remission occurs. Therefore, it is customary to continue treatment despite alleviation of symptoms. This continuation of treatment reduces the likelihood of relapse. For example, in a multicentre trial, 92 patients with a primary depressive illness which had responded to imipramine or amitriptyline, 150 mg daily, were randomly allocated either to continue the tricyclic drug or to switch to placebo (Mindham *et al.* 1973). Of those patients on active treatment, 22 per cent relapsed compared with half the placebo group. In a similar maintenance study, some patients received psychotherapy while others did not. Forty per cent of patients on placebo relapsed, compared with 15 per cent on amitriptyline; psychotherapy did not affect the relapse rate but did improve social adjustment. Adverse life events were more common in those who relapsed, whatever the treatment (Paykel and Tanner 1976).

A recent study has specifically addressed the issue of how long continuation drug therapy should be maintained in major depressive episodes (Prien and Kupfer 1986). The results suggested that the patient should be free of significant symptoms for 4–5 months before treatment is discontinued. Also, mild as well as moderate and severe symptoms should be assessed as they are a good indication that the episode has not run its course. Even after their resolution, however, 4 months or so of further medication is necessary to safeguard against a relapse.

The value of continuation therapy has been shown in formal trials where the treatment adherence rate is likely to be higher than in everyday practice. Once-nightly dosage is more likely to be successful.

Maintenance therapy is usually practised at about half the full therapeutic dose. The time at which discontinuation can be attempted with a high likelihood of success is difficult to predict. Several months is a typical treatment duration for a depressed out-patient although some recover in a matter of weeks and others need drug therapy for over a year. The length of previous episodes is often a fair indicator. Careful questioning of the patient at each out-patient appointment will usually reveal that some symptoms persist, albeit in muted form. Anxiety is one such symptom. Then there comes a time when the patient looks and feels quite normal, and this is a sign that the dosage of antidepressant can be lowered and withdrawn. Of course, if the patient prior to the depressive episode had some personality abnormality or mild chronic anxiety, this condition will persist after the depression remits. On occasion, affective disturbances long antedating the overt episode disappear completely, leaving the patient feeling better than he or she has felt for years. In other patients, residual anxiety proves refractory to both drug and behavioural treatments.

Choice of MAO inhibitor

Comparisons between the MAO inhibitors are difficult because the same drugs have seldom been used in the few comparative studies carried out; also dose and duration of treatment have varied. To judge from crude improvement rates, phenelzine is one of the more effective MAO inhibitors, with isocarboxazid and nialamide rather weaker. Indirect comparisons (against imipramine) would suggest that tranylcypromine is more effective than phenelzine. Comparison of biochemical and clinical effects are not very helpful in view of the low correlation between biochemical and clinical effects.

The side effects of the MAO inhibitors are a major consideration in choosing the optimal one. Phenelzine and tranylcypromine are currently the most frequently used. Of the two, phenelzine is probably the safer, although it is somewhat less effective and slower to act. Newer MAO inhibitors have not been tested sufficiently for their place in therapeutics to be established.

Dosage

The dose of phenelzine is typically 15 mg twice or thrice daily, and for tranylcypromine, 10 mg twice or three times daily. Some practitioners recommend pushing the dose of phenelzine to 60, 75, or even on occasion, 90 mg (Lippmann 1986). Postural hypotension is the most troublesome side effect and often limits the dosage. Thus, the best clinical stratagem is to slowly increase the dose until postural hypotension becomes a problem, and then to lower it slightly. This usually results in a dosage of 45–60 mg a day in divided doses.

Duration of therapy

There is usually a delay between first taking an MAO inhibitor and the onset of clinical response. For phenelzine, this delay may be two weeks or more, but it is usually less for tranylcypromine. Acetylator status has been claimed as important, rapid acetylators taking longer to show a clinical response, but this finding is disputed.

Surprisingly little work has been done to ascertain the length of time MAO inhibitor treatment should be continued once a response has occurred. In most cases, the MAO inhibitor can be tailed off after 6 to 12 months, but some patients require much longer therapy. Indeed, many patients have remained on MAO inhibitors for years because symptoms recur when discontinuation is attempted (Tyrer 1984).

Drug treatment and other therapies

In both general practice and psychiatric practice, the combination of psychotherapy (of some sort) and drug therapy is the commonest form of treatment for the depressed patient (Brandon 1986). Yet very few studies have attempted to evaluate whether such combined treatment has any advantages over either treatment alone or over placebo. A large scale collaborative study has been organized by the National Institute of Mental Health in the USA to test the comparative efficacy of two psychotherapies, interpersonal psychotherapy and cognitive behavioural psychotherapy, administered alone and in combination with imipramine. While this study is in progress, a literature review has been carried out and an attempt made to pool the data (Conte *et al.* 1986). The combined active treatments proved sigificantly more effective than placebo, but only slightly superior to either of the constituent treatments alone.

Earlier predictive indicators of response had been sought in a 16-week controlled trial of amitriptyline, interpersonal psychotherapy, or the two combined (Prusoff *et al.* 1980). Patients with a situational or an endogenous depression responded to combined treatment. Those with endogenous depression did not respond to psychotherapy whereas the situational depressives responded to either treatment alone. Thus, some selection of appropriate treatment can be made, although the authors stress that allocation of a patient to either the endogenous or the situational group is a rather artificial procedure.

Cognitive therapy is becoming a favoured treatment for many depressives (Williams 1984). Several studies have compared cognitive to drug therapy and some have investigated the utility of combined therapy. In one, cognitive variables, mood, and severity all responded together and drug therapy seemed less effective than cognitive or combined therapy in both hospital and a general practice sample (Blackburn and Bishop 1983). Combined therapy was superior to cognitive therapy alone in the hospital patients, but not the general practice patients. By and large and as expected, cognitive factors in depression are particularly improved by cognitive therapy (Rush *et al.* 1982).

Another study in moderately to severely depressed out-patients suggested that either cognitive or drug therapy can be effective and that combining the two affords little advantage (Murphy *et al.* 1984). On one year follow up it was found that patients who had received cognitive therapy with or without antidepressants were less likely to relapse than patients who received drugs alone (Simons *et al.* 1986). Patients with persisting symptoms at termination of the therapy were more likely to relapse. Similar superiority for cognitive therapy was found in a trial comparing it with drug treatment at one year follow up (Kovacs *et al.* 1981).

The implications are important for both psychiatric and general practice. Psychiatrists are well aware of the need to encapsulate drug therapy within the larger context of a psychotherapeutic situation. Within psychotherapy it seems advantageous to address specific abnormal and distorted cognitions because their modification is important both for short-term response and long-term outcome.

In general practice 'a talking cure' is the treatment of first choice (Courtenay 1983). Patients need to talk about their symptoms, then their assumptions and fantasies. Cognitive therapy, or at least supportive psychotherapy based on the principles of cognitive theory, should obviate the use of drug therapy in most of the less severely ill patients. Nevertheless, much more research is needed, both in terms of efficacy, who responds and so on, and in operational matters such as whether to train general practitioners in these techniques or make expert psychological help more easily available.

The treatment of refractory depression

As long as the underlying mechanisms of depression are so poorly understood, treatment must remain empirical by trial and error. Most patients respond to an adequate trial of antidepressant but those that fail to do so form a substantial proportion of psychiatric practice, not so much in numbers but in time and frustrated effort (Mitchell 1987). Accordingly, we have devoted a section to this problem.

Definition of refractoriness

Treatment refractoriness occurs when a patient's depressive illness shows no response to an adequate course of treatment. The term 'adequate' should be explained. First, the medicament must be an appropriate antidepressant of proven effectiveness. The commonest mistake is to overlook the depressive element in a mixed anxiety–depressive state and to treat with a benzodiazepine. Indeed, the patient may become worse as the relief of anxiety uncovers the underlying depression. Secondly, the dose must be adequate. Too often, a small dose, say 50 mg of amitriptyline at night, is given with only a poor effect. Thirdly, the course of treatment at a reasonable dose must have continued for at least 6 weeks before the drug can be deemed a failure (Quitkin *et al.* 1984*a*).

Bias in patient selection

Patients referred to psychiatrists are selected on various factors of which failure to respond is obviously important. Most patients who attend their family physicians with depressive illnesses and are treated with adequate dose of antidepressant recover within 6 months, especially if appropriate social and psychotherapeutic measures are also taken. Those who fail to recover are among those referred to psychiatrists, other factors being intractable social problems and major personality disorders. Consequently, the psychiatrist sees a biased sample of depressed patients, many of whom have already apparently failed to respond to standard antidepressant therapy. As family physicians have become more experienced and confident in dealing with depression and antidepressants, they have treated successfully the straightforward cases.

Compliance

This important factor has been discussed earlier, but it is worth repeating that the commonest cause of failure to respond to antidepressants is failure to take them. Gaining the confidence of the patient, warning him about the immediate onset of side-effects but the delayed onset of therapeutic response, using a simple dosage schedule and being available for help and advice, all help to make the treatment successful (Johnson 1981*b*).

Whether a patient takes medication correctly depends on a complex interaction between the patient, the patient's illness, the psychiatrist, and the medication prescribed. The drug defaulter cannot be detected with certainty. Blood or urine tests may identify the patient who refuses medication but not the one who takes it immediately. One must rely on careful, sympathetic questioning of the patient.

Organic causes of chronic depression

Failure to respond to treatment should lead the psychiatrist to review the patient's history and clinical state for organic factors which might be perpetuating the condition. Any severe physical condition can provoke a reactive depression, but this is usually obvious. Some conditions have been linked more specifically to depression. Hepatitis, viral pneumonia, infective mononucleosis, and brucellosis are often associated with depressive symptoms either during the acute illness or during a protracted recovery phase. Carcinoma of the pancreas has been reported to be related to depressive symptoms with more than the usual frequency of depression accompanying malignant conditions.

Endocrine disturbance may also be associated with depression (Ban *et al.* 1984). Both pituitary underactivity and overactivity produce affective changes. Hypothyroidism may relate to a retarded depression, hyperthyroidism to an anxious or agitated depression. Hyperparathyroidism and poorly controlled diabetes mellitus are also factors inducing or perpetuating affective symptoms.

Several organic states should be considered. In the elderly, early dementia may be difficult to distinguish from depression and indeed often coexists. Temporal lobe epileptics may have complex affective states. Space occupying lesions in the brain may present as depressive syndromes, sometimes refractory to antidepressant therapy. Idiopathic parkinsonism is commonly associated with a chronic depression which may be overlooked because of the akinesia. Multiple sclerosis, classically associated with cheerfulness or even euphoria may induce a reactive depression, as may any neurological condition.

Drug-induced depression

Numerous pharmacological substances during either treatment or withdrawal can be associated with depression. Antihypertensive drugs such as reserpine and methyldopa can induce depression (Ambrosino 1974; Bant 1978), whereas clonidine, guanethidine, and propranolol probably do not. Corticosteroids and oral contraceptives have been implicated in the production of depressive symptoms, although the evidence with respect to the latter drugs is controversial (Parry and Rush 1979). Nevertheless, a depressed woman on the pill could be advised to resort to other means of contraception at least for a trial period of 2–3 months. Alternatively, pyridoxine supplements, 50 mg/day, can be given for a 4-week trial as the mechanism of the depression is believed to involve pyridoxine deficiency.

The vexed question of hormonal replacement therapy in the menopause is germane here (Klaiber *et al.* 1979; Strickler *et al.* 1977). Despite claims based on response in individual cases, the evidence from controlled trials suggests that the only symptoms to respond directly to hormonal replacement therapy are the cardiovascular ones, such as hot flushes. Improvement in psychological symptoms including depression is probably secondary to relief of the somatic symptoms.

Abuse of alcohol can lead to depression or accentuate the pre-existing depression. One should seek the usual signs of covert alcohol use. Other abused drugs sometimes associated with depression include the amphetamines and appetite suppressants, cocaine, the barbiturates and heroin. Sedatives and hypnotics may uncover a depression, and antipsychotic medication in the schizophrenic sometimes induces an akinetic syndrome which may be mistaken for a retarded depression. Less commonly, a true depressive condition supervenes, but the relationship of this to the antipsychotic medication such as fluphenazine decanoate injections is a matter of debate. Depression is a common symptom in both acute and chronic patients not on antipsychotic medication (Johnson 1981*a*).

Psychosocial causes

As well as reviewing the patient's case for organic factors, the psychiatrist should carefully review psychological, environmental, and social factors. It is often helpful to interview another informant about the patient's previous personality and present predicament. In particular, evidence should be sought concerning a possible depressive personality. A further search for precipitating causes, especially of a symbolic nature, should be mounted. For example, a patient may become depressed when nearing the age at which a very close relative died. Events concerning loss are particularly relevant. Environmental influences in the home, the family, at work, and during leisure activities may have been overlooked or underestimated at the initial interview. Conversely, an apparent causative factor may have been wrongly identified or over-emphasized, diverting attention from the real problem.

Pharmacokinetic factors

In the search for reasons why a quarter of depressed patients, by and large, fail to respond to antidepressants, much emphasis has been placed on pharmacokinetic variation. Thus, as discussed earlier, attempts have been made to establish a threshold or a range of plasma concentrations associated with a good clinical response. The quest has been long and arduous, and not entirely successful. The situation with nortriptyline is the least obscure. Clinicians with monitoring facilities should aim at a plasma concentration between 50 and 200 ng/ml. Patients failing to respond often have high rather than low concentrations. Indeed, it has been shown that psychiatric clinic patients on average metabolize nortriptyline at half the normal rate. This implies that depressed patients who metabolize the drug at normal rates attain therapeutic concentrations on normal doses as prescribed by their family physician. They recover, whereas slow metabolizers reach supra-therapeutic levels, fail to respond and are referred to a specialist. This interesting finding needs replication and extension to other antidepressants. The situation is less clear with respect to amitriptyline. In our present state of knowledge, it is probably best for the clinician to aim for a total (amitriptyline plus nortriptyline) concentration of 200–250 ng/ml.

An important drug interaction concerns tricyclic antidepressants and other drugs. Some, like phenobarbitone, are capable of inducing microsomal enzymes in the liver, thus accelerating the metabolism of the tricyclic antidepressant so that therapeutic levels are never attained. The psychiatrist should check that the patient is not being prescribed drugs by another practitioner or has illicit access to barbiturates.

Assessment of drug resistance

Once the practitioner has reassured himself that the patient is actually taking the medication as prescribed, are there any ways of deciding whether an inadequate, adequate, or excessive drug concentration has been attained in the body, without resort to the complexities and ambiguities of plasma drug estimations? One approach is to carefully assess autonomic side effects. Persistent drug-related effects such as constipation, dry mouth, and blurring of vision imply the presence of the drug in substantial amounts, at least in the periphery. As antidepressant drugs readily penetrate the blood–brain barrier, brain concentrations should also be high. An objective test is to measure the near point of vision which steadily recedes as drug concentrations increase. Even this strategy cannot be used with some of the new drugs such as mianserin and viloxazine which have few atropine-like effects. The usual, simple dosage strategy is to increase drug dosage until side-effects come on, and then to decrease the dosage a little. Alternatively, if side effects supervene without any therapeutic response, the dose can be slowly but steadily decreased and any signs of incipient response carefully sought.

Practical management

The various topics discussed above earlier in the chapter can be synthesized into a plan of action for the practical management of a patient who fails to respond adequately to the initial course of tricyclic antidepressants. Each patient must be assessed carefully and the management tailored to his particular requirements and problems.

First, the label of 'resistant' depression must be carefully reviewed. Has the patient been prescribed the drug of first choice in an adequate dose; did the medication appear to be completely inert? Were appropriate and relevant social measures taken to optimize the treatment setting, and were psychological factors evaluated and tackled with psychotherapy? If the treatment to date has dealt with all these essentials, then the patient presents a definite problem; if not, then the omissions in treatment must first be rectified (Lydiard 1985).

It is important to enquire about side effects. If no effects are reported, or if they are inordinately troublesome, poor drug compliance may underlie or be contributing to the lack of therapeutic response. Careful, sympathetic questioning on this point will save many fruitless therapeutic forays later. If side-effects are minimal, the dose of the drug should be cautiously increased. If side effects are very prominent, it is probably better to slowly lower the dose, observing closely for any therapeutic response.

If these manoeuvres fail, the patient's history, physical state and psychological factors should be carefully reviewed, in particular any concurrent therapy such as reserpine, barbiturates or the pill. If no cause is found, the present medication should be tailed off over two or three weeks, never abruptly. If a partial or short lived response occurs, it is possible that the patient has been on too high a dosage and the drug should be restarted cautiously. Usually, however, the patient remains depressed as the drug withdrawal proceeds.

Recently, attention has focused on the use of lithium, adding it to the tricyclic antidepressant (Cowan 1988). Providing lithium concentrations are maintained at 0.5–0.8 mmol/litre, a gradual remission occurs in about 50 per cent of patients refractory to tricyclics alone.

The type of the patient's depression dictates the next, that is, second choice treatment. Some psychiatrists would switch to another tricyclic drug or to a newer antidepressant such as mianserin or trazodone. With a patient with a severe endogenous depression, especially if it is intensifying, the possibility of a course of ECT should be considered. A more untypical, phobic, hypochondriacal, or 'hysterical' type of depressive illness is more likely to respond to an MAO inhibitor than to a tricyclic antidepressant (McGrath *et al.* 1987). However, some chronically ill manic depressives respond to an MAO inhibitor (Larsen and Rafaelsen 1980). If the MAO inhibitor alone is only partially effective, L-tryptophan, 3–6 g/day in divided doses can be added. The trial of the MAO inhibitor with or without L-tryptophan should last 4–6 weeks. Some clinicians advocate the adjunctive use of thyroid hormones (Stein and Avni 1988).

If these treatments are ineffective, it is probably best to try a small dose of flupenthixol or perhaps thioridazine. The combination of tricyclic and MAO inhibitor antidepressants has been enthusiastically advocated. There

Table 9.9. Algorithm for the management of obsessive–compulsive disorder

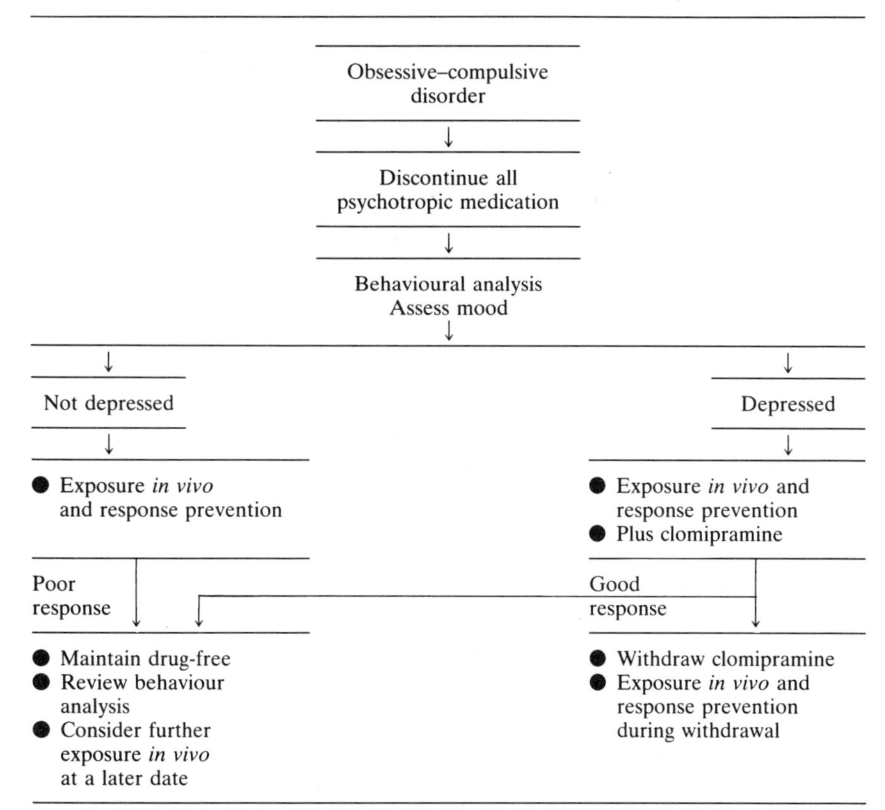

After Lelliott and Monteiro (1986), with permission.

are undoubted dangers if the combination is ill-chosen, and there is no evidence that the combination is more effective than either constituent alone (White and Simpson 1984; Lader 1983; Young *et al.* 1979). Probably by this time, another tricyclic drug will be tried, but using drug after drug unsuccessfully only wearies the patient and saps his confidence in himself and his medical attendant. A policy of 'wait and see' is often best at this juncture, providing it is presented honestly and not despairingly to the patient.

A firm clinical impression exists that some depressed patients (perhaps 5–10 per cent) are genuinely refractory to all forms of antidepressant therapy. Most patients will eventually remit spontaneously. Claims have been made for leucotomy in this situation (see Chapter 17) but only severe, protracted cases should be considered. Meanwhile, careful psychotherapy, attendance in group therapy, or at least a day hospital, may provide sufficient support. Courses of antidepressant drugs can be tried every 6–12 months in an attempt to accelerate a natural remission. However, psychiatrists must acknowledge frankly that there is a minority of depressives whom they cannot cure, and they must become adept in supporting the unfortunate few whose misery drags on.

Other indications

The use of antidepressant medication in the treatment of agoraphobia remains contentious. A number of studies have shown both the tricyclic and MAOI groups of antidepressants to have beneficial effects on certain aspects of the condition. However, in most cases behavioural therapy of some sort was given simultaneously (Telch *et al.* 1983). More recently, studies have been less favourable towards the efficacy of the drugs used alone. Problems in clinical usage include problems with compliance, side effects and relapse when the drug is discontinued.

Obsessive compulsive disorder may also be responsive to antidepressants, although behaviour therapy is the treatment of first choice (Lelliott and Monteiro 1986; Perse 1988). The two types of treatment can be combined (see Table 9.9). Clomipramine has been specifically evaluated in this indication and is efficacious (Jenike *et al.* 1987). The possibility that 5-HT mechanisms are involved in both agoraphobia and obsessive compulsive disorder has been raised (Mavissakalian 1983): the use of 5-HT selective antidepressants might be appropriate (Goodman *et al.* 1989).

References

Abou-Saleh, M.T., and Coppen, A. (1983). Classification of depression and response to antidepressive therapies. *British Journal of Psychiatry* **143,** 601–3.

Ambrosino, S.V. (1974). Depressive reactions associated with reserpine. *New York State Journal of Medicine* **74,** 860–4.

Amsterdam, J., Brunswick, D., and Mendels, J. (1980). The clinical application of tricyclic antidepressant pharmacokinetics and plasma levels. *American Journal of Psychiatry*. **137,** 653–62.

Ananth, J., Pecknold, J.C., Van Den Steen, N., and Engelmann, F. (1979). Double-blind comparative study of chlorimipramine in obsessive neurosis. *Current Therapeutic Research* **25,** 703–9.

Asberg, M., Cronholm, B., Sjoqvist, F., and Tuck, D. (1971). Relationship between plasma level and therapeutic effect of nortriptyline. *British Medical Journal* **3,** 331–4.

Ashcroft, G.W. (1975). Management of depression. *British Medical Journal* **2,** 372–6.

Avery, D., and Winokur, G. (1977). The efficacy of electroconvulsive therapy and antidepressants in depression. *Biological Psychiatry* **12,** 507–23.

Axelrod, J. (1971). Noradrenaline: Fate and control of its biosynthesis. *Science* **173,** 598–606.

Baldessarini, R.J. (1989). Current status of antidepressants: clinical pharmacology and therapy. *Journal of Clinical Psychiatry* **50,** 117–26.

Ball, J.R.B., and Kiloh, L.G. (1959). A controlled trial of imipramine in treatment of depressive states. *British Medical Journal* **2,** 1052–4.

Ban, T.A., Guy, W., and Wilson, W.H. (1984). The psychopharmacological treatment of depression in the medically ill patient. *Canadian Journal of Psychiatry* **29,** 461–5.

Bant, W.P. (1978). Antihypertensive drugs and depression: a reappraisal. *Psychological Medicine* **8,** 275–83.

Bech, P., Allerup, P., Gram, L., Reisby, N. Rosenberg, R., Jacobsen, O., and Nagy, A. (1981). The Hamilton Rating Scale: Evaluation of objectivity using logistic models. *Acta Psychiatrica Scandinavica* **63,** 290–9.

Benfield, P., and Ward, A. (1986). Fluvoxamine—a review of its pharmacodynamic and pharmacokinetic properties and therapeutic efficacy in depressive illness. *Drugs* **32,** 313-34.

Blackburn, I.M., and Bishop, S. (1983). Changes in cognition with pharmacotherapy and cognitive therapy. *British Journal of Psychiatry* **143,** 609–17.

Blackwell, B. (1981*a*). Adverse effects of antidepressant drugs. Part I: Monoamine oxidase inhibitors and tricyclics. *Drugs* **21,** 201–19.

Blackwell, B. (1981*b*). Adverse effects of antidepressant drugs. Part 2: 'Second Generation' antidepressants and rational decision-making in antidepressant therapy. *Drugs* **21,** 273–82.

Blackwell, B., and Simon, J.S. (1986). Second-generation antidepressants. *Drugs of Today* **22,** 611–33.

Boman, B. (1988). L-tryptophan: a rational anti-depressant and a natural hypnotic? *Australian and New Zealand Journal of Psychiatry* **22,** 83–97.

Brandon, S. (1986). Management of depression in general practice. *British Medical Journal* **292,** 287–8.

Braithwaite, R.A., Goulding, R., Theano, G., Bailey, J., and Coppen, A. (1972). Plasma concentration of amitriptyline and clinical response. *Lancet.* **1,** 1297–300.

Brogden, R.N., Heel, R.C., Speight, T.M., and Avery, G.S. (1981). Trazodone: a review of its pharmacological properties and therapeutic use in depression and anxiety. *Drugs* **21,** 401–29.

Browne, B., and Linter, S. (1987). Monoamine oxidase inhibitors and narcotic analgesics. A critical review of the implications for treatment. *British Journal of Psychiatry* **151,** 210–12.

Burley, D., Jukes, A., and Steen, J. (1978). Maprotiline hydrochloride and grand-mal seizures. *British Medical Journal* **2,** 1230.

Burrows, G.D., Davies, B., and Scoggins, B.A. (1972). Plasma concentration of nortriptyline and clinical response in depressive illness. *Lancet.* **2,** 619–23.

Byerley, W.F., Judd, L.L., Reimherr, F.W., and Grosser, B.I. (1987). 5-Hydroxytryptophan: a review of its antidepressant efficacy and adverse effects. *Journal of Clinical Psychopharmacology* **7,** 127–37.

Cazzullo, C., and Silvestrini, B. (eds.) (1989). An antidepressant with adrenolytic activity , *Clinical Neuropharmacology* **12,** Suppl. 1, S1-S59.

Cerletti, U., and Bini, L. (1938). Un nouvo methodi di shock terapia, l'elettroshock. *Bolletino Accademia Medicina, Roma* **64,** 136.

Chambers, C.A., and Naylor, G.J. (1978). A controlled trial of L-tryptophan in mania. *British Journal of Psychiatry* **132,** 555–9.

Chiarello, R.J., and Cole, J.O. (1987). The use of psychostimulants in general psychiatry. A reconsideration. *Archives of General Psychiatry* **44,** 286–95.

Chouinard, G., Young, S.N., and Annable, L. (1985). A controlled clinical trial of L-tryptophan in acute mania. *Biological Psychiatry* **20,** 546–57.

Cocco, G., and Ague, C. (1977). Interactions between cardioactive drugs and antidepressants. *European Journal of Clinical Pharmacology* **11,** 389–93.

Cole, C.E., Patterson, E.M., Craig, J.B., Thomas, W.E., Ristine, L.P., Stahly, M., and Pasamanick, B. (1959). A controlled study of efficacy of iproniazid in treatment of depression. *Archives of General Psychiatry* **1,** 513–18.

Conte, H.R., Plutchik, R., Wild, K.V., and Karasu, T.B. (1986). Combined psychotherapy and pharmacotherapy for depression. A systematic analysis of the evidence. *Archives of General Psychiatry* **43,** 471–9.

Coppen, A., Ghose, K., Montgomery, S., Rama Rao, V.A., Bailey, J., Christiansen, J., Mikkleson, P.L., van Praag, H.M., Van de Poel, F., Minsker, E.J., Kozulja, V.G., Matussek, N., Kungkunz, G., and Jirgensen, A. (1978). Amitriptyline plasma—concentration and clinical effect. A World Health Organization Collaborative Study. *Lancet* **1,** 63–6.

Courtenay, M.J.F. (1983). A general practice approach to depression. *Practitioner* **227,** 45–8.

Cowan, P.J. (1988). Depression resistant to tricyclic anti-depressants. *British Medical Journal* **297,** 435–6.

Cowdry, R.W., and Goodwin, F.K. (1981). Biological and physiological predictors of drug response. In *Handbook of biological psychiatry*, Part VI (eds. H.M. van Praag, M.H. Lader, O.J. Rafaelsen and E.J. Sachar) pp. 263–308. Marcel Dekker, New York.

Crome, P. (1982). Antidepressant overdosage. *Drugs* **23,** 431–61.

Davidson, J., Zung, W.W.K., and Walker, J.I. (1984). Practical aspects of MAOI inhibitor therapy. *Journal of Clinical Psychiatry* **45** (Sec.2), 81–4.

Davies, B. (1973). Diagnosis and treatment of anxiety and depression in general practice. *Drugs*. **6,** 389–99.

d'Elia, G., Hanson, L., and Raotma, H. (1978). L-tryptophan and 5-hydroxytryptophan in the treatment of depression. *Acta Psychiatrica Scandinavica* **57,** 239–52.

d'Elia, G., Lehman, J., and Raotma, H. (1977). Evaluation of the combination of tryptophan and ECT in the treatment of depression. *Acta Psychiatrica Scandinavica* **56,** 303–18.

Disalver, S.C. (1989). Antidepressant withdrawal syndromes: phenomenology and pathophysiology. *Acta Psychiatrica Scandinavica* **79,** 113–17.

Disalver, S.C., and Greden, J.F. (1984). Antidepressant withdrawal phenomena. *Biological Psychiatry* **19,** 237–56.

Disalver, S.C., Feinberg., M., and Greden, J.F. (1983). Antidepressant withdrawal symptoms treated with anticholinergic agents. *American Journal of Psychiatry* **140,** 249–51.

Disalver, S.C., Greden, J.F., and Snider, R.M. (1987). Antidepressant withdrawal syndromes: phenomenology and pathophysiology. *International Clinical Psychopharmacology* **2,** 1–19.

Dorman, T. (1985). Toxicity of tricyclic antidepressants: are there important differences? *Journal of International Medical Research* **13,** 77–83.

Edwards, J.G., Long, S.K., Sedgwick, E.M., and Wheal, H.V. (1986). Antidepressants and convulsive seizures: clinical, electroencephalographic, and pharmacological aspects. *Clinical Neuropharmacology* **9,** 329–60.

Faravelli, C., Ballerini, A., Ambonetti, A., Broadhurst, A.D., and Das, M. (1984). Plasma levels and clinical response during treatment with clomipramine. *Journal of Affective Disorders* **6,** 95–107.

Feighner, J.P., Meredith, C.H., Dutt, J.E., and Hendrickson, G.G. (1982). A double blind comparison of lofepramine, imipramine and placebo in patients with primary depression. *Acta Psychiatrica Scandinavica* **66,** 100–8.

Feighner, J.P., Meredith, C.H., Frost, N.R., Chammas. S., and Hendrickson, G. (1983). A double blind comparison of alprazolam vs imipramine and placebo in the treatment of major depressive disorder. *Acta Psychiatrica Scandinavica* **68,** 223–33.

Folks, D.G. (1983). Monoamine oxidase inhibitors: reappraisal of dietary considerations. *Journal of Clinical Psychopharmacology* **3,** 249–53.

Fuller, R.G. (1930). Expectation of hospital life and outcome for mental patients on first admission (Civil State Hospitals, New York). *Psychiatric Quarterly* **4,** 295.

Garvey, M.J., Schaffer, C.B., and Tuason, V.B. (1984). Comparison of pharmacological treatment response between situational and non-situational depressions. *British Journal of Psychiatry* **145,** 363–5.

Gitlin, M.J., and Gerner, R.H. (1986). The dexamethasone suppression test and response to somatic treatment: a review. *Journal of Clinical Psychiatry* **47,** 16–21.

Glass, R.M., Uhlenhuth, E.H., Hartel, F.W., Matuzas, W., and Fischman, M.W. (1981). Cognitive dysfunction and imipramine in outpatient depressives. *Archives of General Psychiatry* **38,** 1048–51.

Goodman, W.K., Price, L.H., Rasmussen, S.A., Delgado, P.L. Heninger, G.R., and Charney, D.S. (1989). Efficacy of fluvoxamine in obsessive-compulsive disorder. *Archives of General Psychiatry* **46,** 36–44.

Gram, L.F., and Christiansen, J. (1975). First-pass metabolism of imipramine in man. *Clinical Pharmacology and Therapeutics* **17,** 555–63.

Gram, L.F., Sondergaard, I., Christiansen, J., Petersen, G.D., Bech, P., Reisby, N., Ibsen, I., Ortmann, J., Nagy, A., Dencker, S.J., Jacobsen, O., and Krautwald, O. (1977). Steady-state kinetics of imipramine in patients. *Psychopharmacology* **54,** 255–61.

Greden, J.F., and Carroll, B.J. (1981). Psychomotor function in affective disorders: an overview of new monitoring techniques. *American Journal of Psychiatry* **138,** 1441–4.

Green, A.R., and Costain, D.W. (1979). The biochemistry of depression. In *Psychopharmacology of affective disorders* (eds. E.S. Paykel and A. Coppen) pp. 14–40. Oxford University Press, Oxford.

Heel, R.C., Morley, P.A., Brogden, R.N., Carmine, A.A., Speight, T.M., and Avery, G.S. (1982). Zimelidine: A review of its pharmacological properties and therapeutic efficacy in depressive illness. *Drugs* **24,** 169–206.

Hollister, L.E., Overall, J.E., Pokorny, A.D., and Shelton, J. (1971). Acetophenazine and diazepam in anxious depressions. *Archives of General Psychiatry* **24,** 273–8.

Iversen, L.L., and Mackay, A.V.P. (1979). Pharmacodynamics of antidepressants and antimanic drugs. In *Psychopharmacology of affective disorders* (eds. E.S. Paykel and A. Coppen) pp. 60–90. Oxford University Press, Oxford.

Jenike, M.A., Baer, L., and Minichiello, W.E. (1987). Somatic treatments for obsessive-compulsive disorders. *Comprehensive Psychiatry* **28,** 250–63.

Johnson, D.A.W. (1979). A double-blind comparison of flupenthixol, nortriptyline and diazepam in neurotic depression. *Acta Psychiatrica Scandinavica* **59,** 1–8.

Johnson, D.A.W. (1981*a*). Studies of depressive symptoms in schizophrenia. *British Journal of Psychiatry* **139,** 89–101.

Johnson, D.A.W. (1981*b*). Depression: treatment compliance in general practice. *Acta Psychiatrica Scandinavica* **63,** (Suppl. 290), 447–53.

Joyce, P.R. and Paykel, E.S. (1989). Predictors of drug response in depression. *Archives of General Psychiatry* **46,** 89–99.

Jue, S.G., Dawson, G.W., and Brogden, R.N. (1982). Amoxapine: a review of its pharmacology and efficacy in depressed states. *Drugs* **24,** 1-23.

Kathol, R.G., and Petty, F. (1981). Relationship of depression to medical illness. A critical review. *Journal of Affective Disorders* **3,** 111–21.

Klaiber, E.L., Broverman, D.M., Vogel, W., and Kobayashi, Y. (1979). Estrogen therapy for severe persistent depressions in women. *Archives of General Psychiatry* **36,** 550–4.

Kopin, I.J. (1981). Mode of action of antidepressants and central stimulants. In *Handbook of biological psychiatry*, Part IV (eds. H.M. van Praag, M.H. Lader, O.J. Rafaelsen, and E.J. Sachar) pp. 741–66. Marcel Dekker, New York.

Kovacs, M., Rush, A.J., Beck, A.T., and Hollon, S.D. (1981). Depressed outpatients treated with cognitive therapy or pharmacotherapy. A one year follow-up. *Archives of General Psychiatry* **38,** 33–9.

Kragh-Sorensen, P.K., Hansen, E., Baastrup, P.C., and Hvidberg, E.F. (1976). Self-inhibiting action of nortriptyline's antidepressive effect at high plasma levels. A randomised, double-blind study controlled by plasma concentrations in patients with endogenous depression. *Psychopharmacologia* **45,** 305–12.

Kuhn, R. (1958). The treatment of depressive states with G22355 (imipramine hydrochloride). *American Journal of Psychiatry* **115,** 459–63.

Lader, M. (1983). Combined use of tricyclic antidepressants and monoamine oxidase inhibitors. *Journal of Clinical Psychiatry* 44, sec. 2, 20–4.

Lader, M., Lang, R.A., and Wilson, G.D. (1987). *Patterns of improvement in depressed in-patients*. Oxford University Press, Oxford.

Lancaster, S.G., and Gonzalez, J.P. (1989). Lofepramine. A review of its pharmacodynamic and pharmacokinetic properties, and therapeutic efficacy in depressive illness. *Drugs* **37,** 123–40.

Lapierre, Y.D. (1985). Course of clinical response to antidepressants. *Progress in Neuropsychopharmacology and Biological Psychiatry* **9,** 503–7.

Larsen, J.K., and Rafaelsen, O.J. (1980). Long term treatment of depression with isocarboxazide. *Acta Psychiatrica Scandinavica* **62,** 456–63.

Leckman, J.F., Weissman, M.M., Merikangas, K.R., Pauls, D.L., and Prusoff, B.A. (1983). Panic disorder and major depression. Increased risk of depression, alcoholism, panic, and phobic disorders in families of depressed probands with panic disorder. *Archives of General Psychiatry* **40,** 1055–60.

Lelliot, P.T., and Monteiro, W.O. (1986). Drug treatment of obsessive-compulsive disorder. *Drugs* **31,** 75–80.

Lewis, D.A., and Smith, R.E. (1983). Steroid-induced psychiatric syndromes. A report of 14 cases and a review of the literature. *Journal of Affective Disorders* **5,** 319–32.

Lipman, R.S., Covi, L., Rickels, K., McNair, D.M., Downing, R., Kahn, R.J., Lasseter, V.K., and Faden, V. (1986). Imipramine and chlordiazepoxide in depressive and anxiety disorders. I. Efficacy in depressed outpatients. *Archives of General Psychiatry* **43,** 68–77.

Lippmann, S. (1986). Monoamine oxidase inhibitors. *American Family Physician* **7,** 113–19.

Lydiard, R.B. (1985). Tricyclic-resistant depression: treatment resistance or inadequate treatment? *Journal of Clinical Psychiatry* **46,** 412–17.

McCabe, B., and Tsuang, M.T. (1982). Dietary consideration in MAO inhibitor regimens. *Journal of Clinical Psychiatry* **43,** 178–81.

McDaniel, K.D. (1986). Clinical pharmacology of monoamine oxidase inhibitors. *Clinical Neuropharmacology* **9,** 207–34.

McGrath, P.J., Stewart, J.W., Harrison, W., and Quitkin, F.M. (1987). Treatment of tricyclic refractory depression with a monoamine oxidase inhibitor antidepressant. *Psychopharmacology Bulletin* **23,** 169–72.

Marshall, E.F., Mountjoy, C.Q., Campbell, I.C., Garside, R.F., Leitch, I.M., and Roth, M. (1978). The influence of acetylator phenotype on the outcome of treatment with phenelzine, in a clinical trial. *British Journal of Clinical Pharmacology* **6,** 247–54.

Matussek, P., and Feil, W. B. (1983). Personality attributes of depressive patients. Results of group comparisons. *Archives of General Psychiatry* **40,** 783–90.

Mavissakalian, M. (1983). Antidepressants in the treatment of agoraphobia and obsessive-compulsive disorder. *Comprehensive Psychiatry* **24,** 278–84.

Medical Research Council (1965). Clinical trial of the treatment of depressive illness. *British Medical Journal* **1,** 831–6.

Mindham, R.H.S., Howland, C., and Shepherd, M. (1973). An evaluation of continuation therapy with tricyclic antidepressants in depressive illness. *Psychological Medicine* **3,** 5–17.

Mitchell, J.E., and Popkin, M.K. (1983). Antidepressant drug therapy and sexual dysfunction in men: a review. *Journal of Clinical Psychopharmacology* **3,** 76–7.

Mitchell, P. (1987). The pharmacological treatment of tricyclic-resistant depression: review and management guidelines. *Australian and New Zealand Journal of Psychiatry* **21,** 442–51.

Montgomery, S.A., and Asberg, M. (1979). A new depression scale designed to be sensitive to change. *British Journal of Psychiatry* **134,** 382–9.

Morris, J.B., and Beck, A.T. (1974). The efficacy of antidepressant drugs. *Archives of General Psychiatry* **30,** 667–74.

Murphy, G.E., Simons, A.D., Wetzel, R.D., and Lustman, P.J. (1984). Cognitive therapy and pharmacotherapy singly and together in the treatment of depression. *Archives of General Psychiatry* **41,** 33–41.

Nelson, J.C., and Charney, D.S. (1980). Primary affective disorder criteria and the endogenous-reactive distinction. *Archives of General Psychiatry* **37,** 787–93.

Nelson, J.C., and Charney, D.S. (1981). The symptoms of major depressive illness. *American Journal of Psychiatry* **138,** 1–12.

Nelson, J.C., Jatlow, P.I., and Quinlan, D.M. (1984*a*). Subjective complaints during desipramine treatment. Relative importance of plasma drug concentrations and the severity of depression. *Archives of General Psychiatry* **41,** 55–9.

Nelson, J.C., Mazure, C., Quinlan, D.M., and Jatlow, P.I. (1984*b*). Drug-responsive symptoms in melancholia. *Archives of General Psychiatry* **41,** 663–8.

Nies, A., and Robinson, D. (1982). Monoamine oxidase inhibitors. In *Handbook of affective disorders* (ed. E.S. Paykel). Churchill Livingstone, Edinburgh.

Nystrom, C., and Hallstrom, T. (1985). Double blind comparison between a serotonin and a noradrenalin reuptake blocker in the treatment of depressed outpatients. Clinical aspects. *Acta Psychiatrica Scandinavica* **72,** 6–15.

Orme, M.L'E. (1984). Antidepressants and heart disease. *British Medical Journal* **289,** 1–2.

Orsulak, P.J., and Waller, D. (1989). Antidepressant drugs: additional clinical uses. *The Journal of Family Practice* **28,** 209–16.

Pare, C.M.B. (1985). The present status of monoamine oxidase inhibitors. *British Journal of Psychiatry* **146,** 576–84.

Pare, C.M.B., Kline, N., Hallstrom, C., and Cooper, T.B. (1982). Will amitriptyline prevent the 'cheese' reaction of monoamine oxidase inhibitors? *Lancet* **1,** 183–6.

Parker, G., Tennant, C., and Blignault, I. (1985). Predicting improvement in patients with non-endogenous depression. *British Journal of Psychiatry* **146,** 132–9.

Parker, G., Holmes, S., and Manicavasagar, V. (1986). Depression in general practice attenders. 'Caseness', natural history and predictors of outcome. *Journal of Affective Disorders* **10,** 27–35.

Parry, B.L., and Rush, A.J. (1979). Oral contraceptives and depressive symptomatology: biologic mechanisms. *Comprehensive Psychiatry* **20,** 367–58.

Paykel, E.S. (1971). Classification of depressed patients. A cluster analysis derived grouping. *British Journal of Psychiatry* **118,** 275–88.

Paykel, E.S. (1979). Predictors of treatment response. In *Psychopharmacology of affective disorders* (eds. E.S. Paykel and A. Coppen) pp. 193–220. Oxford University Press, Oxford.

Paykel, E.S., and Tanner, J. (1976). Life events, depressive relapse and maintenance treatment. *Psychological Medicine* **6,** 481–5.

Paykel, E.S., Hollyman, J.A., Freeling, P., and Sedwick, P. (1988). Predictors of therapeutic benefit from amitriptyline in mild depression: a general practice placebo-controlled trial. *Journal of Affective Disorders* **14,** 83–95.

Peet, M., and Coppen, A. (1979). The pharmacokinetics of antidepressant drugs: relevance to their therapeutic effect. In *Psychopharmacology of affective disorders* (eds. E.S. Paykel and A. Coppen) pp. 91–107. Oxford University Press, Oxford.

Perse, T. (1988). Obsessive-compulsive disorder: a treatment review. *Journal of Clinical Psychiatry* **49,** 48–55.

Preskorn, S.H. (1986). Tricyclic antidepressant plasma level monitoring: an improvement over the dose-response approach. *Journal of Clinical Psychiatry* **47** (Suppl. 1), 24–30.

Prien, R.F., and Kupfer, D.J. (1986). Continuation drug therapy for major depressive episodes: how long should it be maintained? *American Journal of Psychiatry* **143,** 18–23.

Proudfoot, A.T. (1986). Acute poisoning with antidepressants and lithium. *Prescriber's Journal* **26,** 97–106.

Prusoff, B.A., Weissman, M.M., Klerman, G.L., and Rounsaville, B.J. (1980). Research diagnostic criteria subtypes of depression. Their role as predictors of differential response to psychotherapy and drug treatment. *Archives of General Psychiatry* **37,** 796–801.

Quality Assurance Project. (1983). A treatment outline for depressive disorders. *Australian and New Zealand Journal of Psychiatry* **17,** 129–46.

Quitkin, F.M. (1985). The importance of dosage in prescribing antidepressants. *British Journal of Psychiatry* **147,** 593–7.

Quitkin, F.M., Rabkin, J.G., Ross, D., and McGrath, P.J. (1984*a*). Duration of antidepressant drug treatment. What is an adequate trial? *Archives of General Psychiatry* **41,** 238–45.

Quitkin, F.M., Rabkin, J.G., Ross, D., and Stewart, J.W. (1984*b*). Identification of true drug response to antidepressants. Use of pattern analysis. *Archives of General Psychiatry* **41,** 782–6.

Quitkin, F.M., Rifkin, A., and Klein, D.F. (1979). Monoamine oxidase inhibitors. A review of antidepressant effectiveness. *Archives of General Psychiatry* **36,** 749–60.

Raskin, A., and Crook, T.H. (1976). The endogenous-neurotic distinction as a predictor of response to antidepressant drugs. *Psychological Medicine* **6,** 59–70.

Rees, L., and Benaim, S. (1960). An evaluation of iproniazid (Marsilid) in the treatment of depression. *Journal of Mental Science* **106,** 193–202.

Rickels, K., Weise, C.C., Zal, H.M., Csanalosi, I., and Werblowsky, J. (1982). Lofepramine and imipramine in unipolar depressed outpatients. A placebo controlled study. *Acta Psychiatrica Scandinavica* **66,** 109–20.

Rickels, K., Feighner, J.P., and Smith, W.T. (1985). Alprazolam, amitriptyline, doxepin and placebo in the treatment of depression. *Archives of General Psychiatry* **42,** 134–41.

Risch, S.C., Huey, L.Y., and Janowksy, D.S. (1979*a*). Plasma levels of tricyclic antidepressants and clinical efficacy: review of the literature—Part I. *Journal of Clinical Psychiatry* **40,** 4–16.

Risch, S.C., Huey, L.Y., and Janowsky, D.S. (1979*b*). Plasma levels of tricyclic antidepressants and clinical efficacy: a review of the literature—Part II. *Journal of Clinical Psychiatry* **40,** 58–69.

Risch, S.C., Kalin, N.H., Janowksy, D.S., and Huey, L.Y. (1981). Indications and guidelines for plasma tricyclic antidepressant concentration monitoring. *Journal of Clinical Psychopharmacology* **1,** 59–63.

Robertson, M.M., and Trimble, M.R. (1982). Major tranquillisers used as antidepressants—a review. *Journal of Affective Disorders* **4,** 73–93.

Robertson, M.M., and Trimble, M.R. (1983). Depressive illness in patients with epilepsy: a review. *Epilepsia* **24** (Suppl. 2), S109–S116.

Robinson, D.S., Cooper, T.B., Ravaris, C.L., Ives, J.O., Nies, A., Bartlett, D., and Lamborn, K.R. (1979). Plasma tricylic drug levels in amitriptyline-treated depressed patients. *Psychopharmacology* **63,** 223–31.

Robinson, D.S., Nies, A., Ravaris, L., Ives, J.O., and Bartlett, D. (1978). Clinical pharmacology of phenelzine. *Archives of General Psychiatry* **35,** 629–35.

Rose, S. (1982). The relationship of acetylation phenotype to treatment with MAOIs: a review. *Journal of Clinical Psychopharmacology* **2,** 161–5.

Rudorfer, M.V., and Potter, W.Z. (1989). Antidepressants. A comparative review of the clinical pharmacology and therapeutic use of the 'newer' versus the 'older' drugs. *Drugs* **37,** 713–38.

Rush, J.A., Beck, A.T., Kovacs, M., Weissenburger, J., and Hollon, S.D. (1982). Comparison of the effects of cognitive therapy and pharmacotherapy on hopelessness and self-concept. *American Journal of Psychiatry* **139,** 862–6.

Schuckit, M.A., and Feighner, J.P. (1972). Safety of high-dose tricyclic antidepressant therapy. *American Journal of Psychiatry* **128,** 1456–9.

Segraves, R.T. (1989). Effects of psychotropic drugs on human erection and ejaculation. *Archives of General Psychiatry* **46,** 275–84.

Seppala, T., and Linnoila, M. (1983). Effects of zimeldine and other antidepressants on skilled performance: a comprehensive review. *Acta Psychiatrica Scandinavica* **68,** 135–40.

Settle, E.C., and Ayd, F.J. (1980). Trimipramine: twenty years worldwide clinical experience. *Journal of Clinical Psychiatry* **41,** 266–74.

Shawcross, C.R., and Tyrer, P. (1985). Influence of personality on response to monoamine oxidase inhibitors and tricyclic antidepressants. *Journal of Psychiatric Research* **19,** 557–62.

Simons, A.D., Murphy, G.E., Levine, J.L., and Wetzel, R.D. (1986). Cognitive therapy and pharmacotherapy for depression. Sustained improvement over one year. *Archives of General Psychiatry* **43,** 43–8.

Sommi, R.W., Crismon, M.L., and Bowden, C.L. (1987). Fluoxetine: a serotonin-specific, second-generation antidepressant. *Pharmacotherapy* **7,** 1–15.

Stahl, S.M., and Palazidou, L. (1986). The pharmacology of depression: studies of neurotransmitter receptors lead the search for biochemical lesions and new drug therapies. *Trends in Pharmacological Sciences.* **7,** 349–54.

Stavrakaki, C., and Vargo, B. (1986). The relationship of anxiety and depression: a review of the literature. *British Journal of Psychiatry* **149,** 7–16.

Stein, D., and Avni, J. (1988). Thyroid hormones in the treatment of affective disorders. *Acta Psychiatrica Scandinavica* **77,** 623–36.

Stern, S.L., Rush, A.J., and Mendels, J. (1980). Towards a rational pharmacotherapy of depression. *American Journal of Psychiatry* **137,** 545–52.

Stewart, J.W., Quitkin, F.M., Liebowitz, M.R., McGrath, P.J., Harrison, W.M., and Klein, D.F. (1983). Efficacy of desipramine in depressed outpatients. Response according to research diagnostic criteria diagnoses and severity of illness. *Archives of General Psychiatry* **40,** 202–7.

Stokes, P.E. (1987). DST update: the hypothalamic–pituitary–adrenocortical axis and affective illness. *Biological Psychiatry* **22,** 245–8.

Strickler, R.C., Borth, R., Cecutti, A., Cookson, B.A., Harper, J.A., Potvin, R., Riffel, P., Sorbara, V.J., and Woolever, C.A. (1977). The role of estrogen replacement in the climacteric syndrome. *Psychological Medicine* **7,** 631–9.

Sullivan, E.A., and Shulman, K.I. (1984). Diet and monoamine oxidase inhibitors: a re-examination. *Canadian Journal of Psychiatry* **29,** 707–11.

Task Force on the use of laboratory tests in psychiatry (1985). Tricyclic antidepressants—blood level measurements and clinical outcome: *American Journal of Psychiatry* **142,** 155–62.

Taylor, D.J.E., and Braithwaite, R.A. (1978). Cardiac effects of tricyclic antidepressant medication. A preliminary study of nortriptyline. *British Heart Journal* **40,** 1005–8.

Telch, M.J., Tearnan, B.H., and Taylor, C.B. (1983). Antidepressant medication in the treatment of agoraphobia: a critical review. *Behaviour Research and Therapy* **21,** 505–17.

Thompson, P.J., and Trimble, M.R. (1982). Non-MAOI antidepressant drugs and cognitive functions: a review. *Psychological Medicine* **12,** 539–48.

Thomson, J., Rankin, H., Ashcroft, G.W., Yates, C.M., McQueen, J.K., and

Cummings, S.W. (1982). The treatment of depression in general practice: a comparison of L-tryptophan, amitriptyline, and a combination of L-tryptophan and amitryptyline with placebo. *Psychological Medicine* **12,** 741–51.

Tollefson, G.D. (1983). Monoamine oxidase inhibitors: a review. *Journal of Clinical Psychiatry* **44,** 280–8.

Tyrer, P. (1976). Towards rational therapy with monoamine oxidase inhibitors. *British Journal of Psychiatry* **128,** 354–60.

Tyrer, P. (1979). Clinical use of monoamine oxidase inhibitors. In *Psychopharmacology of affective disorders* (eds. E.S. Paykel and A. Coppen) pp. 159–78. Oxford University Press, Oxford.

Tyrer, P. (1984). Clinical effects of abrupt withdrawal from tricyclic antidepressants and monoamine oxidase inhibitors after long-term treatment. *Journal of Affective Disorders* **6,** 1–7.

Tyrer, P., Candy, J., and Kelly, D. (1973). Phenelzine in phobic anxiety: a controlled trial. *Psychological Medicine* **3,** 120–4.

Tyrer, P., Gardner, M., Lambourn, J., and Whitford, M. (1980). Clinical and pharmacokinetic factors affecting response to phenelzine. *British Journal of Psychiatry* **136,** 359–65.

Vandel, S., Vandel, B., Sandoz, M., Allers, G., Bechtel, P., and Volmat, R. (1978). Clinical response and plasma concentration of amitriptyline and its metabolite nortriptyline. *European Journal of Clinical Pharmacology* **14,** 185–90.

van Praag, H.M. (1981a). Management of depression with serotonin precursors. *Biological Psychiatry* **16,** 291–310.

van Praag, H.M. (1981*b*). Central monoamines and the pathogenesis of depression. In *Handbook of biological psychiatry*, Part IV. (eds. H.M. van Praag, M.H. Lader, O.J. Rafaelsen, and E.J. Sachar) pp. 159–205. Marcel Dekker, New York.

Walinder, J., Skott, A., Carlsson, A., Nagy, A., and Roos, B. (1976). Potentiation of the antidepressant action of clomipramine by tryptophan. *Archives of General Psychiatry* **33,** 1384–9.

Warnock, J.K., and Knesevich, J.W. (1988). Adverse cutaneous reactions to antidepressants. *American Journal of Psychiatry* **145,** 425–30.

West, E.D., and Dally, P.J. (1959). Effects of iproniazid in depressive syndromes. *British Medical Journal* **1,** 1491–2.

White, K., and Simpson, G. (1981). Combined MAOI-tricyclic antidepressant treatment: a reevaluation. *Journal of Clinical Psychopharmacology* **1,** 264–82.

White, K., and Simpson, G. (1984). The combined use of MAOIs and tricyclics. *Journal of Clinical Psychiatry* **45** (Sec. 2), 67–9.

Williams, J.M.G. (1984). Cognitive-behaviour therapy for depression: problems and perspectives. *British Journal of Psychiatry* **145,** 254–62.

Winokur, A., and Rickels, A. (1981). Combination of drugs and psychotherapy in the treatment of psychiatric disorders. In *Handbook of biological psychiatry*, Part VI. (eds. H.M. van Praag, M.H. Lader, O.J. Rafaelsen, and E.J. Sachar.) pp. 181–13. Marcel Dekker, New York.

Wittenborn, J.R., Plante, M., Burgess, F., and Livermore, N. (1961). The efficacy of electroconvulsive therapy, iproniazid and placebo in the treatment of young depressed women. *Journal of Nervous and Mental Disease* **133,** 316–32.

Young, J.P.R., Lader, M.H., and Hughes, W.C. (1979). Controlled trial of trimipramine, monoamine oxidase inhibitors, and combined treatment in depressed outpatients. *British Medical Journal* **2,** 1315–17.

Zeller, E.A., and Barsky, J. (1952). In vivo inhibition of liver and brain monoamine oxidase by 1-isonicotinyl-2-isopropyl-hydrazine. *Proceedings of the Society for Experimental Biology and Medicine* **81,** 459–61.

Zisook, S. (1985). A clinical overview of monoamine oxidase inhibitors. *Psychosomatics* **26,** 240–51.

10. Manic-depressive illness and lithium

Lithium salts provide one of the most fascinating stories in psychopharmacology and psychiatric treatment. The therapeutic effects of lithium in mania were reported by John Cade in 1949, so pride of place in the modern pantheon of psychotropic drugs must go to this substance. Yet it was 20 years before lithium was licensed in the USA, and only in the 1970s was it the subject of widespread study (Goodwin 1979). Not surprisingly, our knowledge of its properties and effects, wanted and unwanted, is still incomplete, although it has become firmly established on the therapeutic scene. Its main indications remain mania and depression, in their more severe forms.

Manic-depressive illness

The features of depression were discussed in Chapter 9, and cover a variety of features and a range of severity. Kraepelin coined the term 'manic-depressive' psychosis and distinguished it from dementia praecox. In doing so he incorporated a variety of affective illnesses including mania, melancholia, and circular and periodic psychoses. The classification of depression has long been a controversial topic but the natural history, genetic, and family factors, and to some extent response to treatment, have led more recently to a classification in terms of unipolar and bipolar conditions (Silverstone and Cookson 1982). In the former the episodes of illness are solely depressive in nature, in the latter both depression and mania occur at different times. Conditions characterized by manic episodes alone are generally considered bipolar in nature at least from the viewpoint of research. Of course, allocation of a patient to the unipolar category is always subject to revision. Even middle-aged patients with previous episodes all depressive in nature can develop manic attacks, necessitating recategorization.

Features of mania

The mood is euphoric in hypomania and elated in mania. Occasionally, states of ecstasy occur but are more typical of schizophrenia and epileptic psychoses. The patient is jovial, sparkling, benign and happy but anger, irritability, and depression rapidly supervene. Thus, the mood is labile especially if the patient is thwarted. On careful examination the elated mood is sensed to have no depth to it.

The manic patient is excessively satisfied with himself, his achievements and circumstances. He claims he has never felt better and loses insight into his morbid state of abnormal well-being. Talk is rapid and often staccato with flight of ideas where associations are determined superficially by the sound of words, by puns, rhymes and paradoxes and not by the intrinsic meaning. The direction of the flow of words constantly changes and the observer cannot get a word in edgeways. The content is often witty, risque, or even salacious and overt sexual advances may be a problem. Biting but penetrating comments on others may be made. Attention is distractible and concentration is poor and any external stimulus may set off a new train of ideas. The patient is restless and overactive: grandiose schemes are prepared but never executed. All is done to excess: talking, writing, singing. Dress may become extravagant, excessively decorative with baubles hanging everywhere. Women use excessive make-up, usually of garish colours. Money is no object; manic patents may squander and fritter away a lifetime's savings in a few weeks.

Good humour and generosity abound, but in more severe cases irritability and a paranoid state may make the patient very unpleasant to his family, relatives, and friends. Then, attempts to thwart his grandiose money-wasting schemes can provoke hostility and aggressive outbursts. Insomnia is an early symptom which intensifies as the patient worsens; typically the patient stays up late and gets up early to attend to his numerous activities. Physical movement increases with restlessness, overactivity, bursts of aimless scurrying and even agitation as competing plans bemuse the patient. In severe mania, the patient becomes self-neglectful, does not wash, sleep, or eat, and may die from exhaustion (Derby 1933). Frankly psychotic features include delusions of grandeur, exhortatory and congratulatory voices as auditory hallucinations, disorganized and incoherent speech, and grossly paranoid ideas and behaviour. Sexual promiscuity may become extreme, perverted, and violent.

Manic attacks usually develop quickly after a few days of restlessness and irritability. Sometimes, the attack is ushered with a depressive swing or the mania rapidly switches over into severe depression. Broken sleep is a common harbinger of an attack and may warn relatives of an impending recurrence of mania.

Hypomania is a milder form of mania. In other patients or at other times, mania and depression coexist, with rapid mood swings, the patient laughing one minute, weeping the next. Such mixed affective psychoses emphasize the close relationship of mania and depression, with the implication that the term 'bipolar' sets the two conditions in misleading antithesis. Also, as with depression, some patients with recurrent hypomania have their attacks provoked by environmental events, both favourable and unfavourable.

The natural history of manic-depressive psychosis varies from patient to patient. Some have one or two hypomanic episodes and are then free from illness but more typically attacks of both mania and depression occur, the periods of normality becoming shorter with the passage of time. Periodic psychoses with regular affective episodes are rare but such patients can continue cycling for years. The earlier the first episode, especially of mania, the worse the long-term outlook.

Lithium

Historical introduction

Lithium salts were used in the nineteenth century in the treatment of various ailments including gout and mental afflictions. The medication was available as 'Lithia' tablets but was found to produce cardiac toxicity. Lithium salts were reintroduced in the 1940s as a taste substitute for sodium chloride in patients with cardiovascular disease maintained on a salt-free diet. Their use was discontinued following several instances of severe side-effects and a few fatalities.

About this time, John Cade in Australia speculated that mania might be related to an excess of a normal body substance (Cade 1970). He injected the urine of manic patients into guinea pigs who convulsed and then died. The urine of some manic patients seemed more toxic than normal samples, the toxic agent being urea. However, urea concentrations were similar in manic and normal subjects so another factor was involved. Creatinine protected guinea pigs against urea-induced convulsions. But creatinine concentrations were also similar in patients and controls. Next, Cade found that uric acid potentiated urea toxicity. He pretreated animals with lithium urate, the most soluble salt and noted that the animals were unexpectedly sedated. Cade then established that the sedative effect was due to lithium ions. He administered lithium to himself and then to ten manic patients, all of whom responded (Cade 1949).

However, the toxicity of lithium also became established about this time and the use of the drug in psychiatry languished. The credit for verifying the use of lithium in mania and for establishing it as a prophylactic for the prevention of manic and depressive episodes goes to the Danish investigator, Mogens Schou (Schou *et al.* 1954). He has devoted his professional lifetime to this task. Lithium is now established as a therapeutic and preventative agent, with toxicity which is undeniable but which is acceptable providing treatment is carefully supervised.

More recently, the indications for lithium have been widened but many of these claims still await confirmation. Also, fears concerning long-term renal toxicity have been raised but, again, in moderate dosage, lithium is on balance beneficial.

Pharmacokinetics

Ingested lithium is well-absorbed from the gut, less than 1 per cent being detectable in the faeces. Sustained release preparations have become standard medication and have the advantage of smoothing out the peaks in the bodily levels of lithium. However, such preparations vary in their ability to yield smooth serum concentration absorption curves so each one must be evaluated on its merits (Caldwell *et al.* 1971).

Distribution into body tissues is fairly slow, particularly to the brain where peak lithium concentrations (in rats) are not attained until about 24 h after intravenous administration. In humans, lithium is not uniformly distributed thoughout the brain but tends to concentrate in certain areas such as the pons.

Serum concentrations decrease biphasically, a steep fall over the first 6 h or so being followed by a slower rate of elimination over the next 24 h. Lithium is not bound to plasma protein. It is almost entirely excreted by the kidneys where it reaches local concentrations much higher than in the plasma. About half of an administered dose is cleared in 24 h. Elimination may slow with prolonged use (Goodnick *et al.* 1981). Lithium excretion is closely related to sodium balance in the body. Thus, if sodium intake is lowered, for example, with a salt-restricted or faddy diet, lithium excretion is reduced and toxicity may supervene. Thiazide diuretics increase sodium excretion without affecting lithium elimination and can also lead to lithium toxicity if the lithium dosage is not reduced.

Serum lithium estimation

Toxic concentrations of lithium are not much greater than therapeutic concentrations, i.e. the therapeutic index is low. Accordingly, serum concentrations must be monitored frequently when treatment is started, dosage altered, the preparation changed or the patient develops a physical illness especially one affecting the gut or the kidney. A typical schedule is to take samples on the 7th, 4th, 21st, and 28th day of treatment and at intervals of 3–6 weeks thereafter or even less frequently in trustworthy, stabilized patients. The usual range aimed at for prophylaxis is 0.7–1.3 mmol/litre, although many advocate lower levels if possible. There seems no therapeutic advantage in exceeding 1.5 mmol/litre and toxicity generally occurs at levels over 2 mmol/litre.

Lithium estimations should complement clinical observation and not form a blind substitute. Thus, some patients are helped and their frequency of affective episodes substantially reduced despite lithium concentrations below 0.5 mmol/litre; others show signs of incipient toxicity with concentrations hardly exceeding 1 mmol/litre. Concentrations tend to be higher in patients receiving lithium in the treatment of hypomania and mania than in patients on long-term prophylactic lithium.

Nevertheless, high concentrations should be heeded seriously. Patients should not be kept on unnecessarily high levels and, in view of the disquiet concerning long-term toxicity, many practitioners are trying to minimize the dosage used, compatible with a continuing therapeutic effect (Vestergaard and Thomsen 1981; Hwang and Tuason 1980; Vestergaard *et al.* 1979). Levels of 0.6 mmol/litre or even less seem quite effective in most patients and it may be that the time-honoured target of 1 mmol/litre was too high, at least in the prevention of affective episodes.

The blood sample must be taken at a standardized time. This should be just before the dose after the longest inter-dose interval during the 24 h, i.e. generally just prior to the morning dose. This comprises the 'basal level'. Peak levels may be much higher.

The regular, albeit infrequent, estimation of serum concentrations will do little to avoid acute lithium toxicity but the procedure reminds the patient that he is taking an active preparation with powerful and potentially dangerous effects and that interest is being maintained in his welfare and in his taking of the medication. Infrequent estimations will detect the patient whose lithium levels are edging up insidiously. Routine estimations also detect the patient who has stopped his medication or lowered the dosage of his own accord and has determined not to tell his doctor. To this end, many hospitals run 'lithium clinics' where patients receive long term supervision and support.

Biochemical pharmacology

Lithium is a monovalent cation, number 3 in the periodic table and the lightest of all the alkali metals. It competes with sodium and potassium for enzyme sites and also displaces calcium and magnesium. It is thus hardly surprising that its pharmacology is exceedingly complex. Unlike the other cations, lithium is fairly equally distributed between intra and extracellular body compartments. Lithium is transported into the cell as efficiently as sodium but it is pumped out only slowly by the sodium pump. Chronic lithium administration is associated with reduced sodium concentration in various parts of the brain but it does not alter potassium distribution. Inorganic phosphate in muscle and liver is increased but that in bone is reduced. The uptake of magnesium and calcium is also reduced so the bone mineral content drops.

Acetylcholine synthesis and release is reduced by lithium but the most marked effect is an increase in noradrenalin turnover. Many other effects of lithium have been reported, such as increased platelet 5-HT uptake and inhibition of release of 5-HT from platelets. More recently, effects on postsynaptic phosphoinositide metabolism have been described. It is quite unclear which effects are most germane to the clinical actions of lithium in lessening affective morbidity.

Lithium influences carbohydrate metabolism by releasing insulin and increasing transport of glucose and formation of muscle glycogen: this may underlie the weight gain seen in patients on chronic lithium therapy.

Human pharmacology

In normal subjects lithium is almost devoid of discernible activity, at least in short-term administration. Subjective well-being is a little decreased and some cognitive performance is impaired in subjects whose serum lithium concentration is maintained in the clinical range (Judd *et al.* 1977*a*,*b*). Memory functions, however, seem particularly affected and this parallels complaints of poor memory in some patients.

Therapeutic effects

At the present time lithium is used to treat manic and hypomanic patients and to prevent the attacks in patients with recurrent affective disorders—both manic and depressive episodes in bipolar patients, attacks of mania in the recurrent manic and depressive episodes in the unipolar patient (Schou 1986). The usefulness of lithium in schizoaffective states is less well established.

Other conditions for which lithium has been advocated include the acute treatment of depressive illness, epilepsy, aggressive disorder, schizophrenia, alcoholism, premenstrual tension, thyrotoxicosis, Huntington's chorea, and spasmodic torticollis. Although there are some controlled trials which lend support to these claims, e.g. in patients with aggressive impulses and outbursts, no firm consensus has yet emerged concerning their usefulness.

Treatment of mania and hypomania (Shaw 1979)

Cade reported on the effectiveness of lithium in ten manic patients and similar encouraging therapeutic effects were later reported in 29 out of 30 manic patients similarly treated. However, the advent of chlorpromazine and other phenothiazines, and later of haloperidol, attracted attention away from the antimanic effects of lithium. This, together with reports of lithium toxicity, led to a waning of interest in lithium until it was rekindled by the stoic efforts of Schou in Denmark. Even now, over 30 years on, some aspects of lithium usage and toxicity remain controversial (e.g. Dickson and Kendell 1986).

Uncontrolled trials indicate that about 80 per cent of manic patients respond adequately to lithium. There were few early controlled trials comparing lithium with placebo and some used inappropriate cross-over designs. Other trials have compared lithium with chlorpromazine although the efficacy of chlorpromazine for this indication has never been established in a series of formal clinical trials, only by clinical usage and consensus. Most trials were small-scale and failed to establish any difference between the treatments. One large-scale trial assigned 255 manic patients randomly to lithium or chlorpromazine for a three-week period (Prien, Caffey, and Klett 1972). On admission the patients were divided into highly active and mildly active groups. Chlorpromazine was significantly superior to lithium in the highly active patients mainly because more patients dropped out of the lithium group. Chlorpromazine controlled the disturbed behaviour within a few days whereas the therapeutic effects of lithium were often delayed until about the tenth day. Attempts to accelerate control by pushing lithium dosage to yield serum levels above 1.5 mmol/litre only resulted in toxic effects. In mildly ill patients chlorpromazine and lithium were equal in therapeutic effectiveness but lithium produced fewer side effects and left the patient feeling less sluggish and fatigued.

Haloperidol is regarded by many clinicians as the treatment of choice for mania, but comparisons with lithium have been few (Shopsin *et al.* 1975). Combinations of lithium with haloperidol are commonly used (Biederman *et al.* 1979), despite some reports of increased toxicity including a few deaths (Cohen and Cohen 1974). The antipsychotic medication provides effective and immediate control of symptoms while the effects of the lithium build up to the point when the antipsychotic drug can be withdrawn. Lithium has qualitative advantages in that it produces fewer and less severe side-effects and milder sedation than the antipsychotic drugs, and therefore has better patient acceptability.

Treatment of depression

Although the earliest reports suggested that lithium was ineffective in the treatment of acute depression, later reports were more optimistic (Mendels 1976, Noyes *et al.* 1974). One or two uncontrolled trials suggested that about half of depressed patients might respond but in view of the fluctuations in course and the trend towards natural remission in acute depressive illnesses, no firm conclusions were possible. Controlled trials recently concluded indicate that bipolar depressives respond best especially when somatic features are marked. However, in general, lithium is not as effective as the tricyclic antidepressants. The improvement following lithium often seems incomplete, but lithium is worth considering in the refractory depressive, even the unipolar (Doyal and Morton 1984). The combination of lithium and antidepressant remains to be properly evaluated but might possess some advantages over either component alone especially in more chronic or recurrent conditions (Lingjaerde *et al.* 1974).

Prevention of affective illnesses

The usefulness of chronic lithium administration in preventing manic and depressive episodes rather than treating them was established only after much controversy, mainly due to the early lack of controlled studies. The first claims of the prophylactic properties of lithium stemmed from longitudinal studies in which the frequency of attacks in patients maintained on lithium was compared with that in the same patients before treatment. In response to criticisms of this type of study, a different approach was used. Patients maintained satisfactorily on lithium were allocated randomly to either continuing on lithium or switching to placebo. Almost without exception, when numbers in the trial were adequate, lithium continuation was associated with fewer relapses than was placebo. Therefore, patients maintained on lithium with a few relapses do indeed derive benefit from the drug (Baastrup *et al.* 1970; Melia 1970; Hullin *et al.* 1972). However, it is probably not justified to institute prophylactic lithium treatment after just one manic episode (Mander 1986*a*).

The most rigorous type of trial, the controlled prospective evaluation, involves allocating patients randomly to treatment with lithium or placebo. Criteria for inclusion in the trial typically comprise two or more affective episodes requiring hospital attendance or admission within two years. In one study 65 patients were studied for up to 112 weeks. Patients receiving lithium had significantly less illness than those on placebo, as measured by such operational factors as admission to hospital or attendance in out-patients. The amount of additional medication was much less in lithium patients than in those on placebo: for example, none of the lithium patients but almost half of the placebo patients needed ECT. Lithium seemed as effective in patients with unipolar recurrent depression as in patients with manic-depressive disorders (Coppen *et al.* 1973).

Other trials have confirmed such findings (Prien *et al.* 1973; Fieve and Mendlewicz 1972; Stallone *et al.* 1973). Some have included a third group comprising patients maintained on a tricyclic antidepressant (Watanabe *et al.* 1975). This treatment is usually quite effective at preventing depressive attacks but does not lessen the frequency or attenuate the severity of manic episodes. Lithium attenuates both manic and depressive episodes, the former rather more effectively than the latter. Episodes which do occur in patients on lithium are typically much less severe than in untreated patients although the episodes last as long.

The effectiveness of lithium in preventing depressive episodes in unipolar depressives is now more clearly established (Editorial 1979). However, lithium does not seem superior to tricyclic antidepressants such as imipramine or amitriptyline (Fieve *et al.* 1975; MRC Drug Trial Subcommittee 1981; Glen *et al.* 1984). In the latter study involving over 100 patients, both lithium and amitriptyline/nortriptyline plasma concentrations were monitored and dosage manipulated to give optimal serum levels.

The importance of establishing whether lithium is effective in preventing relapses of depression in unipolar patients reflects the frequency of the condition: over 4 per cent of the population suffer from this ailment. Clearly, any drug advocated long-term in this condition must be carefully evaluated not only against placebo but against prophylactic tricyclic antidepressants (Freeman 1984). The superiority of lithium over other active medications is not established.

Bipolar patients with rapidly alternating cycles seem to do worse (Dunner and Fieve 1974). Some practitioners believe that the prophylactic effects of lithium wane in some patients but few published data support this view. Sometimes patients lose their motivation to continue taking lithium as the memory of their disturbed behaviour fades. The term 'prophylaxis' probably overstates the therapeutic effect (Pokorny and Prien 1974). Rather, the episodes are attenuated or aborted so that admission to hospital is avoided or mood swings are transient. This therapeutic effect may be delayed, taking months rather than weeks to become apparent.

Other conditions

Schizoaffective disorders are characterized by affective changes and symptoms more typical of schizophrenia. Both schizomanic and schizodepressive syndromes are seen. Schizoaffective disorders are easily confused with depressive syndromes occurring in schizophrenic patients. Provided the latter patients are excluded, schizoaffective patients have a better prognosis than more typical schizophrenics. Lithium has been shown in some trials to have a prophylactic effect but not in others. The contradictions probably reflect different diagnostic criteria in the selection of patients.

Lithium is not generally appropriate to the treatment of schizophrenia, tardive dyskinesia, cluster headaches, and organic brain syndromes.

The relationship between alcoholism and depression is complex and has led some clinicians to try lithium therapy in alcoholic patients (Kline *et al.* 1974). Some improvement in prognosis has been claimed but probably reflects control of concomitant or contributory depression as well as a direct effect on alcohol dependence itself (Merry *et al.* 1976; Fawcett *et al.* 1987).

Lithium has been used to lessen aggressive behaviour in prisoners. Such patients have episodes of recurrent violence with explosive outbursts in response to provocation. Controlled trials have confirmed a lessening of aggression in antisocial prisoners and also in mentally handicapped patients prone to temper tantrums and unprovoked aggression (Mattes 1986).

Some children and adolescents have been treated with lithium to control behaviour disorders. Reports of efficacy are almost all anecdotal, uncontrolled or lack sufficient information to evaluate properly (Jefferson 1982). It is difficult to identify potential responders.

Prediction of response

Lithium treatment of manic patients is unsuccessful in about a quarter of cases and between a third and half of patients maintained on lithium relapse in a 2-year period. In general, the more typical the manic-depressed patient, the more likely he is to respond to lithium. Pyknic body build is twice as common among responders as non-responders, but neither age, sex, nor marital status has much influence. Therapeutic response to lithium is associated with cyclothymic traits, non-response with withdrawn, anxious and obsessive personalities.

A history of schizoaffective or schizophrenic episodes suggests a worse response than purely affective episodes. Mania of late onset responds poorly. A high frequency of affective episodes, four or more per year in the 2–3 years prior to lithium treatment, is also an indicator of poor prognosis. A feature predictive of good response is the presence of a family history of manic-depressive illness (Ananth and Pecknold 1978).

Compliance is crucial (Van Putten 1975). Following the prescribed course of treatment is important, failures often following poor compliance and being predictive of future failures. Biological variables have been evaluated for their predictive potential. For example, lithium responders have lower pretreatment blood platelet MAO levels than those who do not respond.

In general, however, prediction must be based on a total assessment of the patient (Petursson 1979), hopes being highest in those with typical recurrent manic-depressive illnesses. While the mode of action of lithium remains obscure, little progress will be made to establish predictive variables other than on an empirical clinical basis.

Unwanted effects (Table 10.1)

Short-term effects

Many patients become nauseated, often associated with loose bowel movements. These symptoms are usually harmless and more of a nuisance than a hindrance to treatment; they wane in 2–6 weeks. A large proportion

Table 10.1. Unwanted effects of lithium therapy.

Type	Effect	Action
Transitory, usually initial. Remedial action unnecessary.	Metallic taste in mouth nausea, diarrhoea or constipation, weight gain, dry mouth and thirst.	Reassure
Harmless, persistent during treatment, reversible, Remedial action unnecessary. Reassure and continue therapy.	leukocytosis granulocytosis ECG changes EEG changes	Reassure
Possibly requiring corrective action	tremor	check blood levels; try reducing dosage try propranolol 10 mg three/four times/day
	hypothyroidism	repeat test because low value may be transient; if TSH level persistently raised, give thyroxin 50 mg once or twice daily
	persistent polyuria and polydipsia	check blood levels; reduce dosage
Long-term, probably related	chronic renal toxicity severe polyuria (3.5 litres/24 h)	reduce dosage; dose-consider discontinuation.

of patients complain of fine tremor of the fingers, an exaggeration of normal physiological tremor. It can be a major problem in patients whose work involves delicate manual manipulations. This symptom tends to persist throughout treatment but often responds to a slight reduction in dosage. Propranolol has been used to counteract the lithium-induced tremor but with scant success. Another persistent unwanted effect is polyuria which is dose-dependent. It is due to blockade of the action of antidiuretic hormone in the kidney. Nocturnal polyuria is the most distressing component, the patient often having to rise several times during the night. Some patients tend to slake their thirst with calorie-rich fluids and become obese.

Long-term effects (Vestergaard 1983)

The tremor and polyuria tend to persist and weight gain may be a problem (Vendsborg *et al.* 1976). Another long-term effect is benign goitre, usually with depression of thyroid activity. This is probably due to lithium interfering with the uptake of iodine by the thyroid gland. Routine tests of thyroid function are not useful because the drop in thyroid function is usually sudden. Occasionally, frank hypothyroidism supervenes and may be irreversible, replacement therapy being needed (Lindstedt *et al.* 1977).

Other symptoms complained of by patients include poor memory (Ananth *et al.* 1987), indigestion, generalized aches and pains, and slurred speech. Skin reactions include maculopapular, acneiform and follicular eruptions and exacerbation of psoriasis (Deandrea *et al.* 1982).

Long-term adverse effects on the kidney have been described. In the initial reports, interstitital fibrosis, tubular atrophy, and glomerular sclerosis were found in renal biopsy specimens from patients with acute lithium poisoning or severe lithium-induced polyuria (Hwang and Tuason 1980; Walker *et al.* 1981). These findings have been confirmed but in patients without polyuria or toxicity. Some studies have suggested that the changes are related to the duration of lithium therapy whereas others have not confirmed this (Hansen 1981). The early changes seem to consist of tubular fibrosis followed by focal nephron atrophy with sclerotic glomeruli and atrophic tubules. The practical significance of these changes is not clear and a further problem is that renal function is not usually impaired so detection is difficult (Coppen *et al.* 1980; Hullin *et al.* 1979; Vestergaard and Amdisen 1981). Constant review of the need for lithium and the establishment of a minimal dosage are essential. Otherwise, reduced renal function may eventually become a problem in an increasing number of patients (Bendz 1983), perhaps especially in those taking antipsychotic medication concomitantly (Gelenberg *et al.* 1987).

Nephrogenic diabetes insipidus may occur on long-term treatment and be irreversible. Lithium is not advised during pregnancy, especially the first trimester, but may be unavoidable (see p. 381). Lactating mothers should stop breast-feeding their babies if lithium is instituted. Lithium may potentiate some muscle relaxants, so the anaesthetist should take this into account when giving an anaesthetic, e.g. for ECT.

Toxic symptoms

Diarrhoea, vomiting, increased tremor, dysarthria, weakness especially of the lower jaw, drowsiness, and ataxia are all signs that the safe dose limit is being exceeded. More severe effects include coarse tremor, twitching, fasciculations in limbs, hands and face, drowsiness, impaired concentration, unsteadiness, loss of memory, mild disorientation, and dizziness. Finally, restlessness, confusion, nystagmus, fits, and delirium herald coma and eventually death. Urine flow may fail, aggravating the condition.

Treatment of toxicity

In milder cases, the lithium should be stopped for a few days, with serum level monitoring, and when appropriate reinstituted at a lower dose level.

Factors leading to the toxicity should be sought, physical illness, especially in the elderly, often being present.

In more serious cases, fluids containing sodium (e.g. milk) should be given to accelerate the excretion of lithium. In patients with serum lithium concentrations above 2 mmol/litre, admission is advisable. In cases where the patient is seriously ill with levels over 3–4 mmol/litre, intensive care is necessary with saline infusions, or dialysis if the kidneys are becoming oliguric.

Drug interactions

The side-effects of muscular tremor and rigidity caused by antipsychotic drugs can be enhanced by concomitant lithium therapy. No specifically dangerous properties can be ascribed to the haloperidol–lithium interaction. Sodium-depleting diuretics interact adversely with lithium and must be avoided. The practical clinical importance of interactions of lithium with neuromuscular blocking agents, phenytoin, carbamazepine and methyldopa is only weakly supported by data but in cases of doubt the lithium should be reduced or discontinued (Amdisen 1982; Jefferson *et al* 1981).

Use of lithium

Most contraindications to the use of lithium are relative rather than absolute and include chronic renal failure, hypertension, and previous myocardial infarction. Active renal disease is probably the nearest condition to an absolute contraindication. A physical examination is essential before instituting therapy. Renal function tests such as creatinine clearance or urinary concentration and dilution tests are usual, and are mandatory in any patient with a history of renal disease. Similarly, thyroid function, and ECG and electrolyte tests should be carried out routinely. A lithium clearance is useful in establishing the probable dosage (Srinivasan and Hullin 1980). In any patient with physical illness, the initial dosage of lithium should be very conservative, increase in dosage should be gradual, and serum level monitoring must be thorough.

Sustained release preparations are generally preferred, toxicity being somewhat less than with regular preparations. Dosage every 12 h is optimal if the patient can tolerate the dose; less frequent dosing schedules are associated with sustained high levels after each dose, more side effects and more frequent dosing with poorer compliance. However, constant high levels of lithium may increase the possibility of renal toxicity (Plenge *et al*. 1982). For mania 1000–2000 mg a day of lithium carbonate (or equivalent) is usually required. In the maintenance therapy of recurrent affective disorders, the typical daily dose for a fit adult is about 1000 mg. Dosage adjustment must be prompt, so adequate and rapid monitoring facilities are essential.

It is preferable to institute maintenance therapy when the patient is not acutely ill so that he can co-operate fully in starting the medication and in its continuation. Special lithium clinics are often advantageous in managing patients on long-term therapy (Fieve 1975; 1981). The patient needs to be convinced of the value of the therapy, often regretting the mild, if not the severe, hypomanic episodes which previously added zest to life and are now diluted. Attending a clinic with other patients lifts morale, encourages compliance, and provides some group therapy. The staff are trained to detect early signs of relapse and of incipient toxicity; prompt intervention reassures the patient. Careful records can show when the treatment is successful and best discontinued. The monitoring of serum levels indicates to the patient that there is some rationale in the treatment, and spots the treatment defaulter.

Criteria for starting prophylactic treatment vary from practitioner to practitioner; the most conservative would require repeated episodes of mania with or without depression, say three in a year; the most enthusiastic lithium users would advocate its use after just one definite affective illness. The general consensus is that lithium should be considered after two illnesses in two years or three in three years.

There is no consensus concerning the length of time prophylactic treatment should be continued. Some practitioners advocate a fixed period of time, even as short as a year, before trying withdrawal. Others suggest indefinite medication. The best compromise is to consider lithium as a finite therapy, to review each patient in detail at least once a year and to try withdrawal on a tentative basis when either the complications seem to outweigh the benefits or the patient has remained totally well for so long that a natural remission seems likely to have occurred. Lithium does not improve the long-term prognosis once the lithium is stopped (Mander 1986*b*).

Carbamazepine

This drug has been used for over 20 years in the treatment of epilepsy and trigeminal neuralgia. It is chemically related to imipramine and has recently been used to treat affective disorders, although not licensed for this indication (Woods 1986; Crawford and Silverstone 1987).

In mania, both uncontrolled and controlled studies suggest useful efficacy (Post *et al.* 1985; Okuma *et al.* 1979). In the prophylaxis of recurrent affective disorders, good results have been obtained (Post *et al.* 1985; Okuma 1984). In a recent double-blind controlled trial, carbamazepine was compared to lithium (Watkins *et al.* 1987). Both drugs were effective: whereas lithium doubled the mean time in remission, carbamazepine only increased it by 50 per cent. In another trial, carbamazepine and lithium were equi-effective (Placidi *et al.* 1986).

Other conditions in which carbamazepine has been tried include patients with schizoaffective disorder, chronic schizophrenia and aggressive schizophrenia: results are encouraging (Okuma *et al.* 1989).

Unwanted effects of carbamazepine include dizziness, drowsiness, diplopia and nausea; drug interactions are common (Israel and Beaudry 1988). To minimize unwanted effects, treatment should be started at 400 mg/day in divided doses; the usual maintenance dosage is in the range of 600–1000 mg/day.

Thus, carbamazepine has a place in the management of patients with affective disorder who are resistant to or intolerant of more conventional treatments. Nevertheless, like lithium, the drug requires close monitoring.

References

Amdisen, A. (1982). Lithium and drug interactions. *Drugs* **24,** 133–9.

Ananth, J., Ghadirian, A.M., and Engelsmann, F. (1987). Lithium and memory: a review. *Canadian Journal of Psychiatry* **32,** 312–16.

Ananth, J., and Pecknold, J.C. (1978). Prediction of lithium response in affective disorders. *Journal of Clinical Psychiatry* **39,** 95–100.

Baastrup, P.C., Paulsen, J.C, Schou, M., *et al.* (1970). Prophylactic lithium. Double-blind discontinuation in manic depressive and recurrent depressive disorders. *Lancet* **ii,** 325–30.

Bendz, H. (1983). Kidney function in lithium-treated ipatients. *Acta Psychiatrica Scandinavica* **68,** 303–24.

Biederman, J., Lerner, Y., and Belmaker, R.H. (1979). Combination of lithium carbonate and haloperidol in schizo-affective disorder. *Archives of General Psychiatry* **36,** 327–33.

Cade, J. F. (1949). Lithium salts in the treatment of psychotic excitement. *Medical Journal of Australia* **2,** 349–52.

Cade, J.F.J. (1970). The story of lithium. In *Discoveries in biological psychiatry* (eds. F.J. Ayd and B. Blackwell) pp. 218–19. Lippincott, Philadelphia.

Caldwell, H.C., Westlake, W.J., Conner, S.M., and Flanagan, T. (1971). A pharmacokinetic analysis of lithium carbonate absorption from several formulations in man. *Journal of Clinical Pharmacology* **11,** 349–56.

Cohen, J., and Cohen, H. (1974). Lithium carbonate, haloperidol, and irreversible brain damage. *Journal of the American Medical Association* **230,** 1283–7.

Coppen, A., Peet, M., and Bailey, J. (1973). The effect of long-term lithium treatment on the morbidity of affective disorders. Internal report. *Medical Research Council Neuropsychiatry Unit*, Epsom, Surrey.

Coppen, A., Bishop, M.E., Bailey, J.E., Cattell, W.R., and Price, R.G. (1980). Renal function with lithium and non-lithium treated patients with affective disorders. *Acta Psychiatrica Scandinavica* **62,** 343–55.

Crawford, R., and Silverstone, T. (eds.) (1987). Carbamazepine in affective disorder. *International Clinical Psychopharmacology* **2,** Suppl. 1.

Deandrea, D., Walker, N., Mehlmauer, M., and White, K. (1982). Dermatological reactions to lithium: a critical review of the literature. *Journal of Clinical Psychopharmacology* **2,** 199–204.

Derby, I.M. (1933). Manic-depressive 'exhaustion' deaths. *Psychiatric Quarterly* **7,** 436–49.

Dickson, W.E., and Kendell, R.E. (1986). Does maintenance lithium therapy prevent recurrences of mania under ordinary clinical conditions? *Psychological Medicine* **16,** 521–30.

Doyal, L.E., and Morton, W.A. (1984). The clinical usefulness of lithium as an antidepressant. *Hospital and Community Psychiatry* **35,** 685–91.

Dubovsky, S.L., Franks, R.D., and Allen, S. (1987). Verapamil: A new antimanic drug with potential interactions with lithium. *Journal of Clinical Psychiatry* **48,** 371–2.

Dunner, D.L., and Fieve, R.R. (1974). Clinical factors in lithium carbonate prophylaxis failure. *Archives of General Psychiatry* **30,** 229–33.

Editorial. (1979). America salutes lithium. *Lancet* **ii,** 1168.

Fawcett, J., Clark, D.C., Aagesen, C.A., Pisani, V.D., Tilkin, J.M., Sellers, D., McGuire, M., and Gibbons, R.D. (1987). A double-blind, placebo-controlled trial of lithium carbonate therapy for alcoholism. *Archives of General Psychiatry* **44,** 248–56.

Fieve, R. (1975). The lithium clinic: a new model for the delivery of psychiatric services. *American Journal of Psychiatry* **132,** 1018–22.

Fieve, R.R. (1981). Lithium affective disorder clinics. In *Handbook of biological psychiatry* (eds. H.M. van Praag, M.H. Lader, O.J. Rafaelsen, and E.J. Sachar) Part VI, pp. 135–48. Marcel Dekker, New York.

Fieve, R.R., and Mendlewicz, J. (1972). Lithium prophylaxis in bipolar manic-depressive illness. *Psychopharmacology Abstracts* **26,** 93.

Fieve, R.R., Dunner, D.L., Kumbarachi, T., and Stallone, F. (1975). Lithium carbonate in affective disorders. IV. A double-blind study of prophylaxis in unipolar recurrent depression. *Archives of General Psychiatry* **32,** 1541–4.

Freeman, C.P. (1984). Prophylaxis against unipolar depression. *British Medical Journal* **289,** 512–14.

Gelenberg, A.J., Wojcik, J.D., Falk, W.E., Coggins, C.H., Brotman, A.W., Rosenbaum, J.F., LaBrie, R.A., and Kerman, B.J. (1987). Effects of lithium on the kidney. *Acta Psychiatrica Scandinavica* **75,** 29–34.

Glen, A.I.M., Johnson, A.L., and Shepherd, M. (1984). Continuation therapy with lithium and amitriptyline in unipolar depressive illness: a randomized, double-blind, controlled trial. *Psychological Medicine* **14,** 37–50.

Goodnick, P.J., Fieve, R.R., Meltzer, H.L., and Dunner, D.L. (1981). Lithium elimination half-life and duration of therapy. *Clinical Pharmacology and Therapeutics* **29,** 47–50.

Goodwin, F.K. (ed.) (1979). The lithium ion—impact on treatment and research. *Archives of General Psychiatry* **36,** 833–4.

Hansen, J.E. (1981). Renal toxicity of lithium. *Drugs* **22,** 461–76.

Hullin, R.P., MacDonald, R., and Allsop, M.N.E. (1972). Prophylactic lithium in recurrent affective disorders. *Lancet* **ii,** 1044–7.

Hullin, R.P., Coley, V.P., Birch, N.J., Thomas, T.H., and Morgan, D.B. (1979). Renal function after long-term treatment with lithium. *British Medical Journal* **1,** 1457–9.

Hwang, S., and Tuason, V.B. (1980). Long-term maintenance lithium therapy and possible irreversible renal damage. *Journal of Clinical Psychiatry* **41,** 11–9.

Israel, M., and Beaudry, P. (1988). Carbamazepine in psychiatry : a review. *Canadian Journal of Psychiatry* **33,** 577–84.

Jefferson, J.W. (1982). The use of lithium in childhood and adolescence: an overview. *Journal of Clinical Psychiatry* **43,** 174–7.

Jefferson, J.W., Greist, J.H., and Baudhuin, M. (1981). Lithium: interactions with other drugs. *Journal of Clinical Psychopharmacology* **1,** 124–34.

Judd, L.L., Hubbard, B., Janowsky, D.S., Huey, L.Y., and Attewell, P.A. (1977*a*). The effect of lithium carbonate on affect, mood, and personality of normal subjects. *Archives of General Psychiatry* **34,** 346–51.

Judd, L.L., Hubbard, B., Janowsky, D.S., Huey, L.Y., and Takahashi, K.I. (1977*b*). The effect of lithium carbonate on the cognitive functions of normal subjects. *Archives of General Psychiatry* **34,** 355–7.

Kline, N.S., Wren, J.C., and Cooper, T.B. (1974). Evaluation of lithium therapy in chronic and periodic alcoholism. *American Journal of the Medical Sciences* **268,** 15–22.

Lindstedt, G. *et al.* (1977). The prevalence, diagnosis and management of lithium-induced hypothyroidism in psychiatric patients. *British Journal of Psychiatry* **130,** 452–8.

Lingjaerde, O. *et al.* (1974). The effect of lithium carbonate in combination with tricyclic antidepressants in endogenous depression. A double-blind, multicenter trial. *Acta Psychiatrica Scandinavica* **50,** 233–42.

Mander, A.J. (1986*a*). Is lithium justified after one manic episode? *Acta Psychiatrica Scandinavica* **73,** 60–7.

Mander, A.J. (1986*b*). Is there a lithium withdrawal syndrome? *British Journal of Psychiatry* **149,** 498–501.

Mattes, J.A. (1986). Psychopharmacology of temper outbursts. A review. *Journal of Nervous and Mental Disease* **174,** 464–470.

Melia, P.I. (1970). Prophylactic lithium. A double-blind trial in recurrent affective disorders. *British Journal of Psychiatry* **116,** 621–4.

Mendels, J. (1976). Lithium in the treatment of depression. *American Journal of Psychiatry* **133,** 373–8.

Merry, J., Reynolds, M., Bailey, J., and Coppen, A. (1976). Prophylactic treatment of alcoholism by lithium carbonate. A controlled study. *Lancet* **2,** 481–2.

MRC Drug Trial Subcommittee. (1981). Preliminary report. Continuation therapy with lithium and amitriptyline in unipolar depressive illness: A controlled clinical trial. *Psychological Medicine* **11,** 409–16.

Noyes, R., Dempsey, G., Blum, A., and Cavanaugh, G.L. (1974). Lithium treatment of depression. *Comprehensive Psychiatry* **15,** 187–93.

Okuma, T. (1984). In *Anticonvulsants in affective disorders.* (eds. H.M. Emrich *et al.*) Elsevier, Sweden.

Okuma, T., Inananga, K., Otsuki, S., Sarai, K., Takahashi, R., Hazama, H., Mori, A., and Watanabe, M. (1979). Comparison of the antimanic efficacy of carbamazepine and chlorpromazine: a double-blind controlled study. *Psychopharmacology* **66,** 211–17.

Okuma, T., Yamashita, I., Takahashi, R., Itoh, H., Kurihara, M., Otsuki, S., Watanabe, S., Sarai, K., Hazama, H., and Inanaga, K. (1989). Clinical efficacy of carbamazepine in affective, schizoaffective and schizophrenic disorders. *Pharmacopsychiatry* **22,** 47–53.

Petursson, H. (1979). Prediction of lithium response. *Comprehensive Psychiatry* **20,** 226–41.

Placidi, G.F., Lenzi, A., Lazzerini, F. Cassano, G.B., and Akiskal, H.S. (1986). The comparative efficacy and safety of carbamazepine versus lithium: a randomized, double-blind 3-year trial in 83 patients. *Journal of Clinical Psychiatry* **47,** 490–4.

Plenge, P., Mellerup, E.T., Bolwig, T.G., Brun, C., Hetmar, O., Ladefoged, J., Larsen, S., and Rafaelsen, (1982). Lithium treatment: does the kidney prefer one daily dose instead of two? *Acta Psychiatrica Scandinavica* **66,** 121–8.

Pokorny, A.D., and Prien, R.F. (1974). Lithium in treatment and prevention of affective disorder. *Diseases of the Nervous System* **35,** 327–33.

Post, R.M., Uhde, T.W., Joffe, R.T., Roy-Byrne, P.P., and Kellner, C. (1985). In *The psychopharmacology of epilepsy*, pp. 141–71. John Wiley, Chichester.

Prien, R.F., Caffey, E.M., Jr., and Klett, C.J. (1972). Comparison of lithium carbonate and chlorpromazine in the treatment of mania. *Archives of General Psychiatry* **26,** 146–53.

Prien, R.F., Klett, C.J., and Caffey, E.M. (1973). Lithium carbonate and imipramine in prevention of affective episodes. *Archives of General Psychiatry* **29,** 420–5.

Schou, M. (1986). Lithium treatment: a refresher course. *British Journal of Psychiatry* **149,** 541–7.

Schou, M., Juel-Nielson, N., Stromgren, E., *et al.* (1954). The treatment of manic psychoses by the administration of lithium salts. *J. Neurology, Neurosurgery and Psychiatry* **17,** 250–60.

Shaw, D.M. (1979). Lithium and antimanic drugs: clinical usage and efficacy. In *Psychopharmacology of affective disorders* (eds. E.S. Paykel and A. Coppen) pp. 179–82. Oxford University Press, Oxford.

Shopsin, B., Gershon, S., Thompson, H., and Collins, P. (1975). Psychoactive drugs in mania. A controlled comparison of lithium carbonate, chlorpromazine, and haloperidol. *Archives of General Psychiatry* **32,** 34–42.

Silverstone, T., and Cookson, J. (1982). The biology of mania. In *Recent advances in clinical psychiatry* (ed. K. Granville-Grossman) Vol. 4, pp. 201–41.

Srinivasan, D.P., and Hullin, R.P. (1980). Current concepts of lithium therapy. *British Journal of Hospital Medicine* **24,** 466–70.

Stallone, F., Shelley, F., Mendlewicz, J., *et al.* (1973). The use of lithium in affective disorders. III. A double-blind study of prophylaxis in bipolar illness. *American Journal of Psychiatry* **130,** 1006–10.

Van Putten, T. (1975). Why do patients with manic-depressive illness stop their lithium? *Comprehensive Psychiatry* **16,** 179–83.

Vendsborg, P.B., Bech, P., and Rafaelsen, O.J. (1976). Lithium treatment and weight gain. *Acta Psychiatrica Scandinavica* **53,** 139–47.

Vestergaard, P. (1983). Clinically important side effects of long-term lithium treatment: a review. *Acta Psychiatrica Scandinavica* **67,** Suppl. 305.

Vestergaard, P., and Amdisen, A. (1981). Lithium treatment and kidney function. *Acta Psychiatrica Scandinavica* **63,** 333–45.

Vestergaard, P., and Thomsen, K. (1981). Renal side effects of lithium: the importance of the serum lithium level. *Psychopharmacology* **72,** 203–4.

Vestergaard, P., Amdisen, A., Hansen, H.E., and Schou, M. (1979). Lithium treatment and kidney function. A survey of 237 patients in long-term treatment. *Acta Psychiatrica Scandinavica* **60,** 504–20.

Walker, R.G., Davies, B., Holwill, B., and Kincaid-Smith, P. (1981). Lithium nephrotoxicity: is there cause for concern? *Drugs* **22,** 421–2.

Watanabe, S., Ishino, H., and Otsuki, S. (1975). Double-blind comparison of lithium carbonate and imipramine in treatment of depression. *Archives of General Psychiatry* **32,** 659–68.

Watkins, S.E., Callender, K., Thomas, D.R., Tidmarsh, S.F., and Shaw, D.M. (1987). The effect of carbamazepine and lithium on remission from affective illness. *British Journal of Psychiatry* **150,** 180–2.

Wood, A.J., and Goodwin, G.M. (1987). A review of the biochemical and neuropharmacological actions of lithium. *Psychological Medicine* **17,** 579–600.

Woods, M. (1986). Carbamazepine for bipolar disorder. *Drug Intelligence and Clinical Pharmacy* **20,** 49–52.

11. Psychoses and antipsychotic medication

Syndromes of psychosis

This topic encompasses a large part of psychiatric phenomenology and classification and a detailed account is inappropriate here. The basic division is into the organic psychoses and the functional psychoses, but antipsychotic medication is used to combat disturbed behaviour and psychotic symptoms in whatever context they arise. Thus, the acutely psychotic patient is given large doses of chlorpromazine, haloperidol, or a similar drug whether the underlying psychopathology is mania, brain tumour, epilepsy, agitated depression, or schizophrenia.

Nevertheless, a more specific usage can be postulated in schizophrenia. Both in the treatment and the prevention of the acute relapse, antipsychotic medication appears to have an action over and above a simple calming and tranquillizing effect. This is most obvious in the maintenance treatment of patients with paranoid schizophrenic states of late onset. Often the paranoid delusional system dissolves completely only to recrudesce when medication is stopped.

Within syndromes of psychosis certain symptoms are more responsive to antipsychotic medication than others. Hallucinations, restlessness, irritability, and some delusions show a more gratifying response than do social withdrawal, apathy, inertness and lack of co-operation. Part of this impression of differential responsiveness may reflect the problems of assessing the so-called 'negative' features of psychosis.

Antipsychotic drugs

Definitions

As implied already, the term 'antipsychotic medication' seems most apt, as these drugs are useful in the whole range of psychotic illnesses. Although schizophrenic patients are particularly helped, the term 'antischizophrenic drugs' as proposed by some implies too great a specificity. Another term which has been widely used is 'major tranquillizer', but the widespread use, especially by laymen, of 'tranquillizer' for the benzodiazepines leads to confusion here. Another popular term, especially in Europe, is 'neuroleptic', which refers to the pharmacological attributes of the drugs, specifically the neurological (extrapyramidal) side-effects which they produce. We prefer the neutral term 'antipsychotic drug'.

The main chemical groups of these drugs are the phenothiazines, the thioxanthenes, the phenylbutylpiperidines (butyrophenones) and the substituted benzamides. Several other chemical structures are also associated with antipsychotic activity (Fig. 11.1). Reserpine and tetrabenazine have antipsychotic properties but have a somewhat different pharmacology.

In psychiatry, the main uses of the antipsychotic drugs are (Kessler and Waletzky 1981):

(1) to quieten disturbed patients whatever the underlying pathology but most commonly in acute schizophrenics, manics, and the brain-damaged;

(2) as maintenance therapy to prevent or postpone relapses in the chronic schizophrenic patient in the community;

(3) as maintenance therapy to lessen active symptoms in the chronic hospitalized schizophrenic; and

(4) in low-dosage, as antianxiety agents in certain carefully-selected patients.

Non-psychiatric uses include the treatment of nausea and vomiting, hiccough, pruritus, and in conjunction with analgesics in terminal patients with chronic pain.

History

Phenothiazine, the parent compound, was synthesized in the late nineteenth century and was used in the 1930s as a veterinary anthelminthic. A derivative, promethazine, was found to have antihistaminic and sedative effects. In the search for other antihistaminics, chlorpromazine was synthesized in the Rhone-Poulenc-Spécia laboratories in France. Its antihistaminic properties were poor but it was found to have powerful sedative properties in anaesthesia and surgery, inducing 'artificial hibernation' with tranquillization, marked unconcern and indifference to surroundings and to injuries, and lack of temperature control, coupled with retention of consciousness and mental facilities. This effect was called '*lobotomie pharmacologique*'

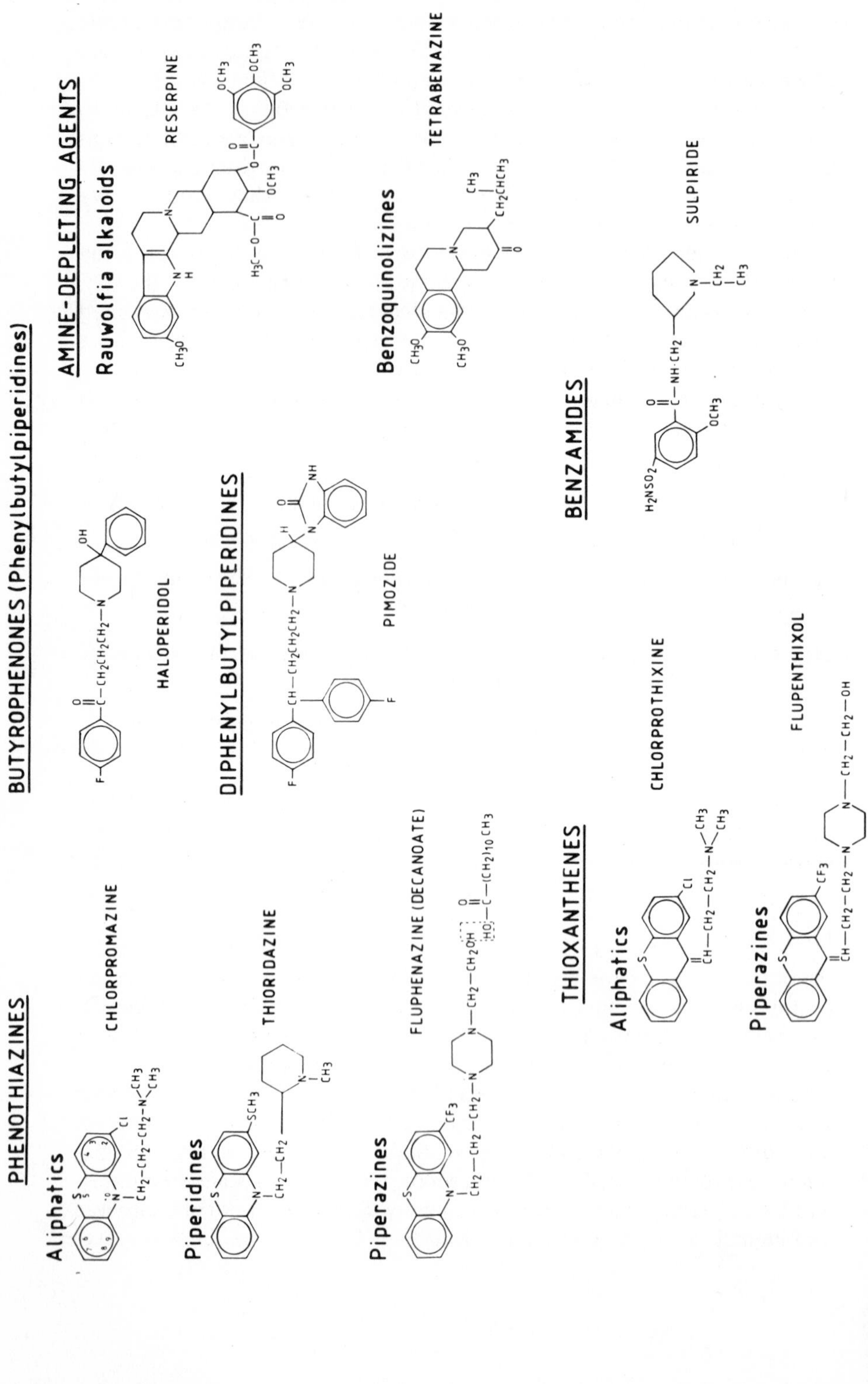

PHENOTHIAZINES

Aliphatics

CHLORPROMAZINE

Piperidines

THIORIDAZINE

Piperazines

FLUPHENAZINE (DECANOATE)

BUTYROPHENONES (Phenylbutylpiperidines)

HALOPERIDOL

DIPHENYLBUTYLPIPERIDINES

PIMOZIDE

AMINE-DEPLETING AGENTS

Rauwolfia alkaloids

RESERPINE

Benzoquinolizines

TETRABENAZINE

THIOXANTHENES

Aliphatics

CHLORPROTHIXINE

Piperazines

FLUPENTHIXOL

BENZAMIDES

SULPIRIDE

and psychiatrists were encouraged to try chlorpromazine first in manic and then in a mixed group of psychotic patients. The unique tranquillizing properties of sedation and antipsychotic activity without clouding of consciousness were quickly recognized but only later were the particular applications to schizophrenia discovered. The drug was also found to have a wide range of other actions, both in the laboratory and the clinic.

Other phenothiazines were synthesized, developed, and marketed. Most were piperazine-type compounds such as trifluoperazine and fluphenazine. A popular piperidine-type compound is thioridazine which was also an early introduction. This typing refers to the nature of the side-chain on the molecule. Chlorpromazine has a dimethylaminopropyl chain and is usually termed an aliphatic phenothiazine. Chlorpromazine has maintained its popularity world-wide although thioridazine is more extensively used in the USA.

In the 1960s, a new type of formulation was developed for fluphenazine in which it was coupled to a long-chain fatty acid and injected in an oily medium as a long-acting depot preparation. This and similar preparations are popular in the UK.

The thioxanthenes are closely related chemically to the phenothiazines and have similar pharmacological properties. The butyrophenones are phenylbutylpiperidines and were developed by modifying the chemical structure of analgesics related to meperidine. They were found to have antipsychotic actions and a pharmacological profile similar to the piperazine phenothiazines. Haloperidol, the prototype, is especially popular in the treatment of mania. A more recent development has been the diphenylbutylpiperidines such as pimozide and the substituted benzamides such as sulpiride. Clozapine is a dibenzodiazepine.

About the same time as the introduction of chlorpromazine, interest was developing in the actions of rauwolfia alkaloids, in particular extracts of *Rauwolfia serpentina*. These substances had long been used in Hindu traditional remedies for several conditions including insanity. Reserpine, the principal alkaloid, was isolated in 1952 and was used as an antihypertensive agent and as an antipsychotic drug. It has fallen into obsolescence in the treatment of hypertension. It was even more rapidly discarded as an antipsychotic agent because its therapeutic effects were usually preceded by a phase of increased disturbance and because retarded, depressive reactions were sometimes induced.

Many other compounds have been synthesized and investigated in the search for new antipsychotic drugs (Meltzer 1986). In particular, the need for effective antipsychotic agents without extrapyramidal effects led pharmacologists to seek drugs with selective actions on the limbic system and lack of effect on the basal ganglia. The increasing problem of tardive dyskinesia has lent additional urgency to this quest.

Pharmacokinetics

Interest has focused on the prototypal compound, chlorpromazine. This is unfortunate because of its metabolic complexity: well over 150 metabolites have been postulated of which nearly 100 have been detected in blood or urine. This complexity would be irrelevant if all the metabolites were psychotropically inactive, but animal and some clinical evidence suggest that 7-hydroxychlorpromazine and perhaps some other metabolites are active. The metabolism of other phenothiazines such as thioridazine and fluphenazine are also complex. Butyrophenones such as haloperidol and thioxanthenes such as fluphenthixol seem less complex and are probably devoid of active metabolites of any practical significance.

Plasma antipsychotic drug concentrations were initially measured using chemical methods and, somewhat later, radioimmunoassays. The ability of these drugs to bind to dopamine receptors has been exploited to develop radioreceptor assays, with the potential advantage that all substances in the plasma drug and active metabolites, should react and be measured. Unfortunately, the technique has proved unexpectedly complex with respect to interpretation of the data (Curry 1985).

Absorption and metabolism

Chlorpromazine and other antipsychotic drugs are highly lipid-soluble and generally rapidly and completely absorbed. Absorption can be impaired by the simultaneous administration of some antacids which tend to adsorb it and by tea and coffee which may precipitate it in an insoluble form. A substantial proportion of chlorpromazine and possibly other phenothiazines are metabolized 'first-pass' in the gut-wall and liver after absorption (Curry *et al.* 1971). The proportion varies from patient to patient but may approach 100 per cent in some. Intramuscular injections of either the regular or the long-acting formulations obviates this first-pass metabolism which explains why the dosage for such forms is less than that for oral administration. Haloperidol and pimozide undergo relatively little first-pass metabolism.

After absorption antipsychotic drugs pass readily to the brain where they tend to accumulate. Chlorpromazine is metabolized by sulphoxidation, hydroxylation, *N*-oxidation, and demethylation, these processes often succeeding each other. Eventually metabolites of low lipophilicity are produced or conjugates are formed and are excreted through the kidney. The sulphoxide is an important inactive metabolite. One interesting study suggested that patients who responded poorly to chlorpromazine had high levels of the sulphoxide while those who responded well had high levels of chlorpromazine or its unconjugated hydroxy metabolites (Sakalis *et al.* 1973). In practical terms, the only inference which can be drawn is that non-response to one drug is best managed by switching to one of a totally different chemical class, although even this is no guarantee that similar metabolic processes are not involved.

Thioridazine is metabolized by sulphoxidation on the ring sulphur to form an inactive metabolite. However, sulphoxidation on the thiomethyl substituent results in active metabolites including mesoridazine. These active metabolites provide much of the antipsychotic activity on chronic administration. Piperazine phenothiazines are metabolized much as is chlorpromazine, sulphoxide formation being the most important. The piperazine ring in the side chain may be opened and further metabolites formed. Thioxanthenes are metabolized similarly although hydroxylation does not occur. Haloperidol is primarily metabolized by splitting into two inactive moieties but there is some recent evidence of hydroxylation to an active metabolite.

The long-acting depot preparations are metabolized by splitting of the ester bond joining the parent drug to its long-chain fatty acid by aliphatic esterase enzymes. The parent drug is slowly released and absorbed from the injection site into the systemic blood stream.

Plasma concentration and clinical response

Chlorpromazine has a fairly short half-life in the plasma (about 8 h) so that fluctuations in plasma concentration following each dose are fairly substantial. However, concentrations of the drug in the brain may fluctuate much less because of the high lipid solubility of the compound. Other phenothiazines also have fairly short half-lives but some diphenylbutylpiperidines have such long half-lives that they can be given once-weekly.

Following acute doses of chlorpromazine, psychiatric patients were sedated while plasma concentrations were high. Both very high concentrations (over 500 ng/ml) and very low concentrations (below 10 ng/ml) were associated with poor response (Curry *et al.* 1970). Inter-patient variation in plasma concentrations after a few weeks treatment with chlorpromazine is substantial. Variations from day to day are also marked as are differences in the peak concentrations attained after each individual dose.

A further complication is that chlorpromazine induces its own metabolism by an effect on liver enzymes. Thus, plasma concentrations reach their peak during the first week or two of treatment and then decline to half or less of these values over the next month, then stabilizing at this lower level.

For these various reasons it is hardly surprising that correlations between plasma concentrations and clinical response have been low and non-significant although generally positive (May and van Putten 1978). For example, in a study of 86 chronic schizophrenic patients given a wide range of oral doses of chlorpromazine, global ratings of improvement were unrelated to plasma concentration. Claims that the concentrations of 7-hydroxychlorpromazine may be important in this respect have not been well substantiated. In acutely psychotic patients, antipsychotic drug concentrations, as measured by a radioreceptor assay, tended to be either high or low in non-responders (Kucharski *et al.* 1984). Low levels also predicted, but only to a weak extent, relapse in chronic schizophrenics (Brown *et al.* 1982). Correlations with side-effects have also been sought. Extrapyramidal syndromes tend to be more common in patients with high plasma drug concentrations than in those with lower levels (Krska *et al.* 1986).

Thus, at present, plasma antipsychotic drug concentrations, however measured, do not usefully predict response in psychotic patients but may have limited application in special situations such as drug toxicity and overdose, apparently inexplicable resistance to drug treatment and idiosyncratic responses (Tang 1985). However, interpretation of the results is by no means straightforward (Curry 1985).

After stopping chlorpromazine, the drug rapidly becomes undetectable in the plasma, as predicted from its short half-life. However, because of its lipophilic nature it tends to remain in lipid organs in the body for some time and to be detectable in metabolite form in the urine. Clinical relapse may also be delayed.

The pharmacokinetics of depot preparations are still poorly worked out, mainly because of the technical problems of measuring the low plasma concentrations produced (Jann *et al.* 1985).

Drug interactions

As well as accelerating its own metabolism by induction effects, chlorpromazine can increase the metabolism of other drugs and, in turn, be metabolized more rapidly by the presence of other drugs such as phenobarbitone. The antiparkinsonian drug, orphenadrine, also reduces chlorpromazine concentrations in the body by inducing liver microsomal oxidizing enzymes. Cigarette smoking may also be associated with induction of liver enzymes and lowering of chlorpromazine drug concentrations. Conversely, some other compounds—for example—steroids, oestrogens and perhaps tricyclic antidepressants—may compete with chlorpromazine for liver enzymes and elevate its levels.

Pharmacology

Biochemical pharmacology

Almost all antipsychotic drugs induce extrapyramidal syndromes. The demonstration that idiopathic parkinsonism was associated with a deficiency of dopamine-containing neurons in the basal ganglia led to a focusing of interest on the interactions of antipsychotic drugs and dopamine mechanisms. The observation that the administration of antipsychotic drugs led to an increase in the turnover of the dopamine metabolite homovanillic acid (HVA) prompted Carlsson (1977) to postulate that these drugs blocked dopamine receptors thus provoking a compensatory increase in the synthesis of dopamine. Dopaminergic blockade also accounts for the extra-pyramidal effects of the antipsychotic drugs. Other effects of dopamine blockade are to inhibit the vomiting centre, thus exerting an antiemetic effect and to interfere with the control of growth hormones and prolactin release. Antipsychotic drugs decrease growth hormone levels and increase prolactin levels leading to neuroendocrine side-effects.

The most direct approach is to assess the affinity of various antipsychotic drugs for the dopamine receptor by measuring their ability to displace radio-labelled haloperidol or a more potent derivative, spiroperidol (Peroutka and Snyder 1980). This can now be done in human subjects using positron emission tomography ('PET scan') (Farde *et al.* 1988). Close correspondence between this property and clinical potency has been claimed (Creese *et al.* 1976). Affinity to muscarinic receptors can also be assessed. Thioridazine has high affinity whereas chlorpromazine has moderate and haloperidol low affinity. The likelihood of extrapyramidal effects appears to increase proportionately. Thioridazine has a low incidence of such effects because it blocks both dopaminergic and cholinergic receptors in the basal ganglia, maintaining the normal balance. Haloperidol and the piperazine phenothiazines block dopamine receptors preferentially with consequent extra-pyramidal effects. At high doses, however, the extrapyramidal syndrome tends to disappear. Presumably, at these dose levels the anticholinergic effect becomes appreciable.

Dopamine receptors may vary in their characteristics in different parts of the brain and some drugs act preferentially in one or other region (Snyder 1981). So far, however, drugs have not been marketed for which there is clear evidence that mesolimbic and mesocortical dopamine receptors are blocked at concentrations which leave the basal ganglia unaffected. As well as dopamine and acetylcholine receptor antagonism, the antipsychotic drugs typically block alpha-adrenergic receptors both peripherally and centrally.

Reserpine and its synthetic analogue, tetrabenazine, act by preventing the storage of amines in the granular vesicles of the presynaptic neuron. Dopamine, noradrenalin and 5-HT are all affected so it is impossible to attribute the antipsychotic action to alterations in the disposition of any one amine.

Some of the clinical and biochemical effects of antipsychotic medication disappear with continued administration while others persist. Thus, the initial drowsiness wears off after a week or two and parkinsonism has usually disappeared within a few months. Conversely, the elevation in prolactin and the clinical effects tend to persist.

Basic pharmacology

The animal pharmacology of chlorpromazine correlates well with its biochemical effects. Dopamine receptor blockade accounts for a powerful antiemetic effect; one of the screening tests for new antipsychotic drugs was the prevention of apomorphine-induced vomiting. Release of prolactin secretion is responsible for a lactogenic effect in animals and other endocrine effects reflect hypothalamic actions. Extrapyramidal effects can be demonstrated grossly by a general reduction in motor activity with diminished motor responsiveness. Animals maintain unnatural positions in which they are placed, so-called 'catalepsy'. A more specific test consists of producing lesions in the basal ganglia of rats on one side only. The animal tends to run round in circles and this can be blocked by giving antipsychotic drugs.

The anticholinergic effects of chlorpromazine and thioridazine can be demonstrated on isolated tissue preparations such as the contraction of the guinea pig ileus. Anti-5-HT actions can also be shown, e.g. on the rat uterus. Although chlorpromazine was originally developed from promethazine, its antihistaminic activity, as assessed by protection of guinea pigs against lethal doses of histamine, is quite weak.

Antiadrenalin properties are quite marked. The lethal effects of adrenalin and noradrenalin in dogs can be prevented by the prior administration of chlorpromazine, although effects of these amines such as hyperglycaemia are not attenuated. In the dog, chlorpromazine produces vasodilatation due to blockade of adrenergic vasoconstrictor impulses, followed by a reflex tachycardia. A decrease in cerebral blood flow occurs but oxygen uptake by the brain is not affected.

Neuropharmacology and behavioural pharmacology

Collateral input from sensory pathways to the cortex is suppressed by antipsychotic drugs, lowering the through-put and consequent diffuse activation of the cortex. Antipsychotic drugs apparently have little direct effect on the cortex. Although dopaminergic pathways have now been traced to the orbital and cingulate cortices, blockade by antipsychotic drugs does not produce obvious effects.

In cats, chlorpromazine increases sociability and decreases hostility. This 'taming effect' is apparent in rhesus monkeys which are normally aggressive, and allows them to be handled. Aggregated mice are made overactive by amphetamine, with subsequent death; isolated mice are much less susceptible. Antipsychotic drugs prevent this toxicity.

Antipsychotic drugs markedly alter learning processes. The conditioned avoidance response involves the coupling of a warning signal with a noxious stimulus, such as footshock. Rats learn to avoid the noxious stimulus when the warning occurs. Antipsychotic drugs suppress this conditioned avoidance response without affecting the unconditioned response, namely jumping away after the footshock.

Clinical pharmacology

Normal humans: A major problem in assessing the effects of antipsychotic drugs on human psychological functions stems from the complex psychotropic effects of these drugs. As well as their primary antipsychotic actions, secondary effects on alertness and other mental functions are very obvious. For example, chlorpromazine is sedative as well as antipsychotic whereas trifluoperazine and flupenthixol are somewhat stimulant. Furthermore, these secondary effects are more evident after single doses and during the first week of chronic administration and in normal subjects.

Tolerance to the acute sedative effects of chlorpromazine can be demonstrated in contrast to a continuing effect when a barbiturate is administered chronically. The antipsychotic effects of chlorpromazine and related drugs which persist after acute sedative or stimulant effects have worn off are of prime clinical interest and these cannot, of course, be demonstrated in normal individuals.

Antipsychotic drugs have characteristic effects on the electroencephalogram. Slow wave, theta, and alpha activity are increased whereas fast activity is somewhat decreased. Paroxysmal activity may increase and fits are more likely.

The autonomic effects of antipsychotic drugs are predictable from their animal pharmacology and easily demonstrated: postural hypotension, reflex tachycardia, stuffy nose, blurring of vision, lowered bowel motility, and pupillary constriction.

Clinical use

Although for the purpose of presentation we have divided the psychiatric uses of antipsychotic medication into separate categories, these indications overlap. For example, the chronic schizophrenic maintained on long-acting depot preparations may nevertheless show an increase in symptoms heralding an exacerbation of the condition for which an increase in dose or frequency of injection is required. Or the relapse may become so obvious that oral medication is required in addition or even so severe that intramuscular injection of the regular formulation is needed to control severely disturbed behaviour. Nevertheless, it is useful to categorize the indications for these drugs.

'Tranquillization'

Chlorpromazine was first used in the management of manic patients but it quickly became evident that disturbed behaviour, of whatever aetiology, responded to the drug. Before this time, the drugs used to quieten noisy, combative, and destructive patients were bromides, barbiturates, paraldehyde, and opiates such as morphine and Omnopon. The drawbacks were that a phase of increased excitation might be induced initially due to removal of inhibition, somnolence might supervene to the point of deep sleep and even coma, toxic confusional psychoses might be produced obscuring the clinical picture and complicating the diagnosis, and withdrawal syndromes might be precipitated or drug dependence initiated. It is a measure of the advantages of chlorpromazine in these various respects that it so quickly supplanted the existing sedatives: there is no paradoxical excitation, no clouding of consciousness, excessive drowsiness or danger of drug-induced psychosis, and dependence and abstinence phenomena are unknown. Thus, it soon became the standard treatment for acutely disturbed patients and, despite expressions of distaste for this 'chemical straitjacket' as it has been pejoratively labelled, it remains a treatment of first choice in admission wards throughout the world. After its introduction, its beneficial effects were quantified quite simply in terms of the decrease in numbers of windows broken, hours patients spent in seclusion, assaults on staff, and use of restraint: in many institutions the padded cell and the straitjacket have become museum-pieces.

An additional factor which should not be underestimated is the increase in confidence of the nursing staff in dealing with disturbed patients. The effectiveness of the antipsychotic drugs is enhanced by firm, purposeful handling of the patient which knowledge of the general effectiveness of the drugs usually produces (Pfeffer 1981).

The indications for the antipsychotic drugs in this non-specific role are accordingly wide. Freyhan (1959) many years ago emphasized these diffuse indications, pointing out that chlorpromazine was mainly effective against symptoms related to hypermotility, abnormal initiative, and increased affective tension, features which he dubbed 'target symptoms'. He listed the following indications for such symptomatic treatment:

(a) Schizophrenia: states of restlessness and excitement, paranoid tension, panic and aggressive outbursts; stereotypical and bizarre activities; noisiness and destructive behaviour.

(b) Affective disorders: hypomanic and manic states; states of agitated depression; paranoid disturbances in involutional psychoses.

(c) Acute brain syndromes; states of intoxication, delirium and hallucinations.

(d) Chronic brain syndromes; states of restlessness, confusional activities, violent outbursts, noisiness and destructive behaviour.

(e) Psychoneurotic and personality disorders; tormenting feelings of tension, aggressive acting out, poor impulse control.

The last category is the most problematical (Klar and Siever 1984; Gunderson 1986). Because diagnosis of personality disorder in particular is a very controversial topic, the administration of powerful drugs like the antipsychotics has led to criticisms; allegations have been made that these drugs are used to quieten inmates of non-medical institutions such as prisons and detention camps.

Treatment of acute schizophrenia

Antipsychotic drugs have now become the mainstay of treatment in acutely ill schizophrenic patients. After 25 years of intensive use it is apparent that antipsychotic medication does not cure schizophrenia, at least in the cases of the severer forms presenting in young adults, especially when the onset is insidious. The condition is kept in check so that the acute, initial attack is cut short and subsequent relapses minimized. The effects of the acute attack on the patient and on his social functioning are ameliorated. Long absences from work may be avoided. Nevertheless, some patients still pursue an inexorable course with deterioration and inevitable relegation to the long-stay wards of the asylum (Mann and Cree 1976).

The effectiveness of antipsychotic medication in the treatment of the acutely ill schizophrenic has been established in hundreds of trials, including some very carefully controlled studies involving hundreds of patients. In one multi-hospital collaborative trial (Casey *et al.* 1960), several phenothiazines (including chlorpromazine, mean dose 635 mg) were more effective than phenobarbitone in the treatment of male patients with acute schizophrenic symptoms. After 12 weeks improvement was noted with respect to belligerence, resistiveness, thinking disturbances, perceptual distortion, paranoid ideas, and withdrawal.

In the large American trial carried out under the aegis of the National Institute of Mental Health (1964), 463 newly admitted acutely schizophrenic patients were randomly allocated to treatment with chlorpromazine, fluphenazine, thioridazine, or placebo. Each drug was given in flexible dosage, that for chlorpromazine averaging 655 mg/day. The psychiatrist-in-charge made global assessments. A total of 344 patients completed 6 weeks of treatment, the majority of drop-outs receiving placebo. Since only the less severely ill patients completed treatment, the results are biased against the phenothiazines. None of the drug-treated patients deteriorated, 5 per cent did not change, 20 per cent improved minimally, but the majority, 75 per cent, improved substantially. Fewer than 40 per cent of those given placebo improved substantially.

The In-patient Multidimensional Psychiatric Scale and the Burdock Ward Behavior Rating Scale provided more detailed information concerning changes in symptom profiles. The phenothiazines produced improvements in a wide range of schizophrenic symptoms and not only in those related to overactivity, so-called 'positive' symptoms. Underactivity and social withdrawal ('negative' features) also improved.

In this trial, differences were not apparent between the three phenothiazines. In another trial, however (Hanlon *et al.* 1965), eight phenothiazines were compared for effectiveness in 322 newly admitted patients with mixed diagnoses, all of whom were considered suitable for phenothiazine therapy. The mean effects of the drug administered in flexible dosage for 30 days did not differ, but three of the phenothiazines—prochlorperazine, perphenazine and fluphenazine—were more effective than the others in the management of the more severely ill patients. By contrast, thioridazine, trifluopromazine, and thiopropazate were more beneficial in the less ill patients. Chlorpromazine was intermediate in effects and trifluoperazine was inconsistent. Clinical experience also suggests that compounds more likely to produce extrapyramidal effects such as the piperazine phenothiazines and the butyrophenones are marginally more effective in the severely disturbed patients than chlorpromazine and thioridazine.

A large scale comparison of five treatment programmes (May 1968) in acute schizophrenia found drug therapy alone to be almost as effective as drug therapy plus psychotherapy, and both these regimens to be more effective than psychotherapy alone, or 'milieu' therapy, i.e. routine ward therapy. Electroconvulsive therapy was more effective than psychotherapy but less so than drugs.

More recently, an evaluation of antipsychotic medication was carried out by a group of Australasian psychiatrists in the project entitled 'Quality Assurance in Aspects of Psychiatric Practice' as part of their treatment outlines for the management of schizophrenia (Quality Assurance Project 1984). To that end, a meta-analysis was carried out of over a hundred trials comparing various treatments. Meta-analysis is a way of combining the results of trials which enables an overall 'effect size' to be calculated in terms of the differences between end-scores of the various treatment groups, standardized statistically. The overall results are depicted in Fig. 11.2 and an explanation of the bar chart is given in the legend.

Hospitalization with usual ward care was the standard basis for comparison. Psychotherapy did not prove additionally beneficial. The two studies of social intervention showed little effect, nor was drug withdrawal associated with much change. However, drug therapy did effect a considerable improvement which was not further increased with psychotherapy. The

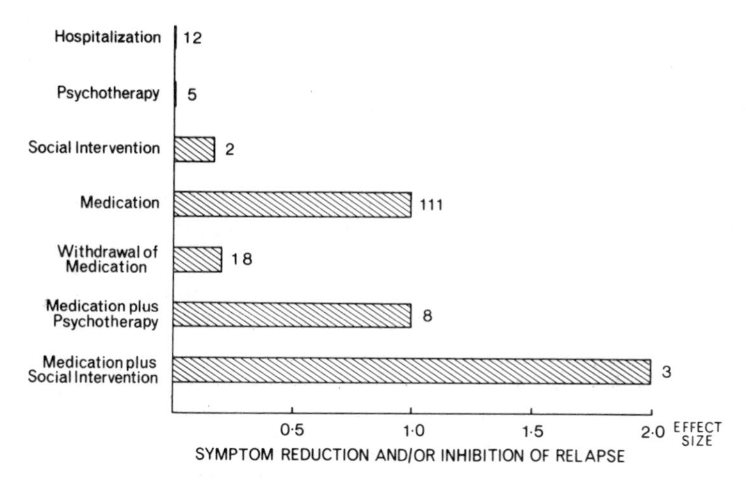

Figure 11.2. A schematic representation in effect size or standard deviation units of the power of 7 treatment regimes used with patients with schizophrenia admitted to hospital. The length of the bars is proportional to the power of the treatment and the number of trials on which each estimate is based is set alongside each bar. (With permission from Australian and New Zealand College of Psychiatrists.)

addition of social intervention did enhance improvement but note that only three trials were involved.

It seems clear that the most helpful therapeutic step in managing acute schizophrenia is to administer antipsychotic medication, thus hastening resolution of the psychotic episode. Whether the 'natural history' of the condition is modified is unclear partly because of the problems of conducting such studies (May 1976). Klein and Davis (1969) assessed a number of controlled studies and concluded that Bleuler's fundamental symptoms—namely, thought disorder, blunt affect, withdrawal and autistic behaviour—were at least as much improved as other less specific symptoms such as auditory hallucinations and paranoid ideation. However, this does not imply that the process of schizophrenia is being modified, merely that the whole spectrum of symptoms is amenable to improvement.

Prevention of relapse

The term 'maintenance therapy' is used to describe the long-term treatment with antipsychotic drugs of schizophrenic patients in remission. Such patients may be living in the community, with relatives or in lodgings, or they may be inmates of a long-stay psychiatric ward. The antipsychotic drugs suppress chronic symptoms such as hallucinations, make delusions less insistent, and generally help prevent the periodic episodes of more acute symptoms which punctuate the course of many schizophrenic illnesses.

Various aspects of patients can be used as indicators of response, including rehospitalization rate, adjustment at work, residual symptoms and social functioning. An analysis of over 20 controlled studies of antipsychotic medication administered for periods longer than one month concluded that patients taking drugs were much less likely to relapse than those maintained on placebo (Davis 1975). For example, Pasamanick and his associates (1964) reported that over 80 per cent of schizophrenics were able to remain outside hospital for 18 months or more when maintained on drugs as compared with a control group given placebo in which half the patients relapsed. The results of various studies differ as to whether maintenance therapy prevents relapse or merely postpones it, the reasons for discrepancies lying in different types of patients studied, the degree of social support provided, type of medication, and so on. On balance, postponement seems to be the type of effect produced: roughly speaking the chance of relapse within a given time is halved by drugs as compared with placebo (Hogarty and Ulrich 1977) (see Fig. 11.3). (Put another way, the 'half-life' of staying out of hospital is doubled.) For haloperidol, but not for propericiazine, relapse prevention was dose-dependent (Nishikawa *et al.* 1984).

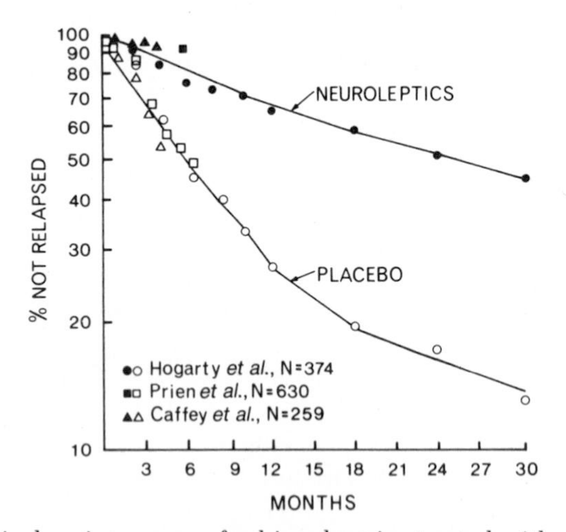

Fig 11.3. Clinical maintenance of schizophrenics treated with a neuroleptic or placebo vs. time. This diagram indicates rates of non-exacerbation ('survival') during follow-up after improvement of patients diagnosed schizophrenic and assigned to continued neuroleptic (phenothiazine) treatment or a placebo. The rate of 'release' (worsening) is remarkably similar in all studies for the placebo groups over at least six months (about 5 to 10 per cent per month). (Reproduced with permission from Baldessarini, R.J., in *The Somatic Therapies* (ed. T.B. Karasu). The American Psychiatric Association on Psychiatric Therapies. American Psychiatric Association, Washington, D.C.).

Leff and Wing (1971) reported that during the course of a year's maintenance therapy with phenothiazines about a third of patients relapsed as compared with four-fifths of those on placebo. No definite clinical predictors of which patients would remain well on placebo were apparent. The authors recommend that patients having a first attack, incorporating depressive features, and having a good previous personality, should not be entered routinely into a standard maintenance programme. In this study, the patient sample was drawn from the middle third of the range of schizophrenic patients with respect to prognosis. Patients excluded from the trial because of their poor prognosis did badly in spite of drug treatment; those with a good prognosis did well without drugs.

A complicating factor in such studies is that an undetermined proportion of patients who relapse either reduce their dosage or cease taking their drugs altogether. Patients may stop their drugs and then relapse or, less commonly, spontaneous relapse may be associated with an increasing reluctance to persist with medication.

Early signs of psychotic relapse were catalogued in a study in which antipsychotic drug withdrawal was followed by relapse in 26 of 32 schizophrenic out-patients (Dencker *et al.* 1986). Important factors included positive psychopathology, motor dysfunction, impaired affect, and sleep disturbance. Relapse could be prevented by re-institution of drug therapy when these prodromata appeared.

The value of social work in relation to continued antipsychotic medication was examined by allocating patients randomly to drug treatment with or without counselling by a social worker or to placebo with or without such help (Hogarty *et al.* 1974*a*, *b*). The counselling was directed towards helping the patient adjust to his or her 'major role' as wage-earner or homemaker. By the end of 2 years, 80 per cent of placebo-treated and 48 per cent of drug-treated patients had relapsed. Effects attributable to social work intervention were much less than the drug–placebo differences but did reduce relapse rates in those patients who remained more than six months in the community. For such patients combining drugs and help from the social worker provided the best treatment. Early relapse was associated with poor premorbid adjustment, longer illnesses and more severe initial symptoms, social instability after discharge, poor interpersonal relationships, and problems in complying with medication regimens. Drugs were most effective in patients with stable family backgrounds and supportive relatives, and in patients who were housewives. Social worker aid was most efficacious when the patient's symptoms had been controlled by medication.

Further insights into the role of relatives in influencing the relapse of schizophrenic patients is provided by the work of Vaughn and Leff (1976). Data were available from 128 schizophrenic patients maintained in the community, of whom 30 per cent relapsed over 9 months. Depending on the number of critical, hostile, and emotionally over-involved comments made about the patient during a standard interview by the relative with whom he lived, the patient's home environment was categorized as high or low in 'Expressed Emotion' (EE). In patients living in a high EE home the relapse rate was 51 per cent as contrasted with only 13 per cent of those in low EE homes. The number of hours the patient spent with the key relative was also a factor: patients in High EE homes who spent less than 35 h per week with their relatives had a much lower rate (28 per cent) than those with more than 35 h of contact (relapse rate 69 per cent). Further protection was provided by regular antipsychotic maintenance therapy. In patients in high EE homes, with less than 35 h/week contact, taking drugs regularly, the relapse rate was the same as that in patients from low EE homes—about 15 per cent. Conversely, the relapse rate was 92 per cent over 9 months in patients in high EE home environments, with over 35 h/week contact and not taking medication. Drug therapy did not affect the prognosis in low EE patients. A 2-year follow-up showed a reverse of this differential protective effect: at that time, drugs lowered the relapse rate in Low EE patients but their effect was no longer evident in high EE patients (Leff and Vaughn 1981). However, a more recent study showed few positive results and the authors concluded that social factors are weak predictors of liability to relapse (MacMillan *et al.* 1986*a*,*b*).

Another factor which was evaluated was life events. Those of an 'independent' nature—that is, outside the patient's control—seemed important in influencing relapse. They tended to cluster in the three weeks immediately prior to relapse and drug therapy was apparently powerless to prevent this.

It has been repeatedly demonstrated that long-acting depot injections are a definite advance over oral medication especially in the maintenance therapy of chronic schizophrenic patients in the community (Johnson 1977, 1982, 1984). One reason for the better results lies in the different mode of administration: The intramuscular injection avoids the first-pass metabolism undergone by much of the orally administered drug.

Another reason relates to the reduction in drug defaulting (Kane 1983). This problem is not peculiar to the schizophrenic or the psychiatric patient but is found in diabetics prescribed insulin and tuberculous patients given chemotherapy. However, the results of drug defaulting in chronic schizophrenics are often dramatically apparent. With oral medication, perhaps as many as a half of schizophrenic patients fail to take their medication as prescribed. When non-psychiatrically trained nurses are responsible for the depot injections and a multiplicity of agents are involved, about a third of patients default. When administrative supervision is simplified to one agency and trained psychiatric nurses give the injections, only 1 in 7 patients default. Thus, as a rough guide, the defaulting rate can be reduced by at least a half by switching them from oral to depot medication. And, of course, defaulters can be immediately identified and followed up.

The benefits from injections have been quantified in several ways (Beresford and Ward 1987). In the earlier trials, patients on oral medication were switched to depot injections: marked clinical gains were apparent ranging between 30 and 70 per cent drop in relapse rate. These gains were attributed by some to non-specific factors such as therapeutic enthusiasm and increased social support. However, fully controlled double-blind trials have demonstrated that the clinical benefits of the depot preparation depended on the drug content.

Nevertheless, the prognosis even with depot injections leaves much room for improvement (Johnson 1976; Stevens 1973; Watt, 1975). About a third of patients are likely to relapse over 2 years. Other less obvious indices of pathology can be used. These drugs have little effect on negative symptoms but do reduce social withdrawal a little and offer some protection against stress.

Chronic hospitalized schizophrenics

An early review of 29 investigations of the therapeutic effects of chlorpromazine in chronic schizophrenic patients concluded that the drug produced a statistically significant global response with particular improvement in such symptoms as anxiety, restlessness, and tension (Heilizer 1960). Positive results tended to be associated with higher dosage and longer duration of treatment; as might be expected, the less chronic the condition the better the therapeutic response. Patients with the highest initial ratings of tension derived the greatest benefit from antipsychotic drug treatment.

Despite this, there is general agreement that these drugs have less effect on the symptoms and behaviour of chronic schizophrenics than those of more acutely ill patients. Some psychiatrists have concluded that the drugs are of little value in the mangement of inert, withdrawn, passive patients whereas others dispute this, finding that overactive patients are also not greatly helped. Various trials show different profiles of action which all suggests that antipsychotic drugs have relatively minor effects in chronic schizophrenics in hospital. Patients with organic brain changes seem particularly unresponsive (Weinberger *et al.* 1980).

The emphasis has changed towards evaluating the interactions of antipsychotic medication and other forms of therapy, particularly social and occupational rehabilitation programmes. Intensive occupational therapy produces improvements which, at least initially, are equal to those produced by chlorpromazine alone, but the administration of the drug enhances the non-specific effects of rehabilitation therapies.

If antipsychotic medication benefits chronic schizophrenics, withdrawal of maintenance therapy should be followed by worsening of symptoms. This is indeed the case, but the relapse is often delayed for up to 6 months after withdrawal. The symptoms which worsen include coherence of speech, stereotyped behaviour, hallucinations and delusions, and the patient's response to the latter. Replacement on therapy usually, but by no means always, results in improvement back to the pre-withdrawal status.

Unwanted effects

Adverse reactions can be roughly divided into two categories: those unwanted effects predictable from the known pharmacological properties of the drug, and those of allergic or idiosyncratic nature, with known or unknown mechanisms peculiar to the patient. In view of the many pharmacological actions of the antipsychotic drugs, it is hardly surprising that many unwanted effects occur (Simpson *et al.* 1981). Also, idiosyncratic responses are common.

The dopamine-blocking effects of antipsychotic drugs are believed to underlie their therapeutic effects. This blockade is also deemed responsible for several different types of neurological disorders secondary to dopamine blockade in the basal ganglia.

Extrapyramidal syndromes

The earliest neurological effect during a course of treatment is *acute dystonia* (Rupniak *et al.* 1986) which may be seen even after a single dose of a high-potency compound such as fluphenazine or haloperidol. It occurs in about 2.5 per cent of patients treated with antipsychotic drugs and it is commoner in men and children than in women. The features are diverse and often bizarre and include torticollis, retrocollis, facial grimaces and distortion, tongue protrusion, dysarthria, opisthotonus, scoliosis, and oculogyric crises. It may be misdiagnosed as tetanus, tetany, or even hysteria but the history of taking an antipsychotic drug usually clinches the diagnosis. Prompt relief usually follows the intravenous injections of diphenhydramine, benztropine, or biperiden. Oral antiparkinsonian drugs may then be needed if the condition threatens to recur. The antipsychotic medication must be discontinued or its dosage reduced.

Akathisia (literally means 'unable to sit') is an uncontrollable motor agitation with fidgeting, inability to sit still, constant pacing and a restless urge to keep on the move (Stahl 1985). It is common (Gibb and Lees 1986). There is a strongly subjective element with unpleasant feelings. Possible subtypes have been suggested. It may be misdiagnosed as a sign of mounting psychotic agitation and treated wrongly by raising instead of lowering the dose of antipsychotic agent. Akathisia is sometimes helped by a benzodiazepine but antiparkinsonian drugs are usually ineffective (Ratey and Salzman 1984). Beta-adrenoceptor antagonists have been used successfully (Adler *et al.* 1989). Akathisia is commonest after a week or two of treatment but it can appear later.

Parkinsonism is the commonest of these neurological conditions. The mildest form is bradykinesia often detectable in the patient's handwriting which becomes minute ('micrographia'). Then akinesia occurs with weakness in muscles used for fine repetitive actions. In the more severe forms, there is loss of associated movements, rigidity, stooped posture, festinant gait, mask-like facies, coarse 'pill-rolling' tremor, excess salivation, and seborrhea. The condition is commoner in women than in men and in patients who have relatives with idiopathic parkinsonism. It is commoner in the elderly and may be mistaken for apathy, depression, or dementia. It usually supervenes in the first month or two of treatment but can be delayed for much longer when it is unlikely to be recognized. Some degree of tolerance develops to this extrapyramidal effect as it tends to disappear after a few months. At modest dosage of chlorpromazine (600 mg/day), its incidence is 15–25 per cent depending on how assiduously it is sought. With thioridazine the incidence is much lower. Antiparkinsonian drugs lessen the tremor more than the akinesia.

A syndrome which may be related to parkinsonism is the 'rabbit' syndrome. The main feature is a perioral tremor and the condition may come on within months or years of the antipsychotic medication being started. Antiparkinsonian agents may help.

Uncommon reactions comprise akinetic mutism and catatonic reactions which may occur on high doses of the potent piperazine phenothiazines and butyrophenones. Withdrawal dyskinesias taking the form of choreo-athetotic reactions lasting a few days have been described when such high doses are abruptly discontinued. Another condition is neuroleptic malignant syndrome with muscular rigidity, hyperthermia and autonomic dysfunction (Caroff 1980). This condition has occasioned concern recently (Szabadi 1984; Editorial 1984). It was first called 'syndrome malin' in the French literature: reported cases have been sporadic and total less than 150 worldwide (Shalev and Munitz 1986). The drugs most often responsible are haloperidol, chlorpromazine, and fluphenazine (Addonizio *et al.* 1987), but tetrabenazine, an amine-depletor, has also been implicated. The rate of increase of drug load seems an important factor in the aetiology. The motor symptoms comprise catatonia, akinesia, tremor, chorea, and changes in muscle tone which may cause dysphagia, dysarthria, and dyspnoea (Gibb and Lees 1985). The most important of the autonomic symptoms is hyperpyrexia but many others have been reported (Abbott and Loizou 1986). The incidence is less than 0.5 per cent of patients taking antipsychotic drugs but the mortality is about 20 per cent. Treatment is to stop the antipsychotic drug and to institute supportive measures. Specific drug measures which have been advocated include dantrolene as a muscle relaxant and bromocriptine to facilitate central dopaminergic mechanisms.

The use of antiparkinsonian medication with antipsychotic drugs is a controversial topic but is also the source of much unthinking prescribing. Too often the psychiatrist admitting a psychotic patient automatically adds antiparkinsonian medication to the patient's antipsychotic drugs. There is no evidence that such routine antiparkinsonian medication will prevent extrapyramidal syndromes developing (Martin 1975). What does occur is a potentiation of the anticholinergic effects. Particularly reprehensible is the further addition of a tricyclic antidepressant as now three anticholinergic drugs are being given. Severe somatic effects such as urinary retention or paralytic ileus have been described and a confusional psychosis is possible. Finally, antiparkinsonian drugs may lessen the effectiveness of antipsychotic medication by interfering with drug absorption or accelerating drug metabolism. For these reasons it is logical prescribing practice to avoid using antiparkinsonian drugs and to rely on a careful reduction in antipsychotic drug dosage (Johnson 1978). The exception is when lowering the dose is followed by an unmanageable increase in symptoms. With the depot neuroleptics, lowering the dose or spacing the injections out more usually lessens extrapyramidal effects. Sometimes antiparkinsonian medication is needed for a few days in each injection cycle, typically the first week. If antiparkinsonian drugs are given, they should be gradually withdrawn after a few months. Parkinsonian effects do not usually recur, although this assertion has been challenged (Manos and Gkiouzepas 1981). Antiparkinsonian drugs available include orphenadrine (50–100 mg three times a day), benztropine (up to 6 mg daily) procyclidine (10–30 mg daily) and benzhexol (up to 5 mg three times a day). Neither levodopa nor amantidine are any use in drug-induced extrapyramidal syndromes.

Tardive dyskinesia

Tardive means belated and these dyskinesias are typically seen after several years of antipsychotic medication. Rarely, tardive dyskinesia may supervene after only a few months of treatment. The prevalence is quite high especially in in-patients on depot antipsychotics where surveys have shown about a 50 per cent prevalence. The figure is about 20–40 per cent in those taking oral medication and about half that for out-patients on oral medication. However, estimates have varied widely (Jeste and Wyatt 1981; Task Force 1980).

Tardive dyskinesia is characterized by co-ordinated, stereotyped involuntary movements, which fluctuate in severity, disappear during sleep and increase during emotional arousal (Klawans 1985). Severity can range from the barely detectable to crippling and rarely life-threatening intensity. A

Table 11.1. Signs of Tardive Dyskinesia

- Ocular Muscles
  - Blinking
  - Blepharospasm
- Facial
  - Spasms
  - Tics
  - Grimaces
- Oral
  - Pouting
  - Sucking
  - Lip smacking
  - Pursing
- Masticatory
  - Chewing
  - Lateral movements
- Lingual
  - Tongue protrusion
  - 'Fly-catching' tongue
  - Writhing movements
- Pharyngeal
  - Palatal movements
  - Swallowing
  - Abnormal sounds
- Neck
  - Retrocollis
  - Torticollis
- Trunk
  - Shoulder shrugging
  - Pelvis rotation or thrusting
  - Diaphragmatic jerks
- Rocking
  - Forced retroflexion
- Limbs
  - Finger movements
  - Wrist torsion and flexion
  - Arm writhing or ballismus
  - Ankle torsion and flexion
  - Foot tapping
  - Toe movements
- Others
  - Generalized rigidity
  - Myoclonic jerks

number of scales exist for the rating of the severity of tardive dyskinesia. Orofacial muscles are most likely to be affected but any muscles may be involved. The signs of tardive dyskinesia are shown in Table 11.1. In most cases the patient tries to hide the abnormal movements and belittles their importance. Nevertheless, the dyskinesia can be very unsightly and, at the very least, add to the problems of rehabilitating the patient in the community. Complications include mucosal ulceration, inability to wear dentures, extrusion of food from the mouth, impaired swallowing, gait, posture and even respiration, weight loss secondary to ceaseless movement, and fractures. The earliest sign of tardive dyskinesia is often a quivering of the tongue or floor of the mouth. Oral movements are most characteristic in the older, limb involvement more in the younger patients.

Dyskinesia can also occur early in treatment, with dystonias or parkinsonism and the lack of clarity in the classification of neurological side-effects of antipsychotic drugs probably stems from this. Also dyskinesias can occur for the first time when medication is discontinued, especially in children and young adults. Some of these dyskinesias are quite transient and are termed 'withdrawal dyskinesias'.

Factors predisposing to tardive dyskinesia vary in the literature. Age is an important factor both in the incidence of the condition and its reversibility:

older patients are more likely to develop an irreversible form. Females have a slightly higher incidence than males. The condition is not confined to schizophrenics. Brain damage is also implicated in a complex way. Although dyskinesias can occur in elderly people who have never taken psychotropic drugs, the relationship to antipsychotic drugs is now well established. Both dosage and duration of therapy have been implicated but no close relationship between either factor and incidence has been proved. It is quite uncertain whether some antipsychotic drugs are more likely to induce tardive dyskinesias than others. Tardive dyskinesias seem more common in patients who developed parkinsonism early in treatment which might suggest thioridazine, with its low incidence of parkinsonism, to be safer than piperazine phenothiazines and butyrophenones. The presence of akathisia also seems to be a predisposing factor (Barnes *et al.* 1983). On the other hand, anticholinergic drugs accentuate tardive dyskinesia but claims that they seem to predispose to it have not been substantiated. Nor is a challenge dose of an anticholinergic drug useful in identifying patients with covert dyskinesias (Gardos *et al.* 1984).

The extent of reversibility of tardive dyskinesia after discontinuing antipsychotic drugs is unclear. In one study, only 1 of 33 patients with tardive dyskinesia completely lost the abnormal movements within 12 months of discontinuing antipsychotic medication (Glazer *et al.* 1984). The median time to first improvement was 7 months. Partial remission of symptoms is, however, encouraging: in patients kept off medication for 18 months, the estimated probability of showing a halving of movements was nearly 90 per cent.

The most popular hypothesis for the pharmacological mechanism underlying this syndrome was that dopaminergic systems in the basal ganglia become hypersensitive to compensate for prolonged blockade of the dopaminergic receptors by the antipsychotic medication (Tarsy and Baldessarini 1977). This may be analogous to a 'denervation supersensitivity'. Thus, the initial extrapyramidal syndrome of impaired dopaminergic transmission, namely parkinsonism, wears off as supersensitivity overcomes the block; later, as the supersensitivity increases, dopaminergic overactivity is manifested as dyskinesias. This hypothesis explains some but not all clinical observations, and new hypotheses have been advanced (Gerlach and Casey 1988). Tardive dyskinesia might reflect blockade of a subset of striatal dopamine receptors or a reduced GABA turnover in striatonigral pathways.

Dyskinesias indistinguishable from neuroleptic-induced syndromes are seen in parkinsonian patients receiving too much levodopa. Withdrawal of neuroleptics uncovers or worsens tardive dyskinesia because dopaminergic overactivity is no longer partly suppressed. Dopamine agonists tend to make the condition worse. Anticholinergic drugs, by upsetting the balance of acetycholine and dopamine in the basal ganglia, worsen tardive dyskinesia; cholinergic drugs such as physostigmine temporarily improve it.

Attempts to treat tardive dyskinesia are generally unsuccessful, at least in the long run, suggesting that dopaminergic supersensitivity continues to increase (Casey 1978). Thus, increasing the dose of antipsychotic medication or substituting a high potency compound such as pimozide effects only a temporary improvement. Similarly, giving a dopamine-depleting drug such as tetrabenazine is only useful for a short while and the dysphoria and depression produced by reserpine-like drugs limit their use. Cholinergic compounds such as the precursor choline and deanol have been disappointing, as has lithium. Gaba-potentiating drugs, including sodium valproate and the benzodiazepines, show minor effects but may act non-specifically as sedatives.

When confronted by a patient developing tardive dyskinesia, the clinician should carefully assess the severity of the abnormal movements and the degree of activation of the psychosis (Simpson *et al.* 1982). Antiparkinsonian drugs should be tailed off. Neuroleptic medication should be slowly lowered in dose until total discontinuation or until the symptoms of the psychosis become troublesome. Addition of a benzodiazepine may allow a little further reduction in dose. It has been claimed that giving a dopamine agonist such as bromocriptine for a few weeks and then discontinuing it is usually followed by remission of the abnormal movements but this approach is still tentative. Similarly, the use of lithium is unestablished.

Prevention should be the goal (Crane 1977; Task Force 1980). The antipsychotic drugs should be restricted to definite major indications especially in the elderly and the brain-damaged. The lowest possible dose should be prescribed. Patients should be examined frequently to detect early signs of tardive dyskinesia, as it is usually reversible at this stage. As the incidence of tardive dyskinesia is appreciably higher in patients receiving depot injections, these should only be used when definite medical indications exist and not for administrative convenience. Antiparkinsonian drugs should be avoided wherever possible, never prescribed routinely, and withdrawn after three months or so. Drug 'holidays' were advocated at one time, when the patient is withdrawn from neuroleptics for 1–2 months every year. However, current sentiment is against such a course because of the hazard of relapse, and the severity of its consequences and evidence that intermittent therapy may predispose towards rather than protect against movement disorders.

Other 'tardive' syndromes have been described and include tardive or rebound psychosis, tardive Tourette's syndrome, tardive akathisia, and tardive dystonia. The separateness of these entities has not been established (Stahl 1985). As with tardive dyskinesia, the treatment of tardive dystonia is disappointing (Yassa *et al.* 1986).

Autonomic effects

The powerful anticholinergic effects of thioridazine and to a lesser extent chlorpromazine are manifested as dry mouth, blurred vision, difficulty in urination, and constipation. These effects are minimal with the high potency piperazine phenothiazines and butyrophenones. Usually merely troublesome, severe effects including urinary retention, paralytic ileus, and oral infection can occur, especially if the antipsychotic drug is combined with antiparkinsonian and antidepressant therapy.

The sympatholytic actions of antipsychotic drugs are due to alpha-adrenergic blocking actions and comprise orthostatic hypotension with reflex tachycardia, and delayed or inhibited ejaculation.

Endocrine and metabolic effects

The secretion of prolactin is increased by antipsychotic medication due to dopaminergic blockade. Alterations in estrogens and testosterone levels have also been reported. Galactorrhea, often with amenorrhoea, is commonly seen in women but the suggestion that breast cancer is more likely is not supported by clear data. Sexual disturbance with loss of libido may occur in men. Growth hormone levels are lowered but retardation of growth does not seem important in children maintained on phenothiazines or butyrophenones.

Weight gain is often apparent reflecting increased appetite and decreased activity. The mechanisms are complex and include alterations in glucose tolerance and insulin release, possibly mediated via hypothalamic mechanisms.

Psychological effects

Many of the antipsychotic drugs produce excessive sedation which usually wears off fairly rapidly. A few of these drugs, mainly piperazine phenothiazines, are somewhat stimulant. Dizziness and muzziness is usually due to postural hypotension.

The induction of depression by antipsychotic medication is a complex and controversial topic. Irrespective of medication, schizophrenic patients may show pronounced affective swings (Johnson 1981*a*). Schizophrenia may present initially as a depressive syndrome and suicide is 50 times more common in schizophrenics than in the general population. The relationship of affective changes to antipsychotic medication is therefore difficult to clarify. Further, the akinesia of extrapyramidal origin can be mistaken for depression. Withdrawal effects may follow the discontinuation of low-potency antipsychotic drugs such as chlorpromazine; they include insomnia, anxiety and restlessness (Chouinard *et al.* 1984).

Adverse effects

The antipsychotic drugs are associated with a long list of adverse effects, most of which, fortunately, are uncommon. Indeed some of these adverse effects have become less common over time since the introduction of the phenothiazines, cholestatic jaundice being a case in point. This syndrome is probably allergic in type as fever, eosinophilia, and rashes accompany the jaundice. An interaction between the drug and protein constituents of the bile underlies the reaction which can occur with other tricyclic drugs such as the antidepressants. The jaundice is almost always benign, remitting when the drug is stopped. Rarely, biliary cirrhosis may supervene. Routine liver function tests are a waste of time in view of the rarity of cholestatic jaundice.

Agranulocytosis is also rare, occasional cases having followed the use of chlorpromazine and thioridazine; it is almost unknown with the high potency piperazine phenothiazines, thioxanthenes, and butyrophenones. It is a particular problem with clozapine, so that weekly WBC counts are mandatory. Comprehensive monitoring systems have been set up in some countries.

Thioridazine in high dosage (over 600 mg/day) carries the risk of inducing pigmentary retinopathy and blindness. This is totally distinct from the accumulation of chlorpromazine and related compounds in cornea, lens and skin, forming purple-grey pigmentation. This effect is more common in sunny climates.

The phenothiazines, especially thioridazine, produce abnormal T-waves in the electrocardiogram perhaps by altering potassium disposition in the myocardium. Life-threatening arrhythmias are consequently more likely and may contribute to instances of sudden death in patients on phenothiazines (Brown and Kocsis 1984). Certainly, cardiac arrhythmias may occur in patients after overdoses.

Toxicity in overdose

Intentional overdoses with psychotropic drugs are very common, schizophrenic patients often attempting suicide by taking overdoses of antipsychotic medication. Accidental overdosage is seen in children. The toxicity of these drugs is low relative to the barbiturates and the tricyclic antidepressants, with a low mortality rate.

The earliest signs of overdose are drowsiness with or without agitation and confusion. Dystonias, twitching, and fits may be seen. The EEG shows prominent slow waves. Hypotension is often profound and cardiac arrhythmias may supervene. Hypothermia is common and may be profound. Anticholinergic effects are especially common with thioridazine and worsen the prognosis. Extrapyramidal reactions are usually not a problem, perhaps because they are counteracted by the anticholinergic actions of the drug.

Treatment is essentially symptomatic. The body temperature must be carefully maintained by warm blankets and heat cradles but it is easy to overcompensate, with resultant hyperthermia. Fits must be controlled with anticonvulsants despite the additional CNS depressant effects of these drugs. Dialysis is of little use because most antipsychotic drugs are highly protein bound. Gastric lavage is useful because gastric emptying may have been delayed. Hypotension is difficult to counteract, noradrenalin being relatively ineffective because of the alpha adrenergic blockade. Drugs acting directly on the blood vessels such as angiotensin have been suggested.

Management of psychosis

Choice of drug

There are now over 20 antipsychotic drugs available in the UK, and elsewhere, some of which are listed in Table 11.2. Despite thousands of comparative trials, few firm decisions can be made concerning the choice of drug in any one particular patient. Rather, a few guidelines only can be suggested. A very detailed account is given in Mason and Granacher (1980).

The therapeutic efficacy of these drugs varies very little among compounds, once dosage is taken into account (Wyatt and Torgow 1976). The major exception is promazine which is not a fully effective compound in controlling psychosis. It is none the less a useful tranquillizer in elderly confused patients. Mepazine also seems weak in its actions.

The Royal Australian and New Zealand College of Psychiatrists' Quality Assurance team broke down their data on drug trials cited earlier in terms of individual drugs. Their relative effectiveness is set out in Fig. 11.4. Obviously, where the number of trials involved is very small, conclusions as to efficacy must be tentative. However, the depot formulation of fluphenazine decanoate seems superior to some of the oral preparations including fluphenazine itself.

A similar exercise for maintenance therapy was carried out. The numbers of trials were very small but the depot preparation again had the largest effect size.

The assessment of effectiveness is itself complex. Among the many criteria are behavioural variables such as combativeness, retardation, and agitation; social variables such as fitness to live in the community, social integration and contact, and work adjustments; administrative variables operationally defined in terms of discharge and readmission rates; and psychopathological features such as thought disorders, ideas of reference and hallucinations. Schizophrenic and other psychotic patients vary in their symptom and behavioural profiles and attempts have been made to relate these differences to different profiles of drug activity. Thus, it is held by some

Table 11.2. Daily dosage ranges of some antipsychotic drugs

Drug	Out-patients	In-patients
Phenothiazines		
Chlorpromazine	75–450	200–1200
Thioridazine	75–450	150–600
Prochlorperazine	25–100	75–150
Perphenazine	8–24	12–48
Trifluoperazine	5–20	10–30
Fluphenazine decanoate	12.5–50 every 15–30 days	25–50 every 15–30 days
Thioxanthenes		
Chlorprothixene	30–60	75–400
Flupenthixol decanoate	20–80 every 15–30 days	40–80 every 15–30 days
Butyrophenones		
Haloperidol	2–10	4–200
Benzamides		
Sulpiride	400–800	800–2400

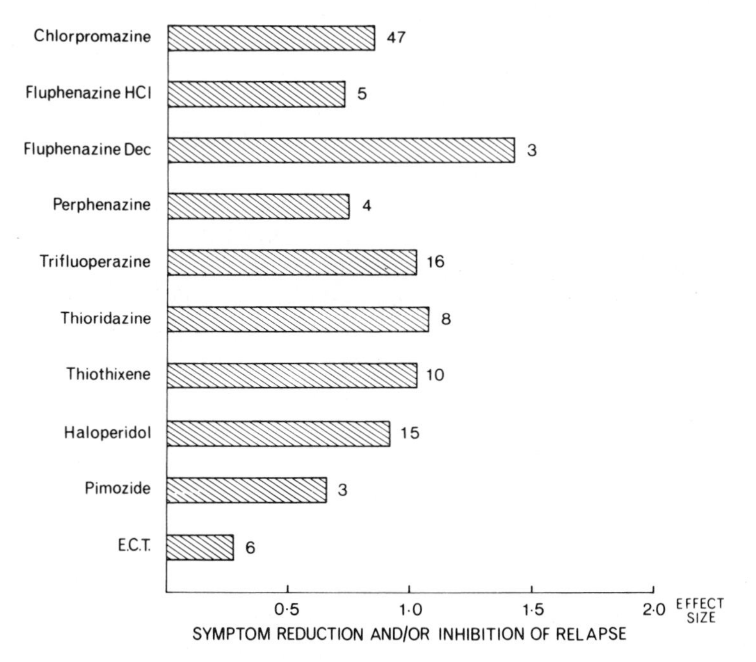

Fig 11.4. A schematic representation in effect size or standard deviation units of the power of 10 treatments used with patients with schizophrenia admitted to hospital. The length of the bars is proportional to the power of the treatment and the number of trials on which each estimate is based is set alongside each bar. (Drawn from data with permission from the Australian and New Zealand College of Psychiatrists.)

that the sedative aliphatic phenothiazines such as thioridazine and chlorpromazine are more effective against 'positive' symptoms of overactivity, hostility, anxiety, etc., whereas the more stimulant high potency compounds are useful in counteracting 'negative' featuress including passivity, social withdrawal and affective blunting. Controlled observations lend little support to this belief (Galbrecht and Klett 1968).

The most obvious differences among antipsychotic drugs concerns their unwanted effects (Richelson 1985). Chlorpromazine possesses the unfortunate combination of extrapyramidal and autonomic symptoms. Thioridazine is almost devoid of neurological problems but has major autonomic effects and is sedative; haloperidol, as a commonly used example of a high potency compound, has marked extrapyramidal effects but few sedative or autonomic effects. Patients vary in their tolerance of their unwanted effects, some finding autonomic effects a great nuisance, others responding adversely with dystonias and parkinsonism. The practitioner should become expert in the use of a few antipsychotic drugs from different regions of the spectrum of side-effects. If one drug proves intolerable to the patient then he can be switched to another type.

The substituted benzamides such as sulpiride are claimed to have less extrapyramidal side effects than conventional neuroleptics. They are also believed to be quite effective in combatting negative symptoms of schizophrenia. Although the clinical evidence is not compelling (Editorial 1984), sulpiride is worth considering in patients at particular risk of developing tardive dyskinesia.

The other decision is whether to use a depot injectable drug. If the patient's compliance is poor, fluphenazine decanoate, flupenthixol decanoate or haloperidol decanoate should be considered as the chance of relapse will be lessened by the use of a depot preparation. Compliance is assured, or if the patient defaults, that fact comes to notice; first-pass metabolism of the drug in the liver is obviated; and social support can be organized more easily from a special clinic devoted to depot injection use. Nevertheless, patients well-maintained on oral medication have little to gain from switching to depot medication and may have more chance of developing tardive dyskinesia.

Dosage

The correct dosage is that which adequately controls the patient's psychopathological state and behaviour with minimal side-effects. As the intensity of many psychotic illnesses waxes and wanes, frequent adjustment of dosage is usually necessary.

There is good evidence that quite low doses of antipsychotic medication (say 300 mg/day of chlorpromazine or equivalent) are effective in many patients (Ortiz and Gershon 1986). Consequently, one should not resort to doses higher than these until the patient has manifestly failed to respond. However, in young, male patients with severe illnesses of short duration, higher doses are usually required (Gardos *et al.* 1973).

Very high doses have been advocated by some authors especially for young acutely psychotic in-patients with relatively good prognosis. Sometimes the doses used have been astronomical, e.g. over a gram a day of haloperidol. A survey of the published controlled trials concluded that no general advantage accrued from such high doses but that unwanted effects were definitely increased (Aubree and Lader 1980). Further trials have supported this conclusion (e.g. Neborsky *et al.* 1981; van Putten and Marder 1986). High (but never very high) doses should be reserved for patients who have proved refractory to moderate doses. Thus, haloperidol 100–150 mg/day or chlorpromazine 1200–1600 mg/day represent the upper dose limits. Thioridazine should *never* be given in high dose (over 800 mg/day).

Although the plasma half-lives of some antipsychotic drugs are relatively short, once-daily dosage is still feasible, presumably because the drugs bind to central sites of action. Initially, however, divided dose schedules are preferable in order to lessen side-effects.

The dosage of depot neuroleptics can be adjusted both with respect to amount per injection and to dosage interval. Some patients require moderate dosage at long intervals, others do better on smaller doses given more frequently. Very high doses of depot neuroleptics have been used without much overall benefit compared with normal dosage (McClelland *et al.* 1976; Kane *et al.* 1986), although occasional patients seem only to respond to high doses such as 100 mg fluphenazine decanoate weekly.

The disturbed patient

'It is imperative to tranquillize the hostile, aggressive, agitated, noisy, destructive patient as quickly as possible' (Gershon and Bassuk 1980). The longer the difficult behaviour continues the more fraught become the nursing attendants, and this tension communicates itself to the patient, increasing his agitation. Calming and confident nursing is especially necessary in elderly confused patients and in schizophrenic patients with florid and terrifying symptoms (Conn and Lion 1984).

Before the antipsychotic drugs, large doses of paraldehyde, barbiturates, or opiates were administered almost to the point of anaesthesia. Some psychiatrists in developing countries with a shortage of trained staff use large doses of diazepam intravenously to rapidly quieten the patient. In Western hospital conditions chlorpromazine or haloperidol are generally used. The dosage required is difficult to predict but tends to be lower in patients not already on antipsychotic medication. Chlorpromazine 50 mg or haloperidol

5 mg intramuscularly repeated every 4 h for 24 h may then be sufficient. Some very ill patients who have relapsed while on antipsychotic medication may require very high doses. Chlorpromazine 100–200 mg or haloperidol 5–20 mg IM may need to be repeated every 2–4 h. The patient should be nursed in bed and postural hypotension may need treating by raising the foot of the bed; antiparkinsonian drugs may be needed by injection to relieve dystonias which occasionally occur.

After 12–24 h the patient is usually sufficiently co-operative to take drugs orally. The change to oral medication should be done as soon as possible to obviate the battles involved with each injection. It is important to keep the oral dosage high, usually above the intramuscular because of the wastage due to first-pass metabolism. Liquid preparations such as chlorpromazine elixir are preferable to tablets which can be hidden in the mouth and later spat out. Any difficulties with oral medication or recrudescence of disturbed behaviour will necessitate recourse to a further few injections.

The acute schizophrenic

The acutely schizophrenic patient may present in a very disturbed state or his illness may be more insidious. Withdrawal and inactivity with emotional blunting characterizes some patients; elaborate delusional systems with escape from imaginary pursuers is seen in other patients; some shout back exasperatedly at their voices; others are distraught at the weird things happening in their minds and their inability to control their thoughts, feelings and behaviour. Despite this great variety of symptom and behavioural presentations, antipsychotic drug treatment is routinely indicated, although the more detailed management of the patient depends on his type of illness (Farmer and McGuffin 1988).

Assessment of the patient is a continuing process. The diagnosis of schizophrenia is often a matter for debate, especially when the patient is suffering his first attack of psychosis. The possible precipitants of the episode should be sought and related to the content and progress of the psychosis. Prognosis depends on several factors including the presence of precipitants, the degree of preservation of affective tone, the insight of the patient, acuteness of onset and previous personality and functioning. An acute psychosis which is already subsiding on admission to hospital may not require drug therapy. The family situation, the social pressures on the patient, relationships with others, and job satisfaction are all factors which influence eventual outcome and success of reintegration into the community. They also affect management in the hospital.

Three features about schizophrenic illnesses should be borne in mind. The acute illness, especially the first one, is extremely frightening to the patient. He is overcome by foreign thoughts, he feels compelled to act strangely, he hears voices, the world becomes an alien and hostile place. Puzzlement and anxiety are therefore extreme. Secondly, there is dissolution of ego boundaries, that is, the patient is no longer sure of his own separate being. His thoughts and feelings no longer seem his own and his uniqueness as an individual is threatened. Thirdly, the senses are overloaded with a constant, confusing press of noises, sounds and smells. The outside world becomes a jumbled chaos of impressions, often frightening or inexplicable.

Management strategies must take note of these phenomena. A supportive framework is essential with the patient having a set routine to which he is made to conform. Meals should be supervised, occupational therapy encouraged and recreational activities organized. Permissiveness and lack of a coherent daily programme may hinder the patient's recovery. A closed ward is often a mercy, not a restriction of the patient's rights. He is not tempted to run away and is spared all the busy traffic of an open ward. Indeed, relapse may occur if the patient is transferred to an open ward too soon.

The staff dealing with the patient should reassure him concerning his bewildering and frightening symptoms. He must be told that his symptoms will lessen and that recovery is possible quite soon. One or two of the staff should attempt to establish a close relationship without resorting to cloying paternalism or arrogant condescension. This may be difficult especially when the patient is withdrawn or suspicious but perseverance is usually rewarded by the patient's trust and confidence. The hostile, aggressive patient must know precisely what the limits of acceptable conduct are otherwise he will establish them by trial-and-error.

The dissolution of ego boundaries may result in social withdrawal and this should be managed sympathetically. Constant exhortations to participate actively in social activities or in ward group therapy sessions may upset the patient. Visits by relatives may help in maintaining a sense of continuity with home and the outside world but can further disturb the patient.

Antipsychotic drugs help in various ways as detailed earlier. In particular they attenuate the sensory overload. The drug dosage should be established by trial-and-error. Unless the patient is becoming more disturbed the dosage can build up gradually over a week or two. Chlorpromazine or thioridazine 300 mg/day, trifluoperazine 30 mg/day or haloperidol 15 mg/day are usual initial dosages. The eventual dose is usually up to 3 times these doses (except thioridazine). Occasionally, some patients require much higher doses or the addition of a benzodiazepine before symptoms are controlled and the symptoms may recur if the dosage is lowered. Dystonia should not occur with gradual elevation of dose and parkinsonism is usually not troublesome. If it does inconvenience the patient, antiparkinsonian medication (e.g. orphenadrine 50–100 mg thrice daily; benzhexol, up to 5 mg thrice daily; procyclidine 10–30 mg daily) should be added for a few weeks. Liquid formulations are preferable to tablets especially in paranoid patients and those who are reluctant to take medication.

Improvement is manifested first by subtle modifications in symptoms. For example, delusions will yield a little to pressure and become less adamantine. Voices are heard less distinctly or become less censorious. Ego-boundaries begin to reform and the patient begins to concentrate a little better. Social contacts are less brusquely avoided, impulses better controlled. The dosage should be maintained at this level for a week or two and then slowly reduced according to the clinical state; if symptoms recur, the dose is increased; if they do not or if akathisia or drowsiness appear, the dosage is further reduced.

Failure to respond is not uncommon (Gelder and Kolakowska 1979). Often this is due to failure to take medication; tablets are thrown away or fed to the ward cat. Or the dosage may be insufficient perhaps because severe side-effects have precluded attainment of adequate dosage. Another antipsychotic drug may be more successful (Tuma and May 1979). Sometimes, response is delayed a little while so the doctor may urge patience on the nursing attendants if he detects early signs of improvement (Hogan *et al.* 1985).

Clozapine has recently been licensed in several countries for the treatment-resistant patients. Impressive efficacy data were obtained in a large-scale US study (Kane *et al.* 1988). Clozapine has a low incidence of EPS but a high incidence of blood dyscrasias (see p. 241). Its wider use will be followed with great interest.

Partly because of concern over the long-term effects of antipsychotic medication, attention has been focused on attempts to predict who will respond and who will not benefit from drug therapy. The area of prediction remains contentious but some pointers have emerged in the literature. The positive symptoms of schizophrenia such as delusions, hallucinations, and incoherence of speech are indicators of better response than negative symptoms such as anergia and withdrawal (Seeman 1985). Where intellectual and neurological impairment is present response is often poor. Where CT scan appearances are abnormal with widening of cortical sulci, cerebellar atrophy, third ventricular enlargement and reversed hemispheric assymetry, response is particularly unimpressive (Bird 1985). Adverse effects may be more marked in such patients who comprise about a half of chronic schizophrenics and upto 20 per cent of acute cases.

Women, especially premenopausal, tend to respond better to antipsychotic medication than do men. This seems to be related to oestrogen levels with some evidence that oestrogens antagonize dopamine in the brain (Seeman 1985). Some patients fail to respond apparently because previous courses of antipsychotic treatment have left them 'supersensitive' in their dopamine mechanisms, a psychiatric equivalent to tardive dyskinesia

(Chouinard and Jones 1980; Csernansky *et al.* 1985). However, by and large, in most schizophrenic patients antipsychotic therapy remains on a trial-and-error basis (Awad 1985).

Total withdrawal of antipsychotic medication may be appropriate in patients experiencing their first episode, with an acute onset, precipitating circumstances and preservation of affect. In other cases, maintenance therapy may be appropriate.

Prevention of relapse

About 20–30 per cent of patients recover from their first attack of schizophrenic-type illness without any recurrence. Consequently, it has generally been accepted that a patient who has recovered completely, is functioning normally and has been out of hospital for a few months should be withdrawn completely from medication. After subsequent attacks or if the symptoms do not resolve completely, maintenance medication should be considered. However, the value of prophylactic antipsychotic medication has been re-evaluated in the large Northwick Park Study of first episodes of schizophrenia. The interval between onset of symptoms and admission to hospital varied widely but often exceeded a year and caused great problems in the family (Johnstone *et al.* 1986). On discharge, 120 of these first-episode schizophrenics entered a randomized placebo-controlled trial of maintenance therapy. Of those on placebo, 62 per cent relapsed over the next two years or so; the figure for the drug group was 46 per cent. Long duration of illness prior to drug treatment was associated with relapse, presumably reflecting the insidious onset of the illness. However, the alternative explanation is that early intervention lessens the risk of subsequent relapse (Crow *et al.* 1986). Thus, generally speaking, outcome was poor (MacMillan *et al.* 1986*a*).

The danger of relapse varies greatly, social and interpersonal factors often being important. The consequences of relapse also sometimes vary. Some patients maintaining a precarious existence outside hospital will lose their job, lodgings, acquaintances and social support if they develop yet another episode of florid psychosis. Others with supportive families, private means and sympathetic friends may be less in jeopardy, although this state of affairs is the exception. Some schizophrenic patients deteriorate in a step-wise way and postponement of relapse may slow this process down.

Assessment of social factors, in the home, in the family and at work is a prerequisite of management. The pressure on the patient must be carefully identified and gauged. But one must not fall into the trap of ascribing all the patient's difficulties to an unsympathetic spouse or employer. The patient may have residual symptoms or behaviour deficits which make him prickly or simply ineffectual. Simple counselling of patient and family, either separately or jointly, may lessen the strains and obviate eventual relapses.

Long-term supervision should be entrusted to an experienced psychiatrist or family physician. Special supportive clinics help provide continuity and a life-line of help in emergency or when trouble brews. Medication should be entrusted to one agency to prevent confusion.

As the patient often remains well for quite long periods he has to be persuaded of the necessity of continuing medication (Soskis and Jaffe 1979). Also, relapse may be delayed some time after drug withdrawal so the patient believes the medication is irrelevant to his condition. A false sense of security may grow if the patient manages a short while without drugs despite previous such experiments culminating in relapse and readmission. Antipsychotic drugs have unpleasant effects such as tension and akathisia, and failure to modify the dosage when the patient complains of definite side effects may be followed by poor compliance (van Putten 1974).

Other patients have persistent symptoms such as auditory hallucinations or excessive fatigue. They become discouraged as to the effectiveness of the medication or may ascribe their symptoms to the drugs and not to the disease. Careful explanations are necessary to both patient and relatives.

The problem of tardive dyskinesia needs facing upto honestly. The possibility of this complication may be known to the patient who becomes reluctant to take medication. The total lack of addictive potential of the antipsychotic drugs should be emphasized as both patient and relatives may be worried by this.

If oral medication schedules are not adhered to, depot injections should be substituted. Roughly speaking, the initial dose per two weeks should be about twice the daily dose of the equivalent amount of oral fluphenazine. Thus, chlorpromazine 600 mg/day is about equal to 12 mg/day of oral fluphenazine and to 25 mg of fluphenazine decanoate injection every 2 weeks. Adjustment of both dosage and dosage interval will be necessary to stabilize the patient on the lowest effective dose. Regular attendance at the clinic is then essential and many hospitals employ special nurses to follow-up patients who default.

Patients with paranoid schizophrenic illnesses of late onset often have their symptoms completely suppressed by regular antipsychotic medication. The need for indefinite therapy should be impressed on the patient.

Depressive illnesses are a particular therapeutic problem in schizophrenic patients (Johnson 1981*a*). In view of the serious and chronic nature of the schizophrenic illness, it is hardly surprising that many patients become depressed, often chronically. Antipsychotic medication is also suspected of contributing to these affective downswings. Increase in dosage may help if the patient is really depressed but may exacerbate matters if the problem is primarily an akinesia. Sometimes change in antipsychotic medication is helpful, flupenthixol being advocated in this situation. Tricyclic antidepressants are commonly given to schizophrenic patients who become depressed, but are of limited value. Strongly anticholinergic antidepressants such as amitriptyline should be avoided if the patient is taking chlorpromazine or thioridazine already. The danger of suicide must be borne in mind. Fixed combinations of antipsychotic and antidepressant drugs are available but are not recommended because of their inherent inflexibility.

Chronic schizophrenia

Patients with chronic schizophrenia may have relapses into periods of acute symptoms as discussed above or they present persistent but not florid symptoms. They may be maintained in institutions or in the community, although the latter situation may be just as unsatisfactory with respect to the secondary handicaps of institutionalization.

The residual symptoms and handicaps are varied. One of the most difficult from the point of view of rehabilitation is anergia. The patient spends hours lying in bed or sitting in a chair, unoccupied, inert, and complaining constantly of fatigue and tiredness. Nothing interests him or motivates him to activity. Patients cannot think or talk coherently, or make any realistic plans. They see no future, remember little of the past and are uninterested in the present. Elaborate and energetic schemes to 'get them moving' such as upgrading the ward, token economies, and work ability assessment results in improvement but as soon as these efforts are relaxed, the patient relapses into torpor. Affective blunting is closely related to this state.

Other patients have a more active psychopathology. They still hear voices or harbour delusional ideas but have learned to avoid talking back to the voices or acting on the delusions. Others still do respond and are characterized by peculiar, stereotyped behaviour.

Drug therapy may help the more positive symptoms but only occasionally will a patient become activated on treatment. Nevertheless, it does occur and rehabilitation may become feasible after decades of frustration. Drug therapy must be combined with careful manipulation of the patient's environment (Freeman 1980; Quality Assurance Project 1984). Rehabilitation is a very slow process, on a time-scale of months and years rather than weeks. Discharge from hospital must be to a proper environment: too often patients are merely transferred to boarding houses in decaying seaside resorts where they relapse into their passive schizophrenic defect states. The social environment must be matched to the patient's capabilities and any remaining personality or occupational assets of the patient fully exploited (Bebbington and Kuipers 1982). Demands and stress must be optimized: too much and the patient relapses into active illness; too little and anergia supervenes. Wherever the patient is, he should feel a sense of asylum without that of neglect.

References

Abbott, R.J., and Loizou, L.A. (1986). Neuroleptic malignant syndrome. *British Journal of Psychiatry* **148,** 47–51.

Addonizio, G., Susman, V.L., and Roth, S. D. (1987). Neuroleptic malignant syndrome: review and analysis of 115 cases. *Biological Psychiatry* **22,** 1004–20.

Adler, L.A., Angrist, B., Reiter, S., and Rotrosen, J. (1989). Neuroleptic-induced akathisia: a review. *Psychopharmacology* **97,** 1–11.

Aubree, J. C., and Lader, M. H. (1980). High and very high dosage antipsychotics: a critical review. *Journal of Clinical Psychiatry* **41,** 341–50.

Awad, A.G. (1985). Prediction of response to neuroleptic drug therapy in schizophrenia. *Canadian Journal of Psychiatry* **30,** 241–2.

Barnes, T.R.E., Kidger, T., and Gore, S.M. (1983). Tardive dyskinesia: a 3-year follow-up study. *Psychological Medicine* **13,** 71–81.

Bebbington, P., and Kuipers, L. (1982). Social management of schizophrenia. *British Journal of Hospital Medicine* 396–403.

Beresford, R., and Ward, A. (1987). Haloperidol decanoate. A preliminary review of its pharmacodynamic and pharmacokinetic properties and therapeutic use in psychosis. *Drugs* **33,** 31–49.

Bird, J.M. (1985). Computed tomographic brain studies and treatment response in schizophrenia. *Canadian Journal of Psychiatry* **30,** 251–5

Brown, R.P., and Kocsis, J.H. (1984). Sudden death and antipsychotic drugs. *Hospital and Community Psychiatry* **35,** 486–91.

Brown, W.A., Laughren, T., Chisholm, E., and Williams, B.W. (1982). Low serum neuroleptic levels predict relapse in schizophrenic patients. *Archives of General Psychiatry* **39,** 998–1000.

Carlsson, A. (1977). Does dopamine play a role in schizophrenia? *Psychological Medicine* **7,** 583–97.

Caroff, S. N. (1980). The neuroleptic malignant syndrome. *Journal of Clinical Psychiatry* **41,** 79–83.

Casey, D.E. (1978). Managing tardive dyskinesia. *Journal of Clinical Psychiatry* **39,** 753–68.

Casey, J. F., Lasky, J. J., Klett, C. J., and Hollister, L.E. (1960). Treatment of schizophrenic reactions with phenothiazine derivatives. *American Journal of Psychiatry* **117,** 97–105.

Chouinard, G., and Jones, B.D. (1980). Neuroleptic-induced supersensitivity psychosis: clinical and pharmacological characteristics. *American Journal of Psychiatry* **137,** 16–21.

Chouinard, G., Bradwejn, J., Annable, L., Jones, B.D., and Ross-Chouinard, A. (1984). Withdrawal symptoms after long-term treatment with low-potency neuroleptics. *Journal of Clinical Psychiatry* **45,** 500–2.

Conn, L.M., and Lion, J.R. (1984). Pharmacologic approaches to violence. *Psychiatric Clinics of North America* **7,** 879–86.

Crane, G. E. (1977). The prevention of tardive dyskinesia. *American Journal of Psychiatry* **134,** 756–8.

Creese, I., Burt, D. R., and Snyder, S. H. (1976). Dopamine receptor binding predicts clinical and pharmacological potencies of antischizophrenic drugs. *Science* **192,** 481–3.

Crow, T.J., MacMillan, J.F., Johnson, A.L., and Johnstone, E.C. (1986). A

randomised controlled trial of prophylactic neuroleptic treatment. *British Journal of Psychiatry* **148,** 120–7.
Csernansky, J.G., Kaplan, J., and Hollister, L.E. (1985). Problems in classification of schizophrenics as neuroleptic responders and nonresponders. *Journal of Nervous and Mental Disease* **173,** 325–31.
Curry, S.H. (1985). The strategy and value of neuroleptic drug monitoring. *Journal of Clinical Psychopharmacology* **5,** 263–71.
Curry, S. H., D'Mello, A., and Mould, G. P. (1971). Destruction of chlorpromazine during absorption in the rat *in vivo* and *in vitro*. *British Journal of Pharmacology* **42,** 403–11.
Curry, S. H., Marshall, J. H. L., Davis, J. M., and Janowsky, D. S. (1970). Chlorpromazine plasma level and effects. *Archives of General Psychiatry* **22,** 289–96.
Davis, J. M. (1975). Overview; Maintenance therapy in schizophrenia. 1. Schizophrenia. *American Journal of Psychiatry* **132,** 1237–65.
Dencker, S.J., Malm, U., and Lepp, M. (1986). Schizophrenic relapse after drug withdrawal is predictable. *Acta Psychiatrica Scandanavica* **73,** 181–5.
Editorial (1984). Neuroleptic malignant syndrome. *Lancet* **1,** 545–6.
Editorial (1984). Sulpiride: an advance in neuroleptics? *Drug and Therapeutics Bulletin* **22,** 31–2.
Farde, L., Wiesel, F.-A., Halldin, C., and Sedvall, G. (1988). Central D2-dopamine receptor occupancy in schizophrenic patients treated with antipsychotic drugs. *Archives of General Psychiatry*, **45,** 71–6.
Farmer, A., and McGuffin, P. (1988). The pathogenesis and management of schizophrenia. *Drugs* **35,** 177–85.
Freeman, H.L. (1980). Coping with schizophrenia. *British Journal of Hospital Medicine* **23,** 54–8.
Freyhan, F. A. (1959). Therapeutic implications of differential effects of new phenothiazine compounds. *American Journal of Psychiatry* **115,** 577–85.
Gaind, R. N., and Barnes, T. R. E. (1981). Depot neuroleptic clinics. In *Handbook of Biological Psychiatry*, Part VI (eds H. M. van Praag, M. H. Lader, O.J. Rafaelsen, and E. J. Sachar) pp. 149–79. Marcel Dekker, New York.
Galbrecht, C. R., and Klett, C. J. (1968). Predicting response to phenothiazines: the right drug for the right patient. *Journal of Nervous and Mental Disease* **147,** 173–83.
Gardos, G., Cole, J. O., and Orzack, M. H. (1973). The importance of dosage in antipsychotic drug administration—A review of dose-response studies. *Psychopharmacologia* **29,** 221–30.
Gardos, G., Cole, J.O., Rapkin, R.M., LaBrie, R.A., Baquelod, E., Moore, P., Sovner, R., and Doyle, J. (1984). Anticholinergic challenge and neuroleptic withdrawal. *Archives of General Psychiatry* **41,** 1030–5.
Gelder, M., and Kolakowska, T. (1979). Variability of response to neuroleptics in schizophrenia: clinical, pharmacologic, and neuroendocrine correlates. *Comprehensive Psychiatry* **20,** 397–408.
Gerlach, J., and Casey, D.E. (1988). Tardive dyskinesia. *Acta Psychiatrica Scandinavica* **77,** 369–78.
Gershon, S., and Bassuk, E. (1980). Psychiatric emergencies: an overview. *American Journal of Psychiatry* **137,** 1–11.
Gibb, W.R.G., and Lees, A.J. (1985). The neuroleptic malignant syndrome—a review. *Quarterly Journal of Medicine* **220,** 421–9.

Gibb, W.R.G., and Lees, A.J. (1986). The clinical phenomenon of akathisia. *Journal of Neurology, Neurosurgery and Psychiatry* **49,** 861–6.

Glazer, W.M., Moore, D.C., Schooler, N.R., Brenner, L.M., and Morgenstern, H. (1984). Tardive dyskinesia: a discontinuation study. *Archives of General Psychiatry* **41,** 623–27.

Gunderson, J.G. (1986). Pharmacotherapy for patients with borderline personality disorder. *Archives of General Psychiatry* **43,** 698–700.

Hanlon, T. E., Michaux, M. H., Ota, K. Y., Shaffer, J. W., and Kurland, A. A. (1965). The comparative effectiveness of eight phenothiazines. *Psychopharmacologia* **7,** 89–106.

Heilizer, F. (1960). A critical review of some published experiments with chlorpromazine in schizophrenic, neurotic and normal humans. *Journal of Chronic Disease* **11,** 102–48.

Hogan, T.P., Awad, A.G., and Eastwood. M.R. (1985). Early subjective response and prediction of outcome to neuroleptic drug therapy in schizophrenia. *Canadian Journal of Psychiatry* **30,** 246–51.

Hogarty, G. E., and Ulrich, R. F. (1977). Temporal effects of drug and placebo in delaying relapse in schizophrenic out-patients. *Archives of General Psychiatry* **34,** 297–301.

Hogarty, G. E. *et al.* (1974*a*). Drug and socio-therapy in the aftercare of schizophrenic patients. II. Two-year relapse rates. *Archives of General Psychiatry* **31,** 603–8.

Hogarty, G. E. *et al.* (1974b). Drug and socio-therapy in the aftercare of schizophrenic patients. III. Adjustment of nonrelapsed patients. *Archives of General Psychiatry* **31,** 609–19.

Jann, M.W., Ereshefsky, L., and Saklad, S.R. (1985). Clinical pharmacokinetics of the depot antipsychotics. *Clinical Pharmacokinetics* **10,** 315–33.

Jeste, D. V., and Wyatt, R. J. (1981). Changing epidemiology of tardive dyskinesia: an overview. *American Journal of Psychiatry* **138,** 297–309.

Johnson, D. A. W. (1976). The expectation of outcome from maintenance therapy in chronic schizophrenic patients. *British Journal of Psychiatry* **128,** 246–50.

Johnson, D. A. W. (1977). Practical considerations in the use of depot neuroleptics for the treatment of schizophrenia. *British Journal of Hospital Medicine* **17,** 546–58.

Johnson, D. A. W. (1978). Prevalence and treatment of drug-induced extrapyramidal symptoms. *British Journal of Psychiatry* **132,** 27–30.

Johnson, D. A. W. (1981*a*). Studies of depressive symptoms in schizophrenia. *British Journal of Psychiatry* **139,** 89–101.

Johnson, D.A.W. (1981*b*). Drug-induced psychiatric disorders. *Drugs* **22,** 57–69.

Johnson, D.A.W. (1982). The long-acting depot neuroleptics. In *Recent advances in clinical psychiatry* (ed. K. Granville-Grossman) pp. 243–60. Churchill Livingstone, Edinburgh.

Johnson, D.A.W. (1984). Observations on the use of long-acting depot neuroleptic injections in the maintenance therapy of schizophrenia. *Journal of Clinical Psychiatry* **45,** sec. 2, 13–21.

Johnstone, E.C., Crow, T.J., Johnson, A.L., and MacMillan, J.F. (1986). The Northwick Park study of first episodes of schizophrenia. I. Presentation of the illness and problems relating to admission. *British Journal of Psychiatry* **148,** 115–20.

Kane, J.M. (1983). Problems of compliance in the outpatient treatment of schizophrenia. *Journal of Clinical Psychiatry* **44 sec. 2,** 3–6.

Kane, J.M., Honigfeld, G., Singer, J., and Meltzer, H. (1988). Clozapine in treatment-resistant schizophrenics. *Psychopharmacology Bulletin*, **24,** 62–7.

Kane, J.M., Woerner, M., and Sarantakos, S. (1986). Depot neuroleptics: a comparative review of standard, intermediate, and low-dose regimens. *Journal of Clinical Psychiatry* **47,** sec. 2, 30–3.

Kessler, K. A., and Waletzky, J. P. (1981). Clinical use of the antipsychotics. *American Journal of Psychiatry* **138,** 202–9.

Klar, H., and Siever, L.J. (1984). The psychopharmacologic treatment of personality disorders. *Psychiatric Clinics of North America* **4,** 791–801.

Klawans, H.L. (1985). Recognition and diagnosis of tardive dyskinesia. *Journal of Clinical Psychiatry*, **46** sec. 2, 3–7.

Klein, D. F., and Davis, J. M. (1969). *Diagnosis and drug treatment of psychiatric disorders*. Williams & Wilkins, Baltimore.

Krska, J., Sampath, G., Shah, A., and Soni, S.D. (1986). Radio receptor assay of serum neuroleptic levels in psychiatric patients. *British Journal of Psychiatry* **148,** 187–93.

Kucharski, L.T., Alexander, P., Tune, L., and Coyle, J. (1984). Serum neuroleptic concentrations and clinical response: a radioreceptor assay investigation of acutely psychotic patients. *Psychopharmacology* **82,** 194–8.

Leff, J., and Vaughn, C. (1981). The role of maintenance therapy and relatives' expressed emotion in relapse of schizophrenia: a two-year follow-up. *British Journal of Psychiatry* **139,** 102–4.

Leff, J.P and Wing, J.K. (1971). Trial of maintenance therapy in schizophrenia. *British Medical Journal* **3,** 599–604.

MacMillan, J.F., Crow, T.J., Johnson, A.L., and Johnstone, E.C. (1986*a*). III. Short-term outcome in trial entrants and trial eligible patients. *British Journal of Psychiatry* **148,** 128–33.

MacMillan, J.F., Gold, A., Crow, T.J., Johnson, A.L., and Johnstone, E.C. (1986*b*). IV. Expressed emotion and relapse. *British Journal of Psychiatry* **148,** 133–43.

McClelland, H.A., Farquharson, R.G., and Leyburn, P., *et al.*, (1976). Very high dose fluphenazine decanoate. A controlled trial in chronic schizophrenia. *Archives of General Psychiatry* **33,** 1435–9.

Mann, S.A., and Cree, W. (1976). 'New' long-stay psychiatric patients: a national sample survey of fifteen mental hospitals in England and Wales 1972/3. *Psychological Medicine* **6,** 603–16.

Manos, N., and Gkiouzepas, J. (1981). Discontinuing antiparkinson medication in chronic schizophrenics. *Acta Psychiatrica Scandinavica* **63,** 28–32.

Martin, I.C.A. (1975). Implications of phenothiazine side effects: a study of antiparkinsonian agents in an older population. *Acta Psychiatrica Scandinavica* **51,** 110–18.

Mason, A.S., and Granacher, R.P. (1980). *Clinical handbook of anti-psychotic drug therapy*. Brunner/Mazel, New York.

May, P.R.A. (1968). *Treatment of schizophrenia: A comparative study of five treatment methods*. Science House, New York.

May, R.R.A. (1976). Schizophrenia—A follow-up study of results of treatment. *Archives of General Psychiatry* **33,** 474–8.

May, P.R.A., and van Putten, T. (1978). Plasma levels of chlorpromazine in schizophrenia: A critical review of the literature. *Archives of General Psychiatry* **35,** 1081–7.

Meltzer, H.Y. (1986). Novel approaches to the pharmacotherapy of schizophrenia. *Drug Development Research* **9,** 23–40.

National Institute of Mental Health Psychopharmacology Service Center Collaborative Study Group (1964). Phenothiazine treatment in acute schizophrenia. *Archives of General Psychiatry* **10,** 246–61.

Neborsky, R., Janowsky, D., Munson, E., and Depry, D. (1981). Rapid treatment of acute psychotic symptoms with high- and low-dose haloperidol. *Archives of General Psychiatry* **38,** 195–9.

Nishikawa, T., Tsuda, A., Tanaka, M., Hoaki, Y., Koga, I., and Uchida, Y. (1984). Prophylactic effect of neuroleptics in symptom-free schizophrenics: a comparative dose–response study of haloperidol and propericiazine. *Psychopharmacology* **82,** 153–6.

Ortiz, A., and Gershon, S. (1986). The future of neuroleptic psychopharmacology. *Journal of Clinical Psychiatry* **47,** sec. 2, 3–11.

Pasamanick, B., Scarpittin, F.R., and Lefton, M., *et al.* (1964). Home vs. hospital care for schizophrenics. *Journal of the American Medical Association* **187,** 177–81.

Peroutka, S.J., and Snyder, S.H. (1980). Relationship of neuroleptic drug effects at brain dopamine, serotonin, α-adrenergic, and histamine receptors to clinical potency. *American Journal of Psychiatry* **137,** 1518–22.

Pfeffer, J.M. (1981). Management of the acutely disturbed patient on the general ward. *British Journal of Hospital Medicine* **26,** 73–8.

Quality Assurance Project (1984). Treatment outlines for the management of schizophrenia. *Australian and New Zealand Journal of Psychiatry* **18,** 19–38.

Ratey, J.J., and Salzman, C. (1984). Recognizing and managing akathisia. *Hospital and Community Psychiatry* **35,** 975–7.

Richelson, E. (1985). Pharmacology of neuroleptics in use in the United States. *Journal of Clinical Pyschiatry* **46,** sec. 2, 8–14.

Rupniak, N.M.J., Jenner, P., and Marsden, C.D. (1986). Acute dystonia induced by neuroleptic drugs. *Psychopharmacology* **88,** 403–19.

Sakalis, G., Chan, T.L., Gershon, S., and Park, S. (1973). The possible role of metabolites in therapeutic response to chlorpromazine treatment. *Psychopharmacologia* **32,** 279–84.

Seeman, M.V. (1985). Clinical and demographic correlates of neuroleptic response. *Canadian Journal of Psychiatry* **30,** 243–5.

Shalev, A., and Munitz, H. (1986). The neuroleptic malignant syndrome: agent and host interaction. *Acta Psychiatrica Scandinavica* **73,** 337–47.

Simpson, G.M., Pi, E.H., and Sramek, J.J. (1981). Adverse effects of antipsychotic agents. *Drugs* **21,** 138–51.

Simpson, G.M., Pi, E.H., and Sramek, J.J. (1982). Management of tardive dyskinesia: current update. *Drugs* **23,** 381–93.

Siris, S.G., van Kammen, D.P., and Docherty, J.P. (1978). Use of antidepressant drugs in schizophrenia. *Archives of General Psychiatry* **35,** 1368–77.

Snyder, S.H. (1981). Dopamine receptor, neuroleptics and schizophrenia. *American Journal of Psychiatry* **138,** 460–6.

Soskis, D.A., and Jaffe, R.L. (1979). Communicating with patients about antipsychotic drugs. *Comprehensive Psychiatry* **20,** 126–31.

Stahl, S.M. (1985). Akathisia and tardive dyskinesia. *Archives of General Psychiatry* **42,** 915–17.

Stevens, B.C. (1973). Role of fluphenazine decanoate in lessening the burden of chronic schizophrenics on the community. *Psychological Medicine* **3,** 161–8.

Szabadi, E. (1984). Neuroleptic malignant syndrome. *British Medical Journal* **288,** 1399–1400.

Tang, S.W. (1985). Prediction of treatment response in schizophrenia: clinical use of neuroleptic blood levels. *Canadian Journal of Psychiatry* **30,** 249–250.

Tarsy, D., and Baldessarini, R.J. (1977). The pathophysiologic basis of tardive dyskinesia. *Biological Psychiatry* **12,** 431–50.

Task Force on Late Neurological Effects of Antipsychotic Drugs (1980). Tardive dyskinesia: summary of a Task Force report of the American Psychiatric Association. *American Journal of Psychiatry* **137,** 1163–72.

Tuma, A.H., and May, P.R.A. (1979). And if that doesn't work, what next . . .? A study of treatment failures in schizophrenics. *Journal of Nervous and Mental Disease* **167,** 566–71.

van Putten, T. (1974). Why do schizophrenic patients refuse to take their drugs. *Archives of General Psychiatry* **31,** 67–72.

van Putten, T., and Marder, S.R. (1986). Low-dose treatment strategies. *Journal of Clinical Psychiatry* **47,** sec. 2, 12–16.

Vaughn, C.E., and Leff, J.P. (1976). The influence of family and social factors on the course of psychiatric illness. *British Journal of Psychiatry* **129,** 125–37.

Watt, D.C. (1975). Time to evaluate long-acting neuroleptics? *Psychological Medicine* **5,** 222–6.

Weinberger, D.R.., Bigelow, L.B., Kleinman, J.E., Klein, S.T., Rosenblatt, J.E., and Wyatt, R.J. (1980). Cerebral ventricular enlargement in chronic schizophrenia. An association with poor responses to treatment. *Archives of General Psychiatry*. **37,** 11–13.

Wyatt, R.J., and Torgow, J.S. (1976). A comparison of equivalent clinical potencies of neuroleptics as used to treat schizophrenia and affective disorders. *Journal of Psychiatric Research* **13,** 91–8.

Yassa, R., Nair, V., and Dimitry, R. (1986). Prevalence of tardive dystonia. *Acta Psychiatrica Scandinavica* **73,** 629–33.

12. Anxiety and antianxiety medication

Anxiety is an ubiquitous emotion within everyone's experience (Sartorius 1980). It is important in psychiatry because it is found in many mental illnesses as a secondary phenomenon as well as constituting a syndrome in its own right, the anxiety state. It presents in many forms and comprises a multitude of symptoms, psychological and somatic. It is an unpleasant emotion, so that many of those who experience it urgently seek relief. It is hardly surprising, therefore, that drugs used to assuage anxiety, the tranquillizers, are among the most widely-used of all drugs (Tyrer 1984).

The management of patients with anxiety requires a judicious mixture of psychotherapy, social help, re-education, and drug therapy, the balance of these components varying from subject to subject according to factors such as the type of anxiety, the personality of the sufferer and his symptom pattern. Before focusing on the drug treatment, an outline of anxiety syndromes will be presented; for a fuller account, reference should be made to Lader and Marks (1971), Fann *et al.* (1979), and Burrows and Davies (1980).

Syndromes of anxiety

Anxiety is a subjective feeling of uneasiness and apprehension about some undefined threat in the future. It is this ineffable character which underlies its unpleasant nature. In particular fears, the threat is physical, with implications of physical harm or even death, or psychological, with especial implications for self-esteem; but when the emotion evoked is anxiety, these threats cannot be identified. If a threat can be found, if the threat is recognizable and if it seems appropriate in size, then the apprehension evoked is labelled 'fear'. Fear is usually easier to cope with, because the threat is obvious. To recapitulate, anxiety is an ineffable feeling of apprehension and dread, for which no precipitating cause is apparent or is out of proportion to the emotion produced (Lewis 1967).

The distinction between normal and neurotic anxiety relates to this factor of precipitant. In anxiety, the individual is responding normally to multiple or diffuse threats, identifiable but less easily defined. These threats are multifarious: imminent redundancy or repeated disappointments in finding a job, trouble with the law, criminal or civil, a sexual entanglement, inability to cope at work with workmates or superiors, desertion of a spouse or discovery of infidelity in a spouse, impending financial ruin, the sudden death of close relatives or friends, the serious illness of a child, sports injuries severe enough to necessitate abandoning that sport, forced marriage due to an unwanted pregnancy, civil or military disturbances , threats of personal physical violence. Sometimes such threats are repeated and it is only after some repetitions that anxiety is evoked; other threats are rare events. The term 'stress' is frequently used in this context but it is so ill-defined a concept with many complex overtones that it is less meaningful than the idea of threat.

Neurotic anxiety is an excessive, inappropriate response to the threat, if one, indeed, can be identified. Thus, internal factors in the individual are important, the anxiety reflecting an interaction between the predisposition in the patient (Torgersen, 1983) and the external event. The anxiety is even more disturbing than normal anxiety because its sources are baffling to the patient. Often he will search around desperately for causes for his disabling symptoms and may be mistaken in his attributions. Neurotic anxiety stems from the special symbolic meaning which an external threat has for an individual. Feelings may be provoked which are conflicting; for example, aggressive or sexual impulses may be provoked by an interpersonal situation which the patient is unable to discuss. Instead of analysing and coming to terms with the situation, and resolving the conflict, the patient with neurotic anxiety remains ambivalent and threatened.

Of course, not everyone with anxiety seeks medical help. Surveys of various sorts have suggested that perhaps as many as 1 in 3 of the adult population suffers from anxiety at some time during the course of each year. About a half (i.e. 15 per cent of adults) will consult their family physician with anxiety and stress-related problems. Of these, less than 5 per cent are referred for a specialist opinion. The definition of clinical anxiety is operational: it is an anxiety which is too severe, too persistent or too pervasive for the person to tolerate so that he seeks medical advice. Personal tolerance is crucial here; some individuals cope with anxiety levels which others would find completely overwhelming. Women preponderate 2:1 (Reich 1986).

Further distinctions can be made. One is between state and trait anxiety. State anxiety refers to anxiety at a particular instant in time; trait anxiety implies an enduring personality predisposition, the anxious temperament. The factors underlying marked trait anxiety are uncertain but genetic, developmental, and emotional learning experiences are all important to differing extents in different individuals. The clinical version of state anxiety comprises the person who is normally calm but then suffers attacks of anxiety for which he seeks help. Clinical trait anxiety is recognized in the person of an anxious disposition who finds the life-long worries becoming increasingly unbearable. Typically, the two types of syndromes coexist. External events interact with the anxious temperament to produce symptoms.

Anxiety may be 'free-floating', i.e. present fairly constantly no matter where and when, or situational (phobic) when panics are elicited by certain situations, often social, or particular objects. The two types often occur together, a background level of free-floating anxiety being exacerbated by particular situations. The patient quickly learns to avoid these obvious precipitants but is nonplussed by the high level of meaningless, apparently spontaneous background anxiety. But in some patients even the panic attacks seem without cause.

Finally, an almost infinite variety of symptom patterns are found in anxious patients. A useful dichotomy is into psychological and physiological symptoms. Many of the latter can be understood as manifestations of excessive activity of the symptomatic nervous system, particularly affecting the heart (Skerritt 1983). Indeed, from time to time, cardiac abnormalities are regarded as important in the causation of anxiety states. The most recent of these 'discoveries' is the attempt to relate some symptoms of anxiety to mitral valve prolapse of the heart. As most instances of mitral valve prolapse are variants of normal, the relationship to anxiety remains unproved (Oakley 1984). Accordingly, as shown in Table 12.1, almost every organ system in the body can be affected. Palpitations, tremor, and gastro-intestinal symptoms are the commonest physical symptoms; apprehension, irritability, depersonalization, and fear of collapse are the most usual psychological symptoms. Any symptom can form the focus of the patient's anxiety state. Thus, a diffuse anxiety state can become increasingly specific both with respect to the apparent precipitants and the selective nature of the symptoms. Ultimately, patients may become monosymptomatic, complaining of palpitations or tension in the head. Patients referred for investigation of chest pain in whom investigations are negative are often anxious and depressed (Channer *et al.* 1985).

Antianxiety drugs

Definitions

The term 'sedative' originally meant that which has the property of allaying, assuaging, or calming. More recently it has come to imply feelings of drowsiness or torpor, a state originally called 'oversedation', and often attributed to the barbiturates and other older drugs such as chloral. In place of sedative, the term 'tranquillizer' has been introduced in an attempt to distinguish

Table 12.1. Symptoms of Anxiety

	Symptoms	Differential diagnosis
Psychological	Anxiety Nervousness Fear Panic Apprehension and anticipation of the worst	Early schizophrenia Drug abuse, especially amphetamine and cocaine Excessive use of caffeine Temporal lobe epilepsy
Cardiovascular	Palpitations Rapid heart beat Tightness in chest Face flushing	Cardia dysrrhythmias Angina, hypertension Pheochromocytoma
Respiratory	Breathlessness Air hunger Paresthesiae	Asthma Respiratory failure Neurological conditions
Gastrointestinal	Difficulty swallowing Nausea and vomiting Diarrhoea	Oesophageal pathology Gastric pathology Ulcerative colitis
Genitourinary	Frequency of micturition Impotence and premature ejaculation Frigidity	Bladder pathology Neurological conditions
Skin	Sweating	Thyrotoxicosis
Somatic	Aches and pains Headache Restlessness Fatigue Tremors	Rheumatology conditions Migraine Chronic infections e.g. TB Neurological conditions
Sleep Nightmares	Insomnia	Specific syndromes (see p. 306)
General/metabolic	Dizziness Faintness	Hypoglycaemia Adrenal insufficiency

Derived from items in Zung (1975), and Hamilton (1959) Anxiety Scales.

in the practitioner's schema of drugs between the older sedatives and the newer drugs, particularly the benzodiazepines. But this distinction is mainly specious as, apart from safety in overdosage, the benzodiazepines sufficiently resemble the barbiturates to justify sharing the same class. Sometimes the word 'tranquillizer' is qualified by the adjective 'minor' to distinguish these drugs from the 'major tranquillizers' or antipsychotic drugs. However, the minor tranquillizers are certainly not minor in their extent of usage or in their value to the truly anxious.

Another term enjoying some popularity is 'anxiolytic', a word of dubious etymology. In line with the antidepressants and the antipsychotic drugs, we will use the term 'antianxiety medications' while deprecating the unnecessary change in usage of 'sedative'.

History

The use of anxiety-allaying drugs goes back thousands of years to the discovery that grape-juice (and grain-mash further north) was fermentable and that alcohol possessed beguiling psychotropic properties. Opium derivatives were known in the Middle and Far East and to the ancient Greeks. Other herbal remedies were discovered but opium and alcohol remained the mainstays of treatment until the last century, being used as anaesthetics, to subdue disturbed lunatics, to allay anxiety and to induce sleep.

The nineteenth century saw the development of inorganic, and later, organic chemistry. Bromides were introduced as sedatives and became widely used. Their poor effectiveness, cumulative toxicity and potential abuse became apparent by the 1930s. Even so, 20 years ago some mental hospitals routinely screened all newly admitted patients for serum bromide levels to detect the occasional bromide-induced toxic psychosis, and bromides have only recently been removed from the UK market.

Organic chemists in the second half of the nineteenth century developed anaesthetics such as ether and chloroform and sedatives such as chloral and paraldehyde. Chloral still has some therapeutic usefulness but paraldehyde is unpleasant to take, prone to abuse and may induce psychotic states. The last of the important nineteenth century sedatives were the barbiturates. Many different compounds were introduced, divided into the ultra-short acting (e.g. anaesthetic induction agents such as thiopentone), short-acting (e.g. quinalbarbitone), medium-acting (e.g. butobarbitone) and the long-acting (e.g. phenobarbitone). In fact, it is now apparent that thiopentone owes its short action to its redistribution phase in the body after intravenous administration, and apart from a few long-acting compounds such as phenobarbitone the rest are of medium duration with half-lives of 16 h or so.

As with the bromides, it has taken over 50 years for the disadvantages of the barbiturates to become apparent. The side-effect of drowsiness, tolerance to their effects, dangers of overdose, and the likelihood of physical and psychological dependence with consequent dangerous withdrawal syndromes led to a growing dissatisfaction with these drugs (Allgulander 1986). Thus the scene was set for the phenomenal short-lived success of meprobamate. This drug was developed from mephenesin, which was a muscle relaxant with its primary action on the spinal cord (Berger 1970). Meprobamate was introduced as the first of the tranquillizers but its advantages over the barbiturates proved nugatory. It is still used as a sedative and muscle relaxant. Other non-barbiturate sedatives and hypnotics were developed including glutethimide, methyprylon, ethchlorvynol, and the ill-fated thalidomide. The eager acceptance of these newer drugs evinced the growing dissatisfaction with the barbiturates, but in turn dissatisfaction with the non barbiturate substitutes set in.

The discovery of the benzodiazepines provides yet another instance of serendipity with psychotropic agents. In the 1930s, Sternbach in Poland became interested in the heptoxdiazepines, compounds with seven-membered rings (Cohen 1970). Twenty years later, by then working for Roche Laboratories, Sternbach decided to screen these compounds for biological activity. He soon found that the compounds as synthesized were actually quinazoline derivatives with six-membered rings. Forty derivatives were synthesized but were biologically inert. The last compound, a methylamine derivative, was not tested but labelled RO 5–0690 and put aside. In 1957, this compound was finally tested after a clean up at the laboratory and was found to have similar actions to meprobamate in cats but with several times the potency. Further evaluation followed but it was some time before the chemical structure of this compound, called chlordiazepoxide, was established. It turned out to have a seven-membered ring, the methylamine being incorporated into the quinazoline ring to form a 1:4 benzodiazepine. Well over a thousand benzodiazepines and related compounds have been synthesized, including diazepam, the most widely used of all (Fig. 12.1).

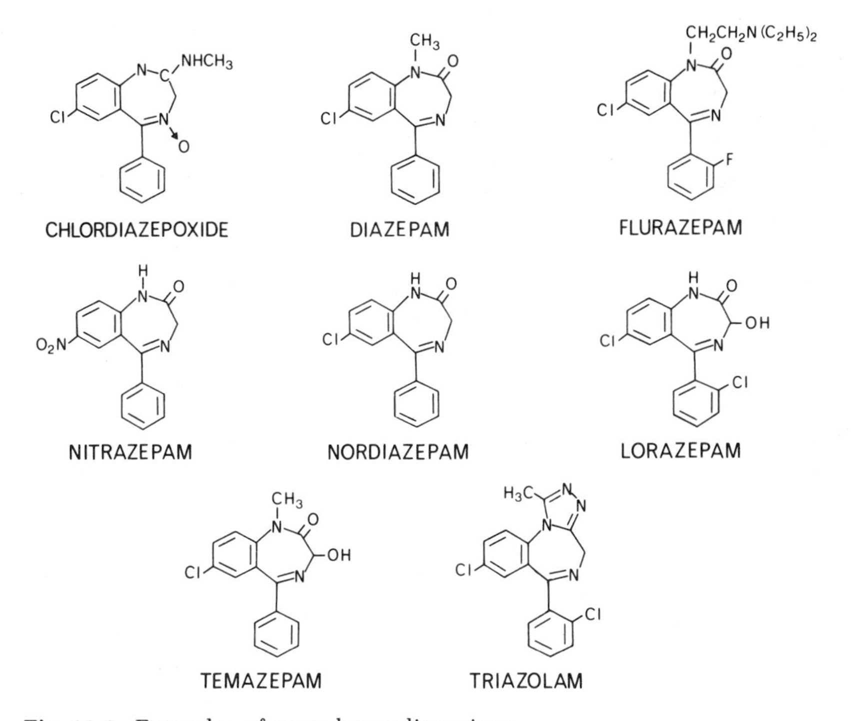

Fig. 12.1. Formulae of some benzodiazepines.

The benzodiazepines

The use of barbiturates as antianxiety agents has declined steadily to the point where they can be judged obsolescent and superceded by the benzodiazepines. The only barbiturate occupying a major therapeutic niche is phenobarbitone in the management of certain forms of epilepsy. Several reasons can be adduced for the ousting of the barbiturates by the benzodiazepines. Of these reasons, that of the safety in overdose of the benzodiazepines as compared to barbiturate toxicity is sufficient for one to prefer the newer drugs.

Nevertheless, a succession of misgivings concerning the benzodiazepines has become evident (Clinthorne *et al.* 1986). Their widespread use, even overuse, (the 'benzodiazepine bonanza', Tyrer 1974) and the possibility of dependence even at normal therapeutic dose led to pleas for greater discretion in prescribing. At the time of writing, however, the prime drug treatment for anxiety remains the prescription of one or other benzodiazepine. These drugs are also widely used by many physicians for patients with depression, circulatory disorders, tension headaches and pains in chest and back and digestive disorders (Lasagna 1977).

Pharmacokinetics

For the prescriber, two aspects of the pharmacokinetics of the benzodiazepine are germane, the speed of onset of action and the duration of action. The speed of onset depends on the mode of administration and the penetration time to the brain. Thus, diazepam enters the brain rapidly so that given intravenously it is a rapidly effective anticonvulsant in the treatment of status epilepticus. Given orally it is rapidly absorbed and exerts a prompt effect in panic states. By contrast, oxazepam is more slowly absorbed and takes some time to penetrate the brain. Clorazepate takes a little longer than diazepam. Lorazepam is also fairly rapid in onset, and although temazepam enters the brain more rapidly than oxazepam, it still takes an appreciable time. With temazepam, formulation is also important: the soft capsules are associated with rapid availability for absorption from the gut, the hard capsules with belated absorption. As with some barbiturates, the redistribution phase is important in determining the duration of action of some benzodiazepines. Examples are diazepam, temazepam, and flunitrazepam whose duration of action is shorter than the elimination half-life would predict.

The metabolic half-lives of the benzodiazepines also vary greatly (Fig. 12.2). The key compound is *N*-desmethyldiazepam (nordiazepam), the major and active metabolite of diazepam. It has a long half-life, about 60 h. Thus, it accumulates over the first month of treatment reaching higher levels than the parent compound. Desmethyldiazepam is also the major

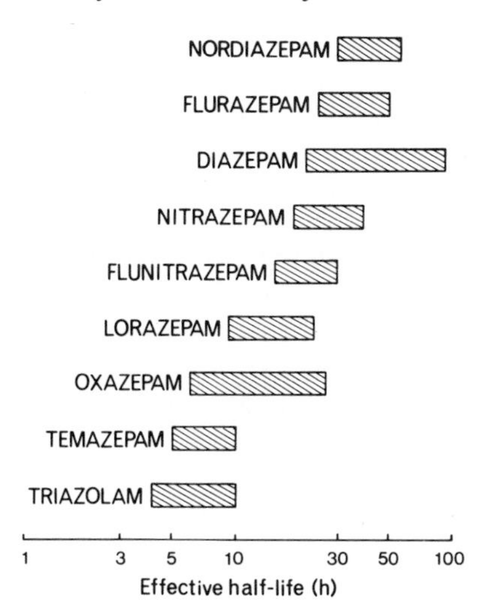

Fig.12.2. Half-lives of some benzodiazepines.

metabolite of clorazepate, medazepam, prazepam, ketazolam, and to a large extent of chlordiazepoxide. Consequently, after the initial week or two of treatment, the clinical effects of these drugs will be similar. Clobazam also has a long-acting metabolite. Metabolism of these drugs is even slower in the elderly and in patients with liver damage (Klotz *et al.* 1975).

In contrast, lorazepam (Ameer and Greenblatt 1981), oxazepam and temazepam have half-lives averaging 12 hours or less. They possess a 3-hydroxyl grouping which permits glucuronide formation and excretion. Liver damage has to be severe before the metabolism of these drugs is affected. Triazolam is even shorter acting, its half life being less than 4 h (Eberts *et al.* 1981). Flurazepam also has a short life but it has an active metabolite, *N*-desalkylflurazepam, which has a half-life of 80 hours or more. Nitrazepam, another hypnotic, also has a fairly long half-life, averaging 30 h.

Both chlordiazepoxide and diazepam are erratically absorbed after intramuscular injection. If sedation is required urgently, slow intravenous injection should be resorted to.

In summary, diazepam and other compounds metabolized to *N*-desmethyldiazepam have a rapid onset of action; some are short in duration of action because of a pronounced redistribution phase; the 3-hydroxy compounds such as oxazepam are fairly short in duration of action; other compounds have long elimination half-lives and accumulate on repeated administration. Some marketed hypnotics are appropriately short-acting but others would be expected to produce 'hangover' and sedative actions during the day, especially on repeated administration. A number of studies have examined the relationship between plasma benzodiazepine concentrations and clinical response but no clinically useful conclusions have been drawn.

Basic pharmacology

The mode of action of the benzodiazepines as with other anxiolytic drugs was obscure until recently. It now seems that the benzodiazepines potentiate the inhibitory neurotransmitter, gamma aminobutyric acid (GABA) (Paul *et al.* 1981). It has been estimated that this transmitter is involved in 40 per cent of all synapses, making it the most ubiquitous of all neurotransmitters. Any drugs potentiating GABA would have widespread inhibitory actions. The mechanism of the potentiation is unclear (Ehlert 1986). Benzodiazepines do not act directly on GABA receptors but have their own receptors. The natural transmitter acting on benzodiazepine-binding receptors has not to date been identified with certainty, although several candidates have been suggested. Barbiturates do not bind to these receptors but have a less specific action on ionic mechanisms in synaptic membranes.

Because of this widespread inhibitory effect, benzodiazepines can alter the turnover of the neurotransmitters such as noradrenalin and 5-hydroxytryptamine. The main sites of action of the benzodiazepines are in the spinal cord where muscle relaxant effects are mediated, the brain stem, perhaps accounting for the anticonvulsant properties, the cerebellum (causing ataxia) and the limbic and cortical areas involved in the organisation of emotional experience and behaviour. Offset actions of the benzodiazepines have been described providing a basis for tolerance (File 1985), rebound and dependence (Haefely 1986).

Although there are close chemical resemblances among many benzodiazepines, particularly the early ones, differences in pharmacological profile do exist. Thus, diazepam has anticonvulsant and muscle-relaxant properties in addition to sedative actions. Chlordiazepoxide is less anticonvulsant and relaxant, desmethyldiazepam less sedative. Clobazam is almost devoid of relaxant and sedative properties. Lorazepam seems particularly potent in producing amnesia especially after intravenous use. Alprazolam has been claimed to have some antidepressant properties.

Recently, a benzodiazepine antagonist, flumazenil, has been introduced (Brogden and Goa 1988). It binds to benzodiazepine receptors preventing the action of the benzodiazepine.

Clinical pharmacology

In normal individuals the depressant effects of single higher doses of the benzodiazepines can be readily detected. At lower doses, however, impairment of psychological functioning is quite difficult to quantify and subjective effects are usually absent. The most systematic work of this type is that by

Nicholson (1979; 1981) who has examined a wide range of benzodiazepines for their immediate effects, their effects on sleep and any residual effects when the subject wakes up. The test system comprises a highly complex sensorimotor task in which the subject is trained to manipulate a joystick control in order to keep a spot on a television screen on target. This task is highly relevant to pilot performance, Nicholson's particular interest. Of the benzodiazepines currently available, impairment of performance in the time after ingestion is highly dose dependent. These data, although derived from a highly specific task, accord well with those of other researchers using a wider range of tasks.

However, in the clinical context with anxious patients and with repeated doses, impairment of functioning is much more difficult to demonstrate. Although some studies have shown decrements in performance after the first dose, by the end of a week of repeated usage, such decrements have generally disappeared and have often been replaced by improvements in functioning in comparison to pre-drug levels (Ghoneim *et al.* 1986). Part of the explanation relates to the well known impairment of performance produced by pathologically high levels of anxiety. Many tasks—perceptual, cognitive, psychomotor, and intellectual—are performed badly by anxious patients. The addition of a sedative drug further depresses performance, at least initially. Then as the antianxiety effects build up, the patient functions better because he is calmer.

A second mechanism concerns tolerance. This is an instance of drug-induced adaptive change (Haefely 1986), and probably reflects several biochemical mechanisms including alteration in number of receptors and uncoupling of the effector systems from the receptors. Tolerance to the benzodiazepines affects some systems much more than others. For example, the subjective sedation associated with benzodiazepines seems to lessen more rapidly than objective psychomotor impairment (Lucki *et al.* 1986). Patients who have a high alcohol intake are tolerant to benzodiazepines.

Volunteer subjects have been used to investigate the dependence potential of benzodiazepines (de Wit *et al.* 1984). Drug preference studies suggested that these drugs are much less preferred than say the amphetamines, implying a low abuse potential for the benzodiazepines. Pharmacokinetic factors related to abuse potential are poorly understood (Busto and Sellers 1986). Differences among benzodiazepines have been documented: for example, oxazepam seems to have less abuse liability than diazepam (Bergman and Griffiths 1986).

Despite the extensive long-term usage of benzodiazepines, few studies have evaluated the chronic effects of these drugs. It is not clear whether therapeutic effects are maintained for longer than a few weeks, let alone whether any psychological impairment can be detected.

Clinical uses

The main use of the benzodiazepines is in the management of anxiety and stress-related conditions especially by family physicians. The indications are often so wide as to be difficult to determine in syndromal terms. Rather, it is the symptom of anxiety, no matter what its context, which is the main indication. As anxiety comes in so many guises, treatment must take account of this. There seems little to choose among the benzodiazepines in terms of effectiveness. Thousands of comparative trials among the benzodiazepines have been carried out, the earlier ones generally using chlordiazepoxide as the standard treatment, more recent ones diazepam. Placebo controls have also been utilized, far more commonly than with the antidepressants. Few differences have been found among the benzodiazepines, although their superiority with respect to placebo and usually to the barbiturates has been established. Usually it is easier to demonstrate superior effectiveness for the benzodiazepines as compared to placebo in acutely anxious patients than in chronically anxious patients. Nevertheless, some scepticism has been expressed concerning the clinical significance of the efficacy of the benzodiazepines (Shapiro *et al.* 1983).

Difficulties abound in assessing antianxiety medications. Anxiety states are very varied in their natural history, some subsiding rapidly over a few weeks, others becoming chronic for no apparent reason. The latter patients tend to be referred to psychiatric out-patients because of the treatment problems they present and because detailed evaluation of the factors sustaining the anxiety state is time consuming. Uncontrolled observations on family practice patients will give a more encouraging impression of antianxiety drugs than will assessment of the more chronic patients attending psychiatric clinics. Even in the latter type of patient, useful symptomatic relief is often obtained without complete resolution of the illness.

The temporal pattern of the anxiety state should suggest the initial choice of benzodiazepine. If the anxiety is sustained at a constant level without marked fluctuations, a benzodiazepine with a long half, life such as diazepam or clorazepate, is appropriate. Because of the long half life, once daily or better, once nightly dosage is sufficient. Nevertheless, many patients prefer divided dosage during the day, apparently because they can detect antianxiety activity and are reassured that drug effects are continuing. For episodic anxiety, shorter acting compounds such as lormetazepam can be used, taken over 30 min or so before entering the anxiety provoking situation (Ameer and Greenblatt 1981). If the panic has already started, lormetazepam can still be given and will exert a fairly prompt action. Oxazepam is also short acting but its absorption rate is too slow for emergency use of this sort.

Many patients suffer increases in anxiety on the background of an already elevated anxiety level. Here the most appropriate drug pharmacokinetically is diazepam. A proportion, say a half, of the daily dose can be given before retiring to bed: this maintains a background level. During the day small additional doses can be given as required. The drug is absorbed and redistributed rapidly so it will have a short lived effect on transient elevations in anxiety.

Recently, benzodiazepines have been assessed as treatment for panic states, preventing the episodes rather than aborting them. Alprazolam, in doses above those used to assuage generalized anxiety, is superior to placebo in preventing panic attacks but is possibly less efficacious than either tricyclic or MAOI antidepressants. Other benzodiazepines for which antipanic actions have been claimed include diazepam and clonazepam.

Other uses for which the short acting benzodiazepines are appropriate are as adjuncts to relaxation therapy, pre-operative medication and deep sedation for minor operative procedures such as dentistry. In the latter use, the drugs render the patient calm, conscious and co-operative, yet there is often total anterograde amnesia for the operation.

However, the most widespread use of the short acting benzodiazepines is in the management of insomnia (see also Chapter 13). The essential criterion for a hypnotic in those relatively few patients in whom insomnia is not a symptom of an affective disturbance is that the drug should not cumulate appreciably. To this end, this half life should not exceed 8–10 h. Temazepam's half life is in this region, that of triazolam is much shorter (less than 4 h). Neither drug has active metabolites. The onset of action of temazepam is a little slow so some patients find it insufficiently positive in its action. Conversely, the very short half life of triazolam may not suit other patients. The choice of hypnotic must be by trial-and-error.

In many patients, initial insomnia is related to a chronic state of anxiety. In these cases, a once nightly dose of diazepam or clorazepate is the most logical therapy. The rapid absorption of the benzodiazepine produces high brain levels which exert an hypnotic effect. The rapid redistribution then allows the patient to wake up without excessive residual effects.

The use of benzodiazepines in alcohol withdrawal is discussed in Chapter 21. These drugs have also been used as skeletal muscle relaxants in the management of acute conditions such as tetanus and chronic conditions such as the relief of spasticity and athetosis in patients with cerebral palsy.

Unwanted effects

The commonest unwanted effect is tiredness, drowsiness and torpor—so called 'over-sedation' (Svenson and Hamilton 1966). The effects are dose- and time-related, being most marked within the first two hours after large doses. Furthermore, drowsiness is most common during the first week of treatment; typically, the over-sedation then disappears probably due to a true tolerance effect. Smokers seem less affected than non-smokers perhaps because they metabolize the drugs more rapidly due to increased liver enzyme activity (Boston Program 1973). Accordingly, patients should be warned of the potential side effects of any prescribed benzodiazepine and the dosage should be cautious initially. Both psychomotor skills and intellectual and cognitive skills are affected. In particular, patients should be advised not to drive during the initial adjustment of dosage. If driving is essential for their livelihood, very cautious dose levels should be used and the patients warned to report any perceived impairment of mental functioning. Important decisions should be deferred during this period because judgement may be upset.

Recently, attention has focused on the effects of benzodiazepines on memory in normal subjects and patients (Curran 1986). Benzodiazepines differ in their propensity to produce memory deficits in normals; lorazepam but not clorazepate impaired recall in one study (Scharf *et al.* 1984). In patients, most benzodiazepines can cause problems, especially in higher doses and in the elderly (Angus and Romney 1984).

Objective psychological tests generally reveal some impairment of functioning after acute dosage in normal subjects. On repeated dosage these deficits tend to disappear. The situation with patients is more complex. Anxiety itself is associated with a decrement in mental functioning. After acute dosage, especially of large amounts, further decrements may ensue. However, on repeated dosage, the anxiolytic effect is accompanied by an improvement in performance unless doses so high as to produce obvious oversedation are utilized. Thus it is a moot point whether it is better for the community to have many of its members driving vehicles while anxious, distractable, and jumpy or sedated by benzodiazepines. On balance, once the patient has been 'titrated' to reach an acceptable dose level, there is little evidence to indicate that such patients constitute any substantial hazard.

As with most depressant drugs, potentiation of the effects of alcohol can occur (Sellers and Busto 1982; Laisi *et al.* 1979). Patients must be warned not to drink alcohol when taking benzodiazepines either chronically or intermittently.

Paradoxical behavioural responses may occur in patients taking benzodiazepines. Such events include increased aggression and hostility (Bond and Lader 1980), acute rage reactions (Tobin and Lewis 1962), 'psychokinetic stimulation' (Ayd 1962), uncharacteristic criminal behaviour such as shop lifting, and uncontrollable weeping (Ashton 1986). This phenomenon is by no means confined to the benzodiazepines: alcohol is a cardinal example of a drug whose ingestion may lead to excessive violence or criminal behaviour. Paradoxical reactions including release of anxiety or hostility are commonest during the initial week of treatment and often resolve spontaneously. If they do not, dose adjustment, usually downwards, is generally successful. It is impossible to predict who will respond adversely (Dietch and Jennings 1988).

In patients with respiratory problems such as chronic bronchitis and emphysema the administration of benzodiazepines can cause respiratory depression. The mechanism involves decreased sensitivity of the respiratory centre to arterial CO_2. Intravenous diazepam seems more hazardous than intravenous lorazepam; indeed, some studies suggest that lorazepam can stimulate the respiratory centre.

Other unwanted effects include excessive weight gain, skin rash, impairment of sexual function, menstrual irregularities and, rarely, agranulocytosis (Edwards 1981). The use of benzodiazepines in pregnancy is unestablished. One report suggested an excess of birth defects among babies born of mothers given meprobamate or chlordiazepoxide during the first 6 weeks of pregnancy (Milkovich and van den Berg 1974). A particular association was suggested between diazepam prenatally and cleft lip, with or without cleft palate (Safra and Oakley 1975). However, a large retrospective survey failed to confirm any such relationship (Hartz *et al.* 1975). A specific syndrome in babies born of mothers who have taken benzodiazepines during pregnancy has been described (Laegreid *et al.* 1987). It comprises slanted eyes, uptilted short nose, dysplastic ears, high arched palate and webbed neck. Further data are awaited. In such a situation of doubt, the prudent prescriber avoids the use of benzodiazepines during the first trimester unless there are compelling reasons such as overwhelming anxiety. Benzodiazepines pass readily into the fetus and have been suspected of producing respiratory depression in the neonate. Withdrawal fits are also a possibility. Finally, benzodiazepines are present in the mother's milk and can oversedate the baby so breast-feeding should be discouraged if benzodiazepines are prescribed, especially in high dose (Kanto 1982).

One of the drawbacks of the barbiturates is that they induce liver enzymes and attenuate the effects of other drugs. In animal experiments benzodiazepines also induce liver enzymes, but this seems of no clinical significance in man. Accordingly, benzodiazepines can be combined with other drugs without complication.

Overdosage

Overdosage with benzodiazepines is extremely common; deaths are mercifully rare (Busto *et al.* 1980). Although fatal overdose statistics contain deaths ascribed to benzodiazepines alone, many such attributions are suspect. Often another drug or alcohol has been taken. Only in children and the physically frail, especially those with respiratory illness, are the benzodiazepines hazardous. Typically, persons who take an overdose, say 100 mg of diazepam, become drowsy and fall into a deep sleep. A few develop dysarthria, rigidity or clonus of limbs or a bullous eruption. Sleep lasts 24–48 h but patients are generally rousable. Plasma benzodiazepine concentrations are often high on admission to hospital and are still very high even though the patient wakes up, seems perfectly conscious, and fit for discharge. This must reflect acute short term tissue tolerance.

The safety of benzodiazepines relative to the barbiturates is sufficient reason to render the latter obsolescent, especially in view of the present pandemic of attempted suicide.

Tolerance and dependence

As outlined previously, acute tolerance effects can be presumed from observations of patients who have taken an overdose when the drug effects wear off despite very high plasma concentrations. In normal subjects it has been shown that subjective effects show tolerance over 2 weeks of administration of moderate doses of benzodiazepines; objective effects, by contrast, do not seem to wane.

Clinically, tolerance has not been studied in any detail. If it occurred escalation of dosage would be apparent. This does occur with the benzodiazepines, but considering the widespread use of these drugs, comparatively rarely. It is our clinical impression that escalation of dose often takes place in a series of steps, each one related to a temporary increase in stressful circumstances. Most patients reduce the dose when the crisis passes but some continue the higher dose to which they presumably develop some tolerance. Patients taking high doses of benzodiazepines have equivalently high plasma concentrations so the tolerance is not pharmacokinetic in nature with accelerated drug metabolism.

Tolerance to clinical effects in patients maintaining moderate doses of benzodiazepines is more controversial. There have been few controlled observations of the efficacy of antianxiety compounds in chronically anxious patients taking the drug for 6 months or so. If medication is withdrawn, symptoms appear resembling those for which the benzodiazepine was originally given, and this is generally taken as evidence that therapeutic benefit still continues. However, newer non benzodiazepines do not show such 'rebound' after long term use.

Undoubtedly, many chronically anxious patients are helped by their benzodiazepines, but many other patients who suffer from recurrent crises take benzodiazepines chronically rather than in response to each crisis. This raises the important question as to the frequency of psychological and physical dependence on the benzodiazepines (Owen and Tyrer 1983). Dependence is easily demonstrable in those patients who have escalated their doses. Rebound and withdrawal symptoms after the long-acting benzodiazepines, diazepam and clorazepate, usually do not supervene until about the sixth day, but onset is correspondingly quicker in patients discontinuing shorter acting benzodiazepines. The mildest symptoms are anxiety, tension, apprehension, dizziness, insomnia, and anorexia. This syndrome is essentially a 'rebound' phenomenon (Power *et al.* 1985; Fontaine *et al.* 1984); Rickels *et al.* 1988*a*). More severe physical dependence is manifested by withdrawal symptoms of nausea and vomiting, tremor, muscle weakness and postural hypotension. Occasionally, hyperthermia, muscle twitches, convulsions and confusional psychoses may occur (Zipursky *et al.* 1985).

The incidence of physical dependence as manifested by escalation of dosage and by withdrawal phenomena after high doses was low (Ladewig 1984). Marks (1978) in a detailed review of the world literature concluded that the incidence of total recorded cases appears to be in the range of one case per 5 million patient-months of drug usage. However, cases have been more frequently reported recently.

Hallstrom and Lader (1981) have identified patients on normal doses of benzodiazepines (e.g. up to 30 mg/day of diazepam or equivalent) who reported difficulty in discontinuing their drugs. On withdrawal, typical symptoms including perceptual changes occurred and the EEG alterations were identical to those seen on withdrawal from high doses. The symptoms seen on withdrawal from normal doses of benzodiazepines are listed in Table 12.2 (Petursson and Lader 1981*a*,*b*, 1984). The proportion of patients taking

Table 12.2. Withdrawal symptoms from benzodiazepines

Symptom	Frequency
anxiety, tension	++++
agitation, restlessness	+++
bodily symptoms of anxiety	++
irritability	++
lack of energy	++
impaired memory and concentration	++
depersonalization, derealization	+
sleep disturbance	++++
tremor, shakiness	+++
headache	+++
muscle pains, aches, twitchings	++
loss of appetite	++
nausea, dry retching	++
depression	+
perspiration	+
metallic taste, hyperosmia	++++
blurred vision, sore eyes, photophobia	+++
incoordination, vertigo	+++
hyperacusis	++
paraesthesias	++
hypersensitivity to touch, pain	++
paranoid reaction	+

benzodiazepines chronically who experience withdrawal symptoms on discontinuation of medication ranges between 27–45 per cent depending on the criteria used (Tyrer *et al.* 1981). Many other studies have now established the reality of normal dose dependence (Busto *et al.* 1986*a*, *b*). Sometimes the withdrawal reactions are very prolonged (Ashton 1984) or depression may supervene (Olajide and Lader 1984).

Since the publicity concerning withdrawal reactions from benzodiazepines, patients have become aware of the difficulties which they may encounter. Pseudo-withdrawal reactions may be seen in which anxiety increases without other symptoms at a time early in the tapering off procedure (Owen and Tyrer 1983).

Management of withdrawal

The most appropriate way to manage patients withdrawing from benzodiazepines is universally accepted to be gradual tapering of the dose (Tyrer and Sievewright 1984). The more severe symptoms of withdrawal such as epileptic fits and confusional episodes are more likely to follow sudden than gradual withdrawal, particularly when shorter-acting compounds have been taken long-term. Views differ as to the rate of withdrawal. Detailed guidelines have been suggested but do not provide a consensus view (Higgitt *et al.* 1985; Editorial 1987). After even a short course of treatment, say 3–4 weeks, a week of half dosage is advisable.

After longer periods of time, especially when a shorter-acting compound has been used, 4 weeks is the minimum period and programmes as long as 16 weeks have been recommended. Indeed, some agencies suggest a month of tapering for every year of benzodiazepine use. There is no evidence to support such a timetable. The regimen may become a morbid focus with the patient becoming obsessed with his symptoms. One strategy is to try a fairly brisk withdrawal, say over 6–8 weeks, and only to resort to more gradual tapering if the symptoms become intolerable.

One can often usefully substitute a long-acting for a short-acting benzodiazepine, say 10 mg of diazepam for 1 mg of lorazepam. After stabilization, the diazepam is then gradually reduced. Whatever the strategy, flexibility in the regimen and constant support are essential. Group therapy is quite helpful (Higgitt *et al.* 1987).

Patients must be carefully followed up because a depressive illness is not uncommon and may need vigorous treatment (Olajide and Lader 1984). Such an illness may be reactive to the stress of withdrawal or be a recurrence of an earlier affective episode. In a few patients, the illness has many biological features such as insomnia and loss of weight.

Adjunctive therapies have been tried. A beta-adrenoceptor antagonist may lessen some symptoms but clonidine is ineffective (Goodman *et al.* 1986). Non-benzodiazepine anxiolytics such as buspirone are non-cross-tolerant with the benzodiazepines and do not help withdrawal (Schweizer and Rickels 1986; Lader and Olajide 1987). Some anecdotal reports have suggested that carbamazepine might be effective (e.g. Ries *et al.* 1989). Phenobarbitone has also been advocated.

Psychological support is most important. The doctor should maintain close contact with the patient during withdrawal, and in the initial stages patients should be seen at least weekly. With in-patients, daily contact has been found to be useful. At these meetings the physician should show that he or she understands the problems of withdrawal and be ready to offer guidance on non-medical as well as medical issues. Patients frequently arrive with numerous misconceptions and negative expectations about tranquillizers and withdrawal; these need to be elicited, identified, and corrected within a broadly educational framework.

Patients need most advice concerning the management of the withdrawal syndrome itself. Most symptoms can be dealt with by reassurance and simple practical advice. With more persistent difficulties, requesting patients to keep diaries so that they may monitor particular symptoms may provide important clues to the source of the difficulty. During the withdrawal period patients are likely to attribute almost all their physical and psychological changes to the withdrawal. This simplistic view must be corrected, for patients may otherwise come to have unrealistic expectations about the likely outcome.

Formal psychological help has not yet been shown to be particularly effective. Relaxation treatment and training in anxiety management skills in the framework of group therapy can boast of only moderate effectiveness (Cormack and Sinnott 1983). Possibly more rigorous administration of such techniques in close co-ordination with withdrawal procedures and with more regard to the specific problems of individual patients might help in group-based withdrawal programmes.

An important determinant of success in withdrawal seems to be the social support received by patients. The process of withdrawal needs to be explained to spouses, and in some cases children, and their support elicited whenever possible. In the absence of (or in addition to) family support some patients find local self help groups a useful adjunct. Unfortunately, but probably inevitably, those members of the community most active in founding support groups for tranquillizer dependence are likely to be those with the worst experiences of withdrawal, who may thus inadvertently set up unnecessarily gloomy expectations in patients.

Other antianxiety drugs

The Quality Assurance Project (1985) team of the Australian and New Zealand College of Psychiatrists have carried out a meta-analysis of treat-

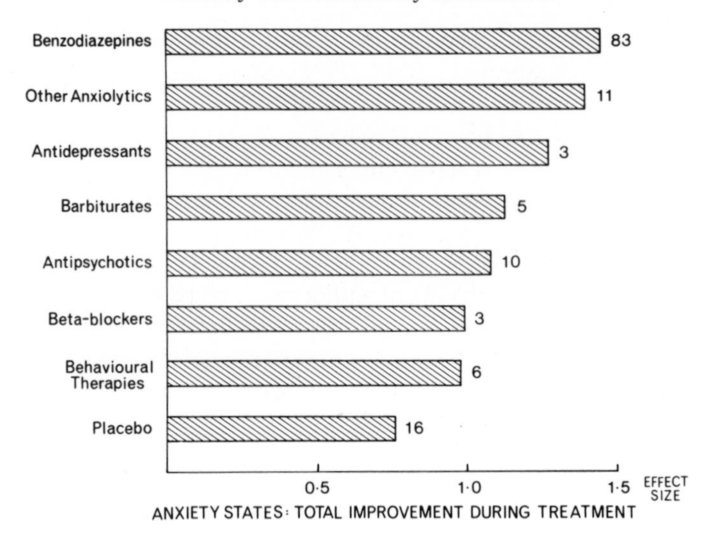

Fig.12.3. A pooled estimate of the improvement with various treatments in anxiety states expressed as a proportion of the initial standard deviation of the severity ratings ('effect size'). The number to the left of each histogram is the number of clinical trials of that treatment included in the meta-analysis (redrawn from Quality Assurance Project 1985, with permission).

ments for anxiety states (see chapter 9 for a further explanation). Figure 12.3 shows schematically the relative improvements. The benzodiazepines about double the improvement associated with placebo. Other anxiolytics and antidepressants are almost as effective as the benzodiazepines. Behavioural therapies and beta-blockers are rather ineffective.

Antipsychotic drugs

Phenothiazines such as chlorpromazine and trifluoperazine and a range of other antipsychotic drugs have been advocated to treat anxiety. The dosage recommended is quite low, typically less than half the initial antipsychotic dose. Sometimes, even at this dosage, the antipsychotic drug is not well-tolerated by the anxious patient because unwanted autonomic effects such as dry mouth and dizziness too closely resemble their own symptoms. Even more disconcerting are extrapyramidal symptoms such as restlessness (mild akathisia) and parkinsonism. However, in the low doses advocated, such unwanted effects are uncommon. It is not clear if there is any real risk of tardive dyskinesia but this possibility should dissuade the practitioner from indiscriminate use of these drugs as anxiolytics.

The chief advantage of this medication is that dependence is virtually unknown so the main indication for their use is in patients with histories of dependence on other CNS depressant drugs such as alcohol or barbiturates. Dosage should be cautious. Extrapyramidal signs should be carefully sought and if detected the dose must be lowered because there is a definite danger of tardive dyskinesia eventually developing.

Tricyclic antidepressants

Several of these drugs such as amitriptyline, doxepin, and mianserin have useful secondary sedative properties. They are the treatment of first choice in depressed patients with anxiety or agitation. Although regarded as not appropriate for patients with primary anxiety states, some clinical trials have showed quite impressive efficacy (Kahn *et al.* 1986, 1987). Fixed combinations of tricyclic antidepressants with anxiolytics or antipsychotic medication have little to commend them as the prescriber loses flexibility of symptom management.

Monoamine oxidase inhibitors

The use of these drugs in the treatment of 'atypical depressives' including those with phobic anxiety is detailed in Chapter 9. In view of the unwanted effects of the MAOIs such as the dietary and drug interactions, they should not be used for minor indications.

Beta-adrenoceptor antagonists

Anxiety states are accompanied by many different bodily symptoms, some of which are mediated by the sympathetic system. In particular, palpitations, tremor, and gastrointestinal upset are related to overactivity of beta-adrenergic pathways. Consequently, blockade of this activity by means of beta-adrenoceptor antagonists might be expected to help patients with anxiety, especially those with the above symptoms.

Many trials have been carried out in the past 15 years using various beta-blockers and the results have been consistent (Tyrer 1980). Only those bodily symptoms mediated by the beta division of the sympathetic nervous system are helped by administration of propranolol or similar drugs. Somatic symptoms not mediated in that way and general psychological symptoms are not consistently improved. Consequently, whether a patient finds relief or not on a beta-blocker depends on his symptom profile. Patients with predominant complaints of palpitations, trembling, and gastrointestinal hurry are often much improved. Even so the improvement may be limited to those symptoms alone and general anxiety symptoms may be unchanged (Hayes and Schulz 1987).

Beta-blockers may be combined with benzodiazepines in an attempt to alter the symptoms peripherally by preventing their mediation and centrally by lowering arousal. Such combinations have to be established by trial and error.

Beta-blockers should not be used in patients with any history of asthma, and a cardiologist's advice should be sought in those with heart disease. A test dose, say 20 mg of propranolol, should be administered to detect undue sensitivity of the patient as shown by bradycardia below 60 beats/min at rest. If no sensitivity is found, the dose can be instituted at 20 mg four times a day and increased over the course of a week or two to 40 mg four times a day. The resting pulse rate should be monitored and used as the 'end-point': dosage should be maintained at that necessary to keep the pulse at normal levels. It is usually unhelpful to push the dose beyond 160 mg/day in total. At these dose levels, the drug predominantly acts peripherally on symptom mechanisms rather than centrally.

Newer drugs

Several non-benzodiazepines are in the process of development. Some of these such as suriclone and alpidem are chemically dissimilar to the benzodiazepines but act on or near to the benzodiazepine receptors. Others are more innovative and appear to act on mechanisms other than those involving GABA (Williams 1983). Such compounds seem inactive in animal models of dependence, tolerance and abuse. They seem as efficacious as the benzodiazepines but with a different profile of side-effects. The leading compound of this type is buspirone, with a novel chemical structure (Editorial 1988). It probably acts on 5-HT$_1$ mechanisms. It produces little or no sedation in its usual clinical dose of 15–30 mg daily (in divided dose), but may be associated with some nausea and headache (Goa and Ward 1986). Buspirone lacks anticonvulsant and muscle relaxant properties. Discontinuation is not accompanied by rebound and withdrawal symptoms (Rickels *et al.* 1988*b*). Another putative anxiolytic acting on 5-HT$_2$ mechanisms is ritanserin (Ceulemans *et al.* 1985). 5-HT$_3$ antagonists may also be anxiolytic.

Management of anxiety states

Conceptual model

In helping patients with anxiety states, it is useful to bear in mind some conceptual model of anxiety such as that outlined in Fig. 12.4. Thus anxiety is regarded as the outcome of an interaction between external events and an internal predisposition resulting in a state of hyperarousal. The latter reflects genetic predisposition and previous learning and contains a symbolic element which distorts and exaggerates the individual's perception of the

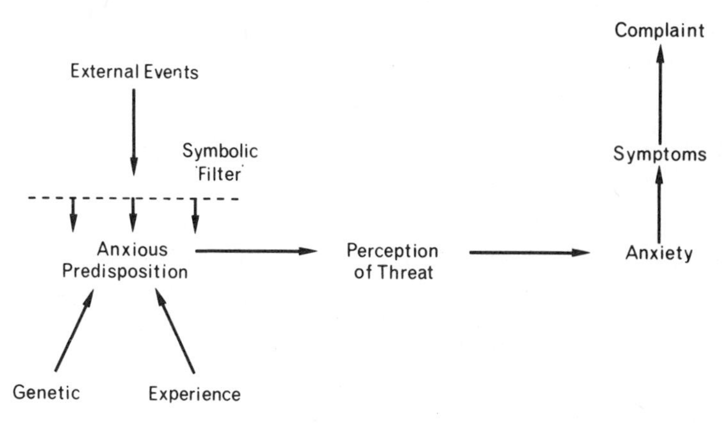

Fig.12.4. A conceptual model of anxiety.

external events. Thus, excessive threat is seen and anxiety, disproportionate to that threat, results.

As well as a model for the onset of anxiety, a conceptual model for the resolution of anxiety is helpful. The excessive arousal interferes with the patient's ability to cope with his own anxiety—he loses mastery over his symptoms. Non-pharmacological therapy such as psychotherapy or relaxation is ineffective at these excessively high anxiety levels because the anxiety prevents the individual co-operating in these therapies. Anxiolytic drugs have to be used, preferably as temporary expedients in order to control the anxiety sufficiently for other therapies to become effective.

History

It is assumed that a careful history is taken if the referring doctor has not already done so. It must be remembered that patients with anxiety states may be seeing a psychiatrist for the first time so reassurance about this is necessary. Trying to elicit a detailed sexual history is often inadvisable at the first interview before rapport has been established and confidence instilled.

Particular attention should be paid to the following points:

1. The apparent precipitants of the present attack should be sought. Care is necessary in evaluating the patient's spheres of functioning (home, work, community, etc.) because patients often attribute causation inaccurately. Commonly a problem produced by the illness is transposed in time to apparently antedate the onset of symptoms and thereby to assume a causative role. A good informant is invaluable here.

2. The patient's previous personality should be assessed, especially the level of anxiety and the ways in which previous crises have been dealt with.

3. The family history may be important, especially if other members have also suffered from anxiety or other neurotic disorders.

4. The current social support, for example, the quality of the marriage often influences the type of treatment recommended and the response to that treatment.

5. The main symptoms—their type, frequency of occurrence, meaning to the patient, etc.—must be carefully recorded. As well as the type and severity, the distress produced by the symptoms and the degrees of interference with personal and social functioning should be carefully enquired about. It is useful to know whether alcohol has been found to assuage these symptoms. Other treatments and responses should be also documented.

6. Finally, the patient's expectations should be evaluated. Is he prepared to admit he needs help? Does a person with life-long high trait anxiety expect a miracle transformation into a phlegmatic stoic? Does the patient think visiting a psychiatrist entails prolonged psychoanalytic therapy? Does he have any confidence in drugs or does he regard them with some trepidation?

Differential diagnosis

Many conditions have features which resemble those of anxiety especially the somatic symptoms. However, only a few present any real problems with respect to differential diagnosis. These are cardiac dysrhythmias, thyrotoxicosis, phaeochromocytoma, and idiopathic hypoglycaemia. Drugs such as excessive caffeine or alcohol use, sympathomimetics (e.g. ephedrine and amphetamine) may produce states of anxiety. As anxiety states are generally conditions arising in the 20s and 30s age groups, the onset of anxiety for the first time in those over 40 needs careful evaluation. It may relate to physical illness such as nutritional deficiencies, hormonal dysfunction or a carcinoma. Organic brain disease such as presenile dementia or a brain tumour may also present initially as anxiety.

Among psychiatric conditions, early schizophrenia is often attended by marked anxiety, often of a socially phobic type. A depressive episode may also be ushered in by symptoms of anxiety. Typically the anxiety is at first free-floating but later becomes more phobic and encapsulated in type before eventually depressive symptoms become obvious. Thus, anxiety presenting for the first time in a stable non-neurotic individual must always be suspected of masking an underlying depression and frequent reassessment is necessary to avoid missing this possibility with its attendant hazard of suicide.

Temporal lobe epilepsy may present as episodes of severe, inexplicable anxiety often somatized to the stomach as part of the aura. The subsequent loss of consciousness establishes the diagnosis but full special investigations may be needed to unravel the problem.

Non-pharmacological measures

Briefly, these comprise explanation, reassurance, crisis intervention, supportive psychotherapy, amelioration of social and work circumstances, relaxation training, group sessions, and so on (Drury 1985). Explanation of symptoms is very important. The anxious patient fears two consequences of his illness. The panic attacks with the extreme somatic symptoms make him fearful that he will die during one of the attacks. Reassurance that this is highly unlikely and that even during a panic his heart is not beating as fast as during moderate exercise relieves him of this worry. Secondly, symptoms such as depersonalization and the total irrationality of the anxious suggest to the patient that he is going mad. Again reassurance on this point alleviates much of the secondary anxiety. Explanation of the various symptoms in simple physiological terms helps the patient set his condition and problems in perspective.

Supportive psychotherapy should be directed towards the patient's immediate problems which should be tackled in a realistic way. Sensible goals for therapy should be established and discussed from time to time to remotivate the patient. Some of the time should be spent discussing any drug therapy prescribed in order to maximize compliance. More searching psychotherapies, including those based on analytic transference, lie outside the scope of this book. Suffice it to say that drug therapy and psychotherapy are not incompatible and may indeed potentiate each other in the hands of skilful practitioners.

Other forms of therapy should also form part of an integrated plan, discussed by therapist and patient, and agreed to as a sensible outline. Psychological treatments are currently being developed for patients with acute reactions to stressful events or chronic anxiety with or without phobic disorder (Gelder 1986). Both generalized and panic anxiety disorders can be approached using psychological methods of treatment (Butler *et al.* 1987). Some patients with social anxiety may benefit from group therapy, others with sexual problems may need referral to more specialized clinics (if they exist) and so on. Whatever means of therapy are decided upon, antianxiety medication if indicated must be integrated into the plan of treatment and not added as an afterthought or as a routine.

The efficacy of non-pharmacological antianxiety measures in comparison with routine benzodiazepine medication was assessed in a study in the Oxford region (Catalan *et al.* 1984*a*,*b*). General practitioners selected 91 patients with new episodes of minor affective disorder who usually would have been given anxiolytic medication. Half were allocated randomly to receive such medication, the other half to a non-drug group. The latter comprised brief counselling by the general practitioner without any attempt at specialized counselling or psychotherapy. It included explanation of symptoms, exploration of personal or other problems and ways of dealing with them, and reasons for not prescribing drugs. Psychiatric and social assessments were made at an initial interview when treatment was started, and one and seven months later. Before treatment the groups were well-matched. On the General Health Questionnaire, 85 per cent of patients were psychiatric 'cases' before treatment, 40 per cent at one month and 30 per cent at seven months. Other measures showed similar changes. No differences were seen in the improvements of the two groups. The non-drug patients did not make increased demands on the doctor's time and neither group increased their consumption of alcohol, tobacco, or non-prescribed drugs. Poor outcome was associated with initial worse measures of psychiatric state and social functioning.

Drug therapy

When to use drugs

Much of this topic has been alluded to already. The fundamental dilemma faced by the therapist is whether the benefits of antianxiety medication outweigh the risks of dependence (physical and/or psychological), the 'medicalizing' of an essentially interpersonal or environmental problem, the facile resort to drugs in future episodes, and so on (Lindsay *et al.* 1987). The main criterion for giving drugs is that the anxiety is so severe as to hinder the patient's coping with both his anxiety and his underlying problems (see Fig. 12.5). Very often it is an acute severe anxiety that requires pharmacological

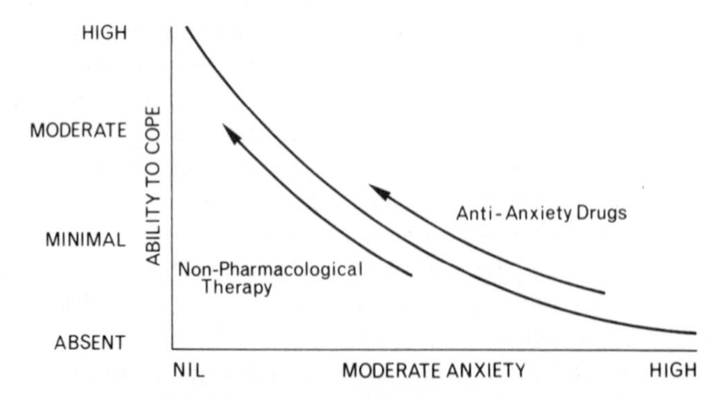

Fig.12.5. Hypothesized relationship between anxiety levels and ability to cope. Antianxiety drugs lower the anxiety levels to the point where some ability to cope is regained and non-drug therapies become effective.

treatment so that the drugs will tide the patient over a week or two of distress while the basic problems are tackled or while the patient adapts to or is re-educated to cope with insoluble problems (Quality Assurance Project 1985). For example, sedation after a particularly tragic bereavement is appropriate but not the routine administration of anxiolytics after a long-expected death in the family. Control of symptoms by prompt and vigorous treatment enables the patient to regain mastery over his own symptoms and to approach his difficulties realistically when the symptoms subside. Although most acute anxiety states subside spontaneously a few become chronic if the symptoms are allowed to persist unabated for more than a week or two. When anxiolytics are given to help combat a crisis, the patient must be warned that the drugs will be given for a limited period and he must agree to this.

A more difficult decision concerns prolonged neurotic episodes (Ballenger 1984). Drug administration will necessarily be long-term, with the risk of dependence. Again the criterion should be the severity of the anxiety and the distress it causes the patient. If the anxiety interferes with everyday functioning thus handicapping the patient in some way, antianxiety drugs are indicated (Marks 1985). Even so such episodes do eventually peter out, or in the younger patient maturation is often accompanied by better coping responses and mastery of anxiety. The practitioner must reassess the patient from time to time to see whether reduction in dosage and eventual discontinuation is feasible.

Yet the most complex decisions concern the patient with life-long personality-bound anxiety. Here the anxiety constantly permeates the individual's existence. Every decision is an agony of doubt, every departure from routine a catalogue of apprehensions, every encounter with a stranger a signal for a panic, and so on. Nevertheless, the individual functions after a fashion; he may be married with children and even be materially successful. To withhold anxiolytics is to make a moral judgment, to resort to 'pharmacological Calvinism'. The essential fact to establish is whether the patient functions better on than off drugs with respect to interpersonal, social, occupational and leisure activities, and is relatively free from anxiety symptoms. If this can be established then long term or indefinite treatment is in the patient's interests. The implications of such chronic treatment should be expounded frankly to the patient. A clue to the probable efficacy of antianxiety therapy may be given by the patient's admission that alcohol helps him greatly; for example, it may prevent a tremor which appears regularly on stressful occasions.

One study from the USA assessed the prevalence and correlates of the long term regular use of antianxiety drugs (Mellinger *et al.* 1984). Long-term use, defined as regular daily use for a year or longer, was found in 15 per cent of all antianxiety drug users, 1.6 per cent of all adults. Such users tended to be older persons with high levels of emotional distress and chronic somatic health problems. Most were women. Similar patterns exist in the UK but the proportion of the adult population who are chronic users is twice as high (Balter *et al.* 1984).

Choice of drug

This follows from the discussion of the pharmacokinetics of the benzodiazepines set out earlier. There is no consistent evidence indicating superiority of one benzodiazepine over another in the reduction of anxiety. Clinicians have their preferences and prescribing fashions do change. For example, diazepam has largely supplanted chlordiazepoxide in hospital practice although family doctors still use the latter quite widely. In general, though, the choice of drug is dictated by the type of anxiety which should be matched to the pharmacokinetic properties of the various drugs, particularly the rate of absorption and duration of action. If a patient requires chronic maintenance therapy to combat a high continuous level of anxiety, a long-acting compound such as diazepam or clorazepate is appropriate. It can be given as one dose at night when it will act as a useful hypnotic. Other patients with intermittent anxiety take a shorter acting benzodiazepine such as oxazepam to provide anxiety relief. Patients who are self-aware and alert to their own internal feelings can be entrusted to take short-acting drugs before they enter anxiety-provoking situations.

The place of buspirone in therapy remains to be established. Its use should be considered in patients who need to be fully alert and in those with previous histories of alcohol or sedative drug dependence. As its onset of action is somewhat delayed, it is not appropriate on its own in patients who need immediate relief.

Beta-adrenoceptor antagonists should be considered when the patient complains of somatic symptoms especially palpitations. Therapeutic results can be gratifying when the symptom assumes overwhelming importance, almost to the point of a monosymptomatic neurosis. Phobic patients may not respond so well as some use their physical symptoms as signals that they are entering a phobic situation: loss of the warning may concern them that they will lose control of themselves.

Dose

The keynote for treatment should be great flexibility to accommodate the individual needs of the patient. If repeated daily doses of a short-acting drug are indicated, it is helpful if the patient keeps a daily log of his panic attacks and of drug usage. This facilitates the adjustment of the dosage which the patient undertakes and increases his sense of participation in a therapeutic process rather than being a passive recipient.

The rules of establishing dosage are to obtain the best clinical response commensurate with the patient's ability to tolerate the side effects. The long-acting drugs are easier to stabilize in this respect although the rapid absorption of diazepam may give rise to a transient peak with concomitant drowsiness. On the other hand, such a rapid and detectable effect may be very reassuring to the patient. Despite the rationale of usage arising from the pharmacokinetics of the various benzodiazepines, too rigid adherence to dosage schedules can be self-defeating. Thus, one patient may manage well on one dose of chlordiazepoxide at night, another on minute doses of diazepam 6 or more times during the day, a third on 8-hourly oxazepam.

Duration of therapy

Short courses of treatment are appropriate to the acutely anxious. As remission is likely to occur anyway, treatment should be planned in terms of 1–2 weeks rather than months. The patient must not be allowed to persist with marginally effective treatment—it must either be made effective by improvement of compliance or dosage manipulation or be discontinued (Nasdahl *et al* 1985). Some patients with recurrent episodes of anxiety keep a store of anxiolytic medicines and are adept at reverting to them for a short course of treatment during a crisis. It is best to encourage this form of self-medication but to ask the patient to inform the doctor when such an episode appears. Disapproval of such a course only leads to the patient taking anxiolytics clandestinely. Such intermittent use is inappropriate for buspirone.

With chronic neurotic anxiety, courses of treatment are obviously prolonged and with the morbidly anxious personality, treatment is indefinite. Nevertheless, the therapist should always be alert to any tendency to escalate the dosage and should seek to lower the dosage when the patient is stabilized in a quiescent period.

One study over 22 weeks suggested that efficacy was maintained (Rickels *et al.* 1983). Most patients started on diazepam did not need medication beyond 2–4 months. At 1 year follow-up, about two-thirds of all improved anxious patients were experiencing symptoms again. Long term benzodiazepine users were frequently chronically anxious or dysthymic patients often with an underlying personality disorder such as passivity or inadequacy. Intermittent medication seemed more appropriate than continuous chronic drug ingestion (Rickels *et al.* 1985).

Response to treatment

Rickels' group in Philadelphia have carried out a large series of studies on response to treatment in anxious patients (Rickels *et al.* 1978). As might be expected anxiety and somatic complaints are the symptom areas most sensitive to anxiolytic drug effects. Depressive symptoms only occasionally and obsessional symptoms rarely respond. Interpersonal sensitivity (i.e. feelings easily being hurt) is also unresponsive. Psychotherapy is more appropriate for patients with excessive sensitivity. Hostility, by contrast, is significantly reduced by antianxiety treatment.

Predictors of response

Rickels' group have also analyzed their extensive data with respect to prognostic variables (Rickels *et al.* 1978). Their replication predictors are set out in Table 12.3. Obviously, some of these factors cannot be altered by the doctor but others can. Thus, establishment of rapport is important and confidence in using drugs maximizes their effect.

Treatment of panic attacks

The traditional treatment for severe panic attacks was sodium amylobarbitone, up to 500 mg, intravenously or intramuscularly. Intravenous diazepam (10 mg) is equally effective and safer, having a short half-life because of redistribution, so prolonged sedation is unlikely.

The prevention of panic attacks is more problematical (Cassano *et al.* 1988). Constant antianxiety therapy may lessen their frequency and/or blunt their severity but many patients complain that the panic attacks often persist despite amelioration of the background anxiety. Antidepressants, both tri-

Table 12.3. Predictors of Good Outcome

Patient:
More educated
Expects drug treatment
Realizes problems are emotional
Female without menopause or hysterectomy
Physician:
Feels comfortable with patient
Likes patient
Considers drug therapy most appropriate
Illness and treatment related:
Acute duration
Diagnosis of anxiety
No previous drugs
Good response to previous drugs
Presenting psychopathology:
Less severe obsessive—compulsive
Less severe interpersonal sensitivity
Less severe depression
More severe anxiety

From Rickels *et al.* 1978.

cyclic and MAOI, have been advocated as antipanic agents. However, significant improvement may be delayed for 4–12 weeks and about 15–30 per cent of patients experience an intensification of anxiety symptoms at the beginning of treatment. Many refuse to continue medication. The antidepressants seem more effective against panic and less against phobic avoidance. Many patients continue to experience anticipatory anxiety, and benzodiazepines are often taken concomitantly to reduce this anxiety.

The whole area of panic attacks and benzodiazepine treatment is currently under intensive investigation (Editorial 1986). In doses up to 10 mg/day in divided doses, i.e. much above the usual anxiolytic doses of 1.5–3 mg/day, alprazolam is fairly effective in lessening the frequency of panic attacks (Dawson *et al.* 1984), and acts more rapidly than imipramine (Charney *et al.* 1986). Some evidence is accruing that other benzodiazepines such as diazepam and clonazepam may also be useful in this indication; again high doses seem necessary (Rickels and Schweizer 1986; Tesar *et al.* 1987). Because of this there is an appreciable risk of rebound and dependence (Fyer *et al.* 1987), and the drugs should eventually be carefully tapered off (Pecknold and Swinson 1986).

The relationship of agoraphobia to panic attacks is the subject of debate. Most agoraphobics date the onset of their illness to a panic attack subsequent to which they start to avoid certain situations associated with panics. Anxiolytic drugs are not regarded by psychiatrists as effective (Levin and Liebowitz 1987), behavioural treatments being preferred (Quality Assurance Project 1982).

Obsessive-compulsive syndromes

Benzodiazepines are generally ineffective in this indication (Lelliott and Monteiro 1986) (see also Chapter 9).

Post-traumatic stress disorder

The symptoms of this disorder consist of recurrent and intrusive recollections of the traumatic events, including nightmares and flashbacks, together with numbing of responsiveness to the outside world and often feelings of detachment and emotional withdrawal. Benzodiazepines lessen insomnia, decrease nightmares and decrease alcohol use. However, habituation is a hazard (van der Kolk 1983).

Sedative-facilitated interviewing

The drugs most commonly used to facilitate interviewing and to produce 'abreactions' are the barbiturates although the amphetamines have also been popular. The most favoured barbiturates are intravenous sodium amylobarbitone or methohexitone. The benzodiazepines provide a safer alternative.

Several uncontrolled trials concluded that barbiturate interviews were useful, but there is only one major controlled trial (Dysken *et al.* 1979). Twenty patients were selected because they were found to have some difficulty communicating with their primary therapist during the initial psychiatric evaluation. Two diagnostic interviews were conducted 6 h apart; before one, chosen randomly, intravenous sodium amylobarbitone was administered, before the other, saline. The patient's primary therapist scored the usefulness of each interview, while blind to the injection. Both saline and barbiturate were equally useful.

This use of sedative-facilitated interview does not seem fruitful but other indications are generally accepted as appropriate. These are:

1. For mobilizing stuporous, catatonic, withdrawn patients;
2. For aiding in the diagnosis of intellectual impairment;
3. For lessening negative affect associated with traumatic and stressful experiences.

In the last, the patient may experience a 'flashback' and relive his experiences, often with extreme affective and behavioural disturbances, shouting, cringing in fear, screaming in anger, etc. Afterwards, there may be little recall of the session but the catharsis is often quite successful in lessening anxiety, panics and especially nightmares.

Sedative-facilitated interviews have also been used in interviewing people suspected of criminal offences—the 'truth drug'. Courts vary in whether they will accept disclosures after the drug as evidence. Although material, incriminating or absolving of guilt may be uncovered, it should also be remembered that fantasy material may be released as well.

References

Allgulander, C. (1986). History and current status of sedative-hypnotic drug use and abuse. *Acta Psychiatrica Scandinavica* **73,** 465–78.

AMA Committee on Alcoholism and Drug Dependence (1974). Barbiturates and barbiturate-like drugs: considerations in their medical use. *Journal of the American Medical Association* **230,** 1440–1.

Ameer, B., and Greenblatt, D.J. (1981). Lorazepam: a review of its clinical pharmacological properties and therapeutics. *Drugs* **21,** 161–200.

Angus, W.R., and Romney, D.M. (1984). The effect of diazepam on patient's memory. *Journal of Clinical Psychopharmacology* **4,** 203–5.

Ashton, H. (1984). Benzodiazepine withdrawal: an unfinished story. *British Medical Journal* **288,** 1135–40.

Ashton, H. (1986). Adverse effects of prolonged benzodiazepine use. *Adverse Drug Reaction Bulletin* **118,** 440–3.

Ayd, F.J. (1962). A critical appraisal of chlordiazepoxide. *Journal of Neuropsychiatry* **3,** 177–80.

Ballenger, J.C. (1984). Psychopharmacology of the anxiety disorders. *Psychiatric Clinics of North America* **7,** 757–71.

Balter, M.B., Manheimer, D.I., Mellinger, G.D., and Uhlenhuth, E.H. (1984). A cross national comparison of anti-anxiety/sedative drug use. *Current Medical Research and Opinion* **8** (Suppl. 4), 5–20.

Berger, F.M. (1970). Anxiety and the discovery of tranquilizers. In *Discoveries in biological psychiatry* (eds. F.J. Ayd, and B. Blackwell) pp. 115–29. Lippincott, Philadelphia.

Bergman, U., and Griffiths, R.R. (1986). Relative abuse of diazepam and oxazepam: prescription forgeries and theft/loss reports in Sweden. *Drug and Alcohol Dependence* **16,** 293–301.

Bond, A., and Lader, M. (1979). Benzodiazepines and aggression. In *Psychopharmacology of aggression* (ed. M. Sandler) pp. 173-82. Raven Press, New York.

Boston Collaborative Drug Surveillance Program. (1973). Clinical depression of the central nervous system due to diazepam and chlordiazepoxide in relation to cigarette smoking and age. *New England Journal of Medicine* **288,** 277–80.

Brogden, R.N., and Goa, K.L. (1988). Flumazenil. A preliminary review of its benzodiazepine antagonist properties, intrinsic activity and therapeutic use. *Drugs* **35,** 448–67.

Burrows, G.D., and Davies, B. (1980). *Handbook of studies on anxiety*. Elsevier, Amsterdam.

Busto, U., and Sellers, E.M. (1986). Pharmacokinetic determinants of drug abuse and dependence. A conceptual perspective. *Clinical Pharmacokinetics* **11,** 144–53.

Busto, U., Kaplin, H.L., and Sellers, E.M. (1980). Benzodiazepine-associated emergencies in Toronto. *American Journal of Psychiatry* **137,** 226–7.

Busto, U., Sellers, E.M., Naranjo, C.A., Cappell, H.C., Sanchez-Craig, M., and Simpkins, J. (1986*a*). Patterns of benzodiazepine abuse and dependence. *British Journal of Addiction* **81,** 87–94.

Busto, U. Sellers, E.M., Naranjo, C.A., Cappell, H., Sanchez-Craig, M., and Sykora, K. (1986*b*). Withdrawal reaction after long-term therapeutic use of benzodiazepines. *New England Journal of Medicine* **315,** 854–9.

Butler, G., Gelder, M., Hibbert, G., Cullington, A., and Klimes, I. (1987). Anxiety management: developing effective strategies. *Behavioural Research Therapy* **25,** 517–22.

Cassano, G.B., Perugi, G., and McNair, D.M. (1988). Panic disorder: review of the empirical and rational basis of pharmacological treatment. *Pharmacopsychiatry* **21,** 157–65.

Catalan, J., Gath, D., Edmonds, G., and Ennis, J. (1984*a*). The effects of non-prescribing of anxiolytics in general practice I. Controlled evaluation of psychiatric and social outcome. *British Journal of Psychiatry* **144,** 593–602.

Catalan, J., Gath, D., Bond, A., and Martin, P. (1984*b*). The effects of non-prescribing of anxiolytics in general practice II. Factors associated with outcome. *British Journal of Psychiatry* **144,** 603–10.

Ceulemans, D.S.L., Hoppenbrouwers, M.-L.J.A., Gelders, Y.G., and Reyntjens, A.J.M. (1985). The influence of ritanserin, a serotonin antagonist, in anxiety disorders: a double-blind placebo controlled study versus lorazepam. *Pharmacopsychiatry* **18,** 303–5.

Channer, K.S., James, M.A., Papouchado, M., and Rees, J.R. (1985). Anxiety and depression in patients with chest pain referred for exercise testing. *Lancet* **2,** 820–2.

Charney, D.S., Woods, S.W., Goodman, W.K., Rifkin, B., Kinch, M., Aiken, B., Quadrino, M.S., and Heninger, G.R. (1986). Drug treatment of panic disorder: the comparative efficacy of imipramine, alprazolam, and trazodone. *Journal of Clinical Psychiatry* **47,** 580–6.

Clinthorne, J.K., Cisin, I.H., Balter, M.B., Mellinger, G.D., and Uhlenhuth, E.H. (1986). Changes in popular attitudes and beliefs about tranquilizers. *Archives of General Psychiatry* **43,** 527–32.

Cohen, I.M. (1970). The benzodiazepines. In *Discoveries in biological psychiatry* (eds. F.J. Ayd, and B. Blackwell) pp. 130–41.

Cormack, M.A., and Sinnott, A. (1983). Psychological alternatives to long-term benzodiazepine use. *Journal of the Royal College of General Practitioners* **33,** 279–81.

Curran, H.V. (1986). Tranquillising memories: a review of the effects of benzodiazepines on human memory. *Biological Psychology* **23,** 179–213.

Dawson, G.W., Jue, S.G., and Brogden, R.N. (1984). Alprazolam. A review of its pharmacodynamic properties and efficacy in the treatment of anxiety and depression. *Drugs* **27,** 132–47.

de Wit, H., Johanson, C.E., and Uhlenhuth, E.H. (1984). The dependence potential of benzodiazepines. *Current Medical Research and Opinion* **8,** 48–59.

Dietch, J.T., and Jennings, R.K. (1988). Aggressive dyscontrol in patients treated with benzodiazepines. *Journal of Clinical Psychiatry* **49,** 184–7.

Drury, V.W.M. (1985). Benzodiazepines—a challenge to rational prescribing. *Journal of the Royal College of General Practitioner* **35,** 86–8.

Dysken, M.W., Chang, S.S., Casper, R.C., and Davies, J.M. (1979). Barbiturate—facilitated interviewing. *Biological Psychiatry* **14,** 421–32.

Eberts, F.S., Philopoulos, B.S., Reineke, L.M., and Vliek, R.W. (1981). Triazolam disposition. *Clinical Pharmacology and Therapeutics* **29,** 81–93.

Editorial, (1986). Panic disorders : a separate entity? *Lancet* **1,** 1014–5.

Editorial, (1987). Treatment of benzodiazepine dependence. *Lancet* **1,** 78–9.

Editorial, (1988). Buspirone—a radical advance in the treatment of anxiety? *Lancet* **1,** 804–6.

Edwards, J.G. (1981). Adverse effects of antianxiety drugs. *Drugs*. **22,** 495–514.

Ehlert, F.J. (1986). 'Inverse agonists', cooperativity and drug action at benzodiazepine receptors. *Trends in Pharmacological Sciences* **?,** 28–32.

Fann, W.E., Karacan, I., Pokorny, A.D., and Williams, R.L. (eds.) (1979). *Phenomenology and treatment of anxiety*. SP Books, New York.

File, S.E. (1985). Tolerance to the behavioral actions of benzodiazepines. *Neuroscience and Biobehavioural Reviews* **9,** 113–21.

Fontaine, R., Chouinard, G., and Annable, L. (1984). Rebound anxiety in anxious patients after abrupt withdrawal of benzodiazepine treatment. *American Journal of Psychiatry* **141,** 848–52.

Fyer, A.J., Liebowitz, M.R., Gorman, J.M., Campeas, R., Levin, A., Davies, S.O., Goetz, D., and Klein, D.F. (1987). Discontinuation of alprazolam treatment in panic patients. *American Journal of Psychiatry* **144,** 303–9.

Gelder, M.G. (1986). Psychological treatment for anxiety disorders: a review. *Journal of the Royal Society of Medicine* **79,** 230–3.

Ghoneim, M.M., Hinrichs, J.V., and Mewaldt, S.P. (1986). Comparison of two benzodiazepines with differing accumulation: behavioral changes during and after 3 weeks of dosing. *Clinical Pharmacology and Therapeutics* **39,** 491–500.

Goa, K.L., and Ward, A. (1986). Buspirone. A preliminary review of its pharmacological properties and therapeutic efficacy as an anxiolytic. *Drugs* **32,** 114–29.

Goodman, W.K., Charney, D.S., Price, L.H., Woods, S.W., and Heninger, G.R. (1986). Ineffectiveness of clonidine in the treatment of the benzodiazepine withdrawal syndrome: report of three cases. *American Journal of Psychiatry* **143,** 900–3.

Haefely, W. (1986). Biological basis of drug-induced tolerance, rebound, and dependence. Contribution of recent research on benzodiazepines. *Pharmacopsychiatry* **19,** 353–61.

Hallstrom, C., and Lader, M. (1981). Benzodiazepine withdrawal phenomena. *International Pharmacopsychiatry* **16,** 235–44.

Hamilton, M. (1959). The assessment of anxiety states by rating. *British Journal of Medical Psychology* **32,** 50–5.

Hartz, S.L., Heinonen, O.P., Shapiro, S. *et al.* (1975). Antenatal exposure to meprobamate and chlordiazepoxide in relation to malformations, mental development, and childhood mortality. *New England Journal of Medicine* **292,** 726–8.

Hayes, P.E., and Schulz, S.C. (1987). Beta-blockers in anxiety disorders. *Journal of Affective Disorders* **13,** 119–30.

Higgitt, A., Golombok, S., Fonagy, P., and Lader, M. (1987). Group treatment of benzodiazepine dependence. *British Journal of Addiction* **82,** 517–32.

Higgitt, A.C., Lader, M.H., and Fonagy, P. (1985). Clinical management of benzodiazepine dependence. *British Medical Journal* **291,** 688–90.

Kahn, R.J., McNair, D.M., Lipman, R.S., Covi, L., Rickels, K., Downing, R., Fisher, S., and Frankenthaler, L.M. (1986). Imipramine and chlordiazepoxide in depressive and anxiety disorders. II. Efficacy in anxious outpatients. *Archives of General Psychiatry* **43,** 79–85.

Kahn, R.J., McNair, D.M., and Frankenthaler, L.M. (1987). Tricyclic treatment of generalized anxiety disorder. *Journal of Affective Disorders* **13,** 145–51.

Kanto, J.H. (1982). Use of benzodiazepines during pregnancy, labour and lactation, with particular reference to pharmacokinetic considerations. *Drugs* **23,** 354–80.

Klotz., U., Avant, G., Hoyumpa, A. *et al.* (1975). The effects of age and liver disease on the disposition and elimination of diazepam in adult man. *Journal of Clinical Investigation* **551,** 347–59.

Lader, M., and Marks, I. (1971). *Clinical anxiety.* Heinemann Medical Books, London.

Lader, M.H., and Olajide, D. (1987). A comparison of buspirone and placebo in relieving benzodiazepine withdrawal symptoms. *Journal of Clinical Psychopharmacology* **7,** 11–15.

Ladewig, D. (1984). Dependence liability of the benzodiazepines. *Drug and Alcohol Dependence* **13,** 139–49.

Laegreid, L., Olegard, R., Wahlstrom, J., and Conradi, N. (1987). Abnormalities in children exposed to benzodiazepines in utero. *Lancet* **1,** 108–9.

Laisi, U., Linnoila, M., Seppala, T., Himberg, J.J., and Mattila, M.J. (1979). Pharmacokinetic and pharmacodynamic interactions of diazepam with different alcoholic beverages. *European Journal of Clinical Pharmacology* **16,** 263–70.

Lasagna, L. (1977). The role of benzodiazepines in non-psychiatric medical practice. *American Journal of Psychiatry* **134,** 656–8.

Lelliot, P.T., and Monteiro, W.O. (1986). Drug treatment of obsessive-compulsive disorder. *Drugs* **31,** 75–80.

Levin, A.P., and Liebowitz, M.R. (1987). Drug treatment of phobias. Efficacy and optimum use. *Drugs* **34,** 504–14.

Lewis, A. (1967). Problems presented by the ambiguous word 'anxiety' as used in psychopathology. *Israel Annals of Psychiatry and Related Disciplines* **5,** 105–21.

Lindsay, W.R., Gamsu, C.V., McLaughlin, E., Hood, E.M., and Espie, C.A. (1987). A controlled trial of treatments for generalized anxiety. *British Journal of Clinical Psychology* **26,** 3–15.

Lucki, I., Rickels, K., and Geller, A.M. (1986). Chronic use of benzodiazepines and psychomotor and cognitive test performance. *Psychopharmacology* **88,** 426–33.

Marks, J. (1978). *The benzodiazepines. Use, overuse, misuse, abuse.* MTP Press, Lancaster.

Marks, J. (1985). Chronic anxiolytic treatment: benefit and risk. In *Chronic treatments in neuropsychiatry*. (eds. D. Kamali and G. Racagni). Raven Press, New York.

Mellinger, G.D., Balter, M.B., and Uhlenhuth, E.H. (1984). Prevalence and correlates of the long term regular use of anxiolytics. *Journal of the American Medical Association* **251,** 375–9.

Milkovich, L.M., and van den Berg, B.J. (1974). Effects of prenatal meprobamate and chlordiazepoxide hydrochloride on human embryonic and fetal development. *New England Journal of Medicine* **291,** 1268–71.

Nasdahl, C.S., Johnston, J.A., Coleman, J.H., May, C.N., and Druff, J.H. (1985). Protocols for the use of psychoactive drugs—Part IV: Protocol for the treatment of anxiety disorders. *Journal of Clinical Psychiatry* **46,** 128–32.

Nathan, R.G., Robinson, D., Cherek, D.R., Sebastian, C.S., and Hack, M. (1986). Alternative treatments for withdrawing the long-term benzodiazepine user: a pilot study. *International Journal of Addiction* **21,** 195–211.

Nicholson, A.N. (1979). Performance studies with diazepam and its hydroxylated metabolites. *British Journal of Clinical Pharmacology* **81,** 39S–42S.

Nicholson, A.N. (1981). The use of short- and long-acting hypnotics in clinical medicine. *British Journal of Clinical Pharmacology* **11,** 61S–69S.

Oakley, C.M. (1984). Mitral valve prolapse: harbinger of death or variant of normal? *British Medical Journal* **288,** 1853–4.

Olajide, D., and Lader, M. (1984). Depression following withdrawal from long-term benzodiazepine use: a report of four cases. *Psychological Medicine* **14,** 937–40.

Owen, R.T., and Tyrer, P. (1983). Benzodiazepine dependence. A review of the evidence. *Drugs* **25,** 385–98.

Paul, S.M., Marangos, P.J., and Skolnick, P. (1981). The benzodiazepine-GABA-chloride-ionophore receptor complex: common site of minor tranquilizer action. *Biological Psychiatry* **16,** 213–29.

Pecknold, J.C., and Swinson, R.P. (1986). Taper withdrawal studies with alprazolam in patients with panic disorder and agoraphobia. *Psychopharmacology Bulletin* **22,** 173–6.

Petursson, H., and Lader, M.H. (1981*a*). Withdrawal from long-term benzodiazepine treatment. *British Medical Journal* **283,** 643–5.

Petursson, H., and Lader, M.H. (1981*b*). Withdrawal symptoms from clobazam. *Royal Society of Medicine International Congress and Symposium Series* **43,** 181–3.

Petursson, H., and Lader, M. (1984). Benzodiazepine dependence, tolerance and withdrawal syndrome. *Advances in Human Psychopharmacology* 89–119.

Power, K.G., Jerrom, D.W.A., Simpson, R.J., and Mitchell, M. (1985). Controlled study of withdrawal symptoms and rebound anxiety after six week course of diazepam for generalised anxiety. *British Medical Journal* **290,** 1246–8.

Quality Assurance Project (1982). A treatment outline for agoraphobia. *Australia and New Zealand Journal of Psychiatry* **16,** 25–33.

Quality Assurance Project (1985). Treatment outlines for the management of anxiety states. *Australia and New Zealand Journal of Psychiatry* **19,** 138–51.

Reich, J. (1986). The epidemiology of anxiety. *Journal of Nervous and Mental Disorder* **174,** 129–36.

Rickels, K., Downing, R.W., and Winokur, A. (1978). Antianxiety drugs: clinical use in psychiatry. In *Handbook of psychopharmacology*, Vol 13. (eds. L.L. Iversen, S.D. Iversen, and S.H. Snyder) pp. 395–430. Plenum Press, New York.

Rickels, K., Case, G.W., Downing, R.W., and Winokur, A. (1983). Long-term diazepam therapy and clinical outcome. *Journal of the American Medical Association* **250,** 767–71.

Rickels, K., Case, W.G., Downing, R.W., and Winokur, A. (1985). Indications and contraindications for chronic anxiolytic treatment: is there tolerance to the anxiolytic effect? In *Chronic treatments in neuropsychiatry* (eds. D. Kamali and G. Racagni) pp. 193–204. Raven Press, New York.

Rickels, K., and Schweizer, M.D. (1986). Benzodiazepines for treatment of panic attacks: a new look. *Psychopharmacology Bulletin* **22,** 93–8.

Rickels, K., Case, W.G., Schweizer, E.E., Swenson, C., and Fridman, R.B. (1986). Low-dose dependence in chronic benzodiazepine users: a preliminary report on 119 patients. *Psychopharmacology* **22,** 407–15.

Rickels, K., Fox, I.L., Greenblatt, D.J., Sandler, K.R., and Schless, A. (1988*a*). Clorazepate and lorazepam : clinical improvement and rebound anxiety. *American Journal of Psychiatry* **145,** 312–17.

Rickels, K., Schweizer, E., Csanalosi, I., Case, G., and Chung, H. (1988*b*). Long-term treatment of anxiety and risk of withdrawal. *Archives of General Psychiatry* **45,** 444–50.

Ries, R.K., Roy-Byrne, P.P., Ward, N.G., Neppe, V., and Cullison, S. (1989). Carbamazepine treatment for benzodiazepine withdrawal. *American Journal of Psychiatry* **146,** 536–7.

Safra, M.J., and Oakley, G.P. (1975). Association between cleft lip with or without cleft palate and prenatal exposure to diazepam. *Lancet* **2,** 478–80.

Sartorius, N. (1980). Epidemiology of anxiety. *Pharmacopsychiatry* **13,** 249–53.

Scharf, M.B., Khosla, N., Brocker N., and Goff, P. (1984). Differential amnestic properties of short- and long-acting benzodiazepines. *Journal of Clinical Psychiatry* **45,** 51–3.

Schweizer, E., and Rickels, K. (1986). Failure of buspirone to manage benzodiazepine withdrawal. *American Journal of Psychiatry* **143,** 1590–2.

Sellers, E.M., and Busto, U. (1982). Benzodiazepines and ethanol: assessment of the effects and consequences of psychotropic drug interactions. *Journal of Clinical Psychopharmacology* **2,** 249–57.

Shapiro, A.K., Struening, E.L., Shapiro, E., and Milcarek, B.I. (1983). Diazepam: how much better than placebo? *Journal of Psychiatric Research* **17,** 51–73.

Skerritt, P.W. (1983). Anxiety and the heart—a historical review. *Psychological Medicine* **13,** 17–25.

Svenson, S.E., and Hamilton, R.G. (1966). A critique of overemphasis on side effects with the psychotropic drugs: an analysis of 18,000 chlordiazepoxide-treated cases. *Current Therapeutic Research* **8,** 455–64.

Tesar, G.E., Rosenbaum, J.F., Pollack, M.H., Herman, J.B., Sachs, G.S., Mahoney, E.M., Cohen, L.S., McNamara, M., and Goldstein, S. (1987). Clonazepam versus alprazolam in the treatment of panic disorder: interim analysis of data from a prospective, double-blind, placebo-controlled trial. *Journal of Clinical Psychiatry* **48,** 10 Suppl., 16–19.

Tobin, J.M., and Lewis, N.D.C. (1960). New psychotherapeutic agent, chlordiazepoxide. *Journal of the American Medical Association* **174,** 1242–9.

Torgersen, S. (1983). Genetic factors in anxiety disorders. *Archives of General Psychiatry* **40,** 1085–9.

Tyrer, P. (1974). The benzodiazepine bonanza. *Lancet* **2,** 709–10.

Tyrer, P.J. (1980). Use of beta-blocking drugs in psychiatry and neurology. *Drugs* **20,** 300–8.

Tyrer, P.J. (1984). Benzodiazepines on trial. *British Medical Journal* **288,** 1101–2.

Tyrer, P., Rutherford, D., and Huggett, T. (1981). Benzodiazepine withdrawal symptoms and propranolol. *Lancet* **i,** 520–2.

Tyrer, P., Owen, R., and Dawling, S. (1983). Gradual withdrawal of diazepam after long-term therapy. *Lancet* **i,** 1402–6.

Tyrer, P.J., and Seivewright, N. (1984). Identification and management of benzodiazepine dependence. *Postgraduate Medical Journal* **60,** Suppl. **2,** 41–6.

van der Kolk, B. (1983). Psychopharmacological issues in posttraumatic stress disorder. *Psychopharmacology* **34,** 683–91.

Williams, M. (1983). Anxioselective anxiolytics. *Journal of Medicinal Chemistry* **26,** 620–8.

Zipursky, R.B., Baker, R.W., and Zimmer, B. (1985). Alprazolam withdrawal delirium unresponsive to diazepam: case report. *Journal of Clinical Psychiatry* **46,** 344–5.

Zung, W.W.K. (1975). A rating instrument for anxiety disorders. *Psychosomatics* **12,** 371–9.

13. Sleep disorders and hypnotic drugs

Sleep

We spend a third of our lives asleep and yet sleep largely remains an enigma. The purpose of sleep has been speculated about repeatedly but, apart from some relationships with hormone secretion, little of note has been discovered. Yet we all know how unpleasant lack of sleep can be, whether this is spontaneous as in insomnia, or self-inflicted. The complaint of insomnia is one of the most frequent encountered by the family physician and it is also one of the commonest reasons for prescribing one group of drugs, namely, the hypnotics.

Although the function of sleep remains obscure, modern electrophysiological and endocrine techniques have provided much information concerning the patterns of normal sleep and how these are disrupted in the various types of insomnia. Drug treatment also alters sleep, and attempts to withdraw hypnotics may in turn produce insomnia. However, the psychiatrist usually deals with insomnia associated with other psychiatric conditions, mainly the affective disorders, anxiety, and depression. Other specific causes of insomnia exist but are relatively uncommon.

In this chapter, we review the physiology of normal sleep, its alterations with insomnia and with drugs. The management of insomnia is discussed with particular emphasis on avoiding the indiscriminate use of hypnotics. As well as insomnia, excessive daytime sleepiness is also dealt with briefly. Sleep deprivation as treatment for depression is not discussed. Reviews are available elsewhere (Tolle 1981; Vogel 1981), and although useful therapeutic effects have been claimed, they have tended to be short-lived in most cases. Further studies are necessary (Rudolf and Tolle 1978; Gerner *et al*. 1979).

Normal sleep

Sleep has been defined as a recurring state of inactivity accompanied by loss of awareness and a decrease in responsiveness to the environment. All night

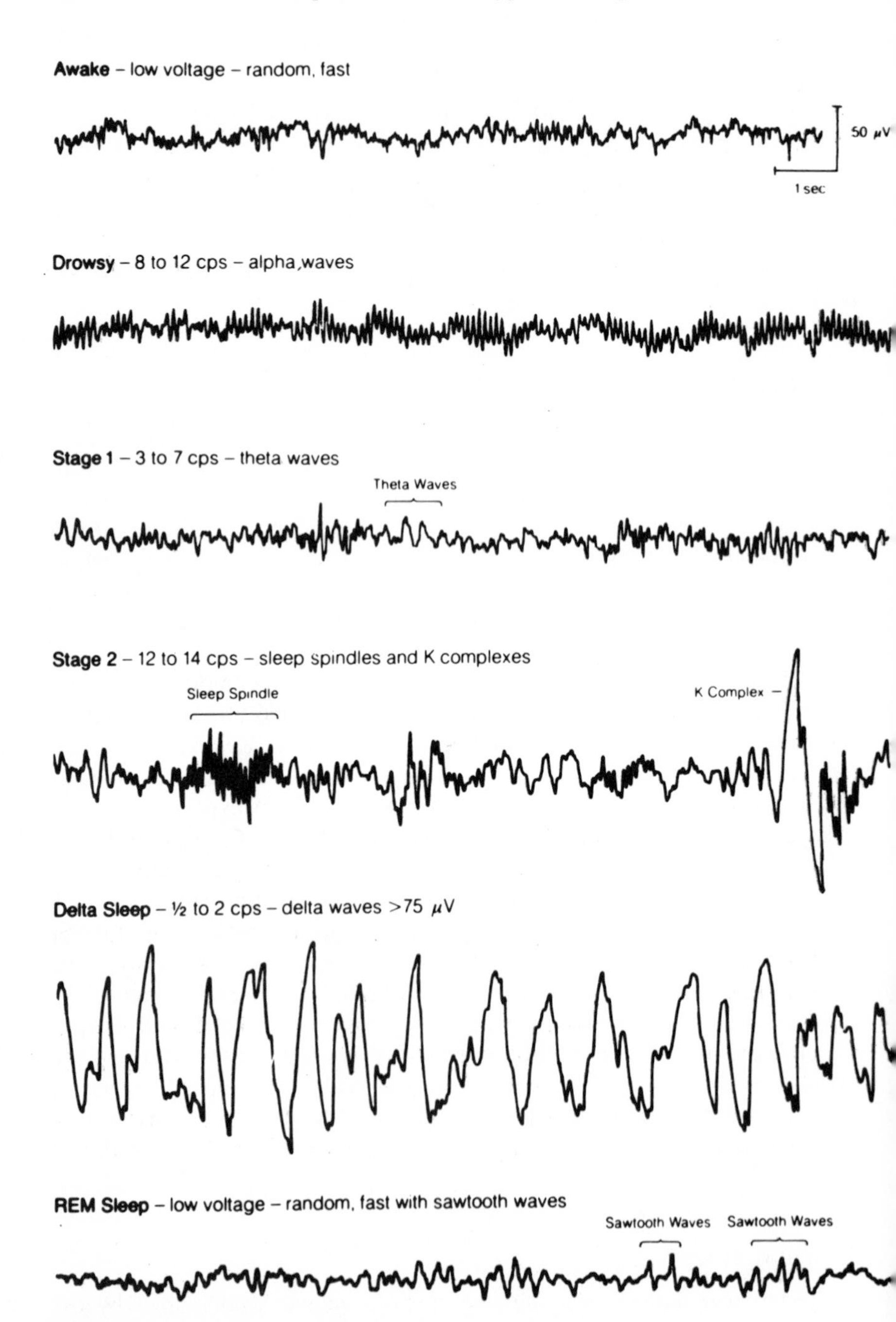

Fig.13.1. Human sleep stages. (With permission, from Hauri 1977.)

recordings of physiological functions, primarily the EEG, have distinguished two main states of sleep (Aserinsky and Kleitman 1953; Dement and Kleitman, 1955) (Fig. 13.1).

1. Rapid eye movement sleep [REM, desynchronized (D-sleep) or paradoxical sleep], characterized by bursts of rapid conjugate eye movements accompanied by a low-voltage electroencephalogram. The muscles are completely relaxed, but autonomic functions such as heart-rate and sweat-gland activity are active and highly variable, and the penis is erect. If the subject is awakened he usually reports dreaming.

2. Non-rapid eye movement sleep (NonREM, orthodox, or quiescent sleep) is classified into 3 or 4 stages:

   Stage 1. This is hard to define but the EEG comprises low-voltage desynchronized activity sometimes together with low-voltage regular 4–6 Hz (cycles per second) waves.

   Stage 2. Shows frequent 13–15 Hz spindle-shaped trains of waves, known as 'sleep spindles'. Also found are high-voltage spikes, '*K*-complexes'.

   Stage 3 is typified by delta waves, high voltage 0.5–2 Hz activity, occurring in bursts.

   Stage 4 is dominated by these waves.

The two deepest stages, 3 and 4, are often amalgamated into one stage termed 'slow-wave sleep', SWS. There are few eye movements in non-REM sleep and bodily functions are quiescent. Dreaming is not generally associated with this state.

Healthy people have fairly standard patterns of sleep throughout the night (Fig. 13.2). As the subject becomes drowsy, the muscles relax and EEG alpha activity disappears. NonREM sleep supervenes and deepens to reach SWS within 30 to 60 min. The pulse rate drops and muscle tone further diminishes. About 90 min after falling asleep, the first REM sleep episode appears. Four to six such periods occur during the night at intervals of 80 to 100 min. Each lasts 5 to 30 min, increasing in duration throughout the night. Conversely, SWS is concentrated into the early part of the night.

The young adult spends about half the night in stages 1 and 2 (mainly 2) and about a quarter each in SWS and in REM sleep. The elderly have much less SWS, sometimes hardly any, and the total sleep time is reduced with frequent awakenings. Rapid-eye-movement periods, both number and duration, are reduced only marginally so that the proportion of sleeping time spent in REM sleep may even increase a little. Conversely, children have larger amounts of SWS (Fig. 13.3).

Many brain systems are involved in sleep mechanisms (Hobson 1984). The pontine reticular formation is important in the generation of REM

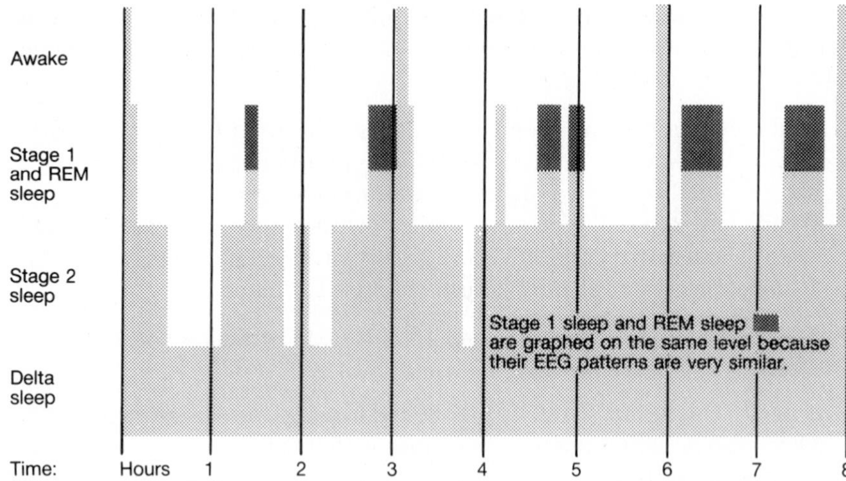

Fig.13.2. Typical sleep pattern of a young human adult. (With permission, from Hauri 1977.)

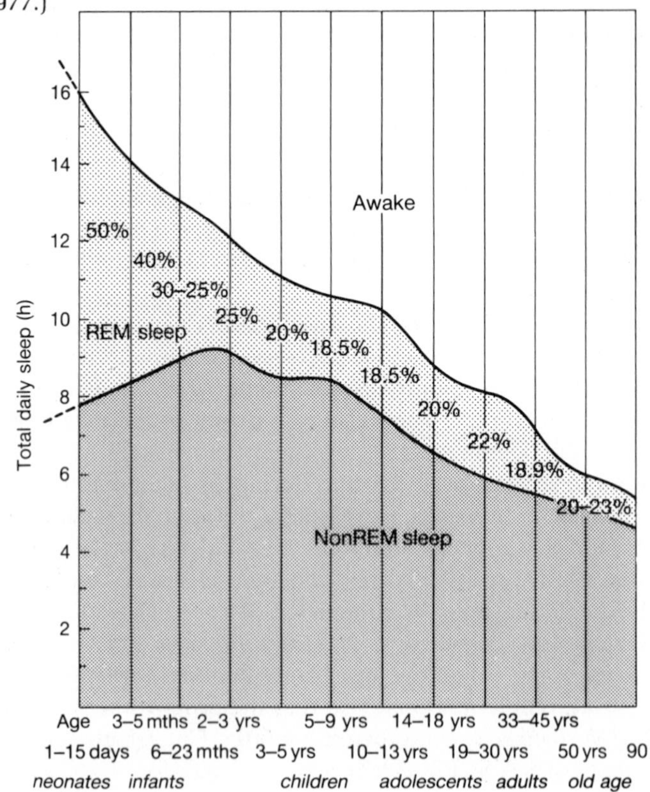

Fig. 13.3. Mean development of human sleep over a lifetime. (With permission, from Hauri 1977.)

sleep, cells in this area increasing their firing just prior to the onset of such episodes. Conversely, serotonergic cells in the dorsal raphé nuclei diminish their firing rate before and during REM episodes. Rats lesioned in the midbrain raphé have diminished sleep and reduced forebrain 5-HT content. Lesioning of noradrenalin tracts such as the ascending dorsal pathway leads to hypersomnia, decreased noradrenalin in the forebrain, but increased 5-HT. This suggests that a sleep–waking cycle is regulated by two interacting ascending systems of adrenergic and serotonergic neurones.

Cholinergic fibres are also involved in both REM and nonREM sleep. Rapid-eye-movement sleep is blocked by atropine and by lesions in various cholinergic tracts in tegmental, pontine, and caudate sites, so that at least two systems may be necessary for the induction of REM sleep.

Sleep hygiene

Before dealing with insomnia, it is useful to outline the strategems which people find useful in inducing sleep. A regular bed-time routine is conducive to sleep and many people carry out almost a ritual before they go to bed. Similarly, a regular arousal time and routine helps to consolidate sleep. Reading before falling asleep is common, although arousing or disturbing material should be avoided. Trying to do mental work or the household accounts at bed-time does not aid sleep.

Relaxation routines are used by some people, especially those who resort to meditative techniques during the day. However, meditation and the induction of sleep are different physiological and psychological processes and it is the muscular relaxation which is more relevant. Simple relaxation exercises in which the person relaxes muscle groups progressively from toes to limbs, trunk, neck and head are appropriate. Behavioural techniques have been advocated in chronic insomnia (see Cleghorn *et al.* 1983*b* for an account).

A bed-time drink may aid sleep. Alcohol tends to disturb sleep during the latter half of the night; however, a modicum of alcohol is helpful to many people. Others rely on a milk-based drink, of which there are many on the market. Tea and coffee, however, may induce insomnia or, at the least, lighten sleep. An excessively warm room disturbs sleep but an excessively cold one does not aid sleep. Sound-attenuating a bedroom near traffic or an airport may help.

Exercise late at night is used by many people to help the onset of sleep, although it is probably the routine which is most important. Moderate exercise earlier in the day makes many people drowsy later on as anyone taking an unaccustomed walking holiday can testify. Heavy exercise, by contrast, may be too exhausting (Horne 1981).

Insomnia

Insomnia is a common complaint. It essentially means the awareness of too much wakefulness. There are two main types: difficulty in falling asleep and difficulty in remaining asleep with broken sleep, early wakening, or unsatisfying sleep (Hartmann 1980). The commonest is inability to fall asleep promptly with consequent feelings of tiredness the next day.

Healthy people often have bouts of sleeplessness at times of mental and physical stresses or sometimes for no apparent reason. Such 'spontaneous' insomnia may evidence some cyclicity. In addition, some people are chronically poor sleepers. Laboratory studies confirm that sleep is indeed delayed and broken with more stage 2 and less SWS and REM sleep. Poor sleepers accumulate more of their SWS early in the night than do good sleepers and tend to be physiologically active—for example, to have higher pulse rates.

People with 'good' sleep cover a wide range of length of sleep. Short sleepers, those with less than 6½ h per night, spend more time proportionately in SWS and REM sleep than do long sleepers (over 8½ h). They also seem to have a higher mortality rate than do long sleepers (Oswald 1984). The long sleepers accumulate more REM sleep during the last two hours of sleep, but do not attain the amount of deep sleep of the short sleepers. One might speculate that short sleepers have a more 'efficient' sleep pattern, although the precise needs of various types of sleep remain obscure.

Many people complain of insomnia. A survey in the USA, conducted in 1979, found that a third of all adults suffered from insomnia at some time during the course of a year (Mellinger *et al.* 1985). About half of these individuals experienced the problem as serious. Women and the elderly are more likely than others to have serious insomnia together with high levels of 'psychic distress' and somatic anxiety, symptoms resembling major depression and multiple health problems. During the year prior to the survey, a medically prescribed hypnotic was used by 2.6 per cent of adults. Use was typically for one or two days at a time or for short courses (less than two weeks) of regular use. However, some people (11 per cent of all users, 0.3 per cent of all adults) used sleeping tablets regularly for over a year.

The distinction between poor sleepers and patients with insomnia is operational, the latter being sufficiently upset by their symptoms to see a doctor. Thus, the causes of poor sleep are often relevant to the management of insomniacs.

Some claims have been made that sleep patterns are related to personality traits. Poor sleepers are supposed to be more prone to anxiety and depression than are good sleepers. Long sleepers may also be mildly anxious and depressed, with a greater number of psychological and social problems than short sleepers. Nevertheless, these relationships are not hard-and-fast features.

The classification of insomnia can be made quite complex. However, a Consensus Conference (1984) was held in the USA to review the use of medications in insomnia. Three main types of insomnia were identified:

1. Transient insomnia caused by a stressful situation or jet-lag.
2. Short-term insomnia usually associated with a situational stress.
3. Long-term insomnia with many antecedents.

No consensus was arrived at concerning treatment and the use of hypnotic drugs, except that benzodiazepines were the hypnotics of choice, but to be used as sparingly as possible.

The following are the types of insomnia encountered by clinicians, although more elaborate schemes have been proposed (Cleghorn *et al.* 1983*a*) (Table 13.1).

Table 13.1. Descriptive classification of insomnia.

Classification
1. Benign variation of normal
(a) Advanced age
(b) Transient situational stress
(c) Sleep–wake cycle disturbance
(d) Short-sleepers
2. Pseudo-insomnia
(a) Misattribution of fatigue
(b) Misinterpretation
(c) Hypochondriasis
(d) Delusion of sleepiness
3. Non-restorative sleep
4. Primary insomnia of childhood and adolescence
5. Early morning awakening
(a) Affective disorder
(b) Preparation for activity requiring alertness
6. Onset insomnia
(a) Acute onset insomnia
(b) Phobia of insomnia
(c) Sleep phobia
(d) Traumatic neurosis
(e) Chronic neurosis
7. Maintenance insomnia
(a) Acute
(b) Secondary
(c) Chronic—no apparent immediate cause—new syndrome, 'true insomnia'
8. Mixed onset and maintenance insomnia

From Cleghorn *et al.* 1983*a*, with permission).

Stress-related insomnia

Life events undoubtedly affect sleep patterns. Stress at work, marital problems, bereavements—all the well-documented life events—may be accompanied by short, unsatisfying sleep, usually with initial insomnia. Conversely, some people sleep longer almost as an escape from life's problems.

More severe and persistent insomnia often leads to the individual seeking medical advice. Generally such complaints are confirmed if laboratory studies are carried out. Sleep onset is delayed, total sleep reduced, and several periods of wakefulness occur during the night. No differences in REM sleep episode duration have been found but there is proportionately less SWS. A marked feature is the great variability in sleep pattern from night to night. Sometimes, however, complaints of insomnia are not substantiated, patients sleeping soundly for seven hours and then denying they slept a wink.

In general, the severity of the sleep disturbance is related to the impact of the stress on the individual. He takes his problems to bed with him, mulling over his difficulties although there is usually little constructive that he can do to tackle them while lying in bed. Often the concentration on these problems can become obsessional in intensity with ruminations that the individual vainly resists. Sometimes the person tries too hard; he has an important appointment the next day for which he wants to feel his best; he goes to bed early but then cannot sleep and becomes increasingly anxious as the hours slip by.

Sleep-rhythm related insomnias

Jet-lag is a well recognized cause of insomnia (McFarland 1975). Because of travelling across time-zones, the body's rhythms are out of phase with local clock time. When it is bed-time for the traveller, it is breakfast time in actuality. Such jet-lag is worse on east-bound than west-bound journeys. After a period of time, depending on the extent and direction of travel, the rhythms re-synchronize themselves. Some insomniacs appear to have a similar desynchrony without having travelled, perhaps finding they do not feel sleepy before 4 a.m. and then sleeping until midday. Treatment is often difficult but consists of attempting to institute a more normal cycle by gradually altering the times of going to bed and getting up.

Habit insomnia

This type of insomnia is believed to be a secondary learned phenomenon. Insomnia in the past, perhaps due to transient anxieties, has become associated with the patient's bed and bedroom. Thus, the patient's bed is experienced as a place to lie awake tossing and turning. In strange surroundings sleep is usually normal, the converse of general experience. Management consists of advising the patient to get up and go to another room unless sleep supervenes soon after lying down. After reading for a while the patient returns to bed and tries again. This is repeated until the patient falls asleep.

Insomnia in physical conditions

In many illnesses sleep is disturbed as a result of pain, cough, pruritus, indigestion, breathlessness, bladder distension, etc. Frequently a borderline pain or discomfort can be ignored in the daytime but becomes disturbing at night. The treatment of insomnia is secondary to the alleviation of the primary symptom. Hypnotics are indicated only if symptom relief is incomplete. Even then hypnotics must be prescribed with care because they may aggravate the primary condition; for example, barbiturates and benzodiazepines may depress respiration and encourage the onset of bronchopneumonia.

Moldofsky and his co-workers (1975; Moldofsky and Scarisbrick 1976) have described an inverse relationship, namely abnormal sleep producing pain. They delineated a group of patients who have musculoskeletal pains, the 'fibrositis' syndrome. Their sleep was punctuated by anomalous episodes of alpha rhythm which was postulated to interfere with the restorative function of sleep and lead to the development of symptoms. Such pains can be induced in normal subjects by depriving them of SWS.

Insomnia in psychiatric conditions

Sleep disturbances are a common feature of many psychiatric conditions. Anxiety states and depressive illnesses are common instances but schizophrenic breakdowns and organic states are also associated with insomnia and disrupted sleep patterns. As detailed in the appropriate chapters, the primary medication can often be chosen for its secondary hypnotic activity and administered as a large dose at night with or without daytime supplements (Karacan *et al.* 1975) although nightmares may be induced (Flemenbaum 1976).

Drug-induced insomnia

Hypnotics induce definite changes in sleep patterns. These have been detailed in many sleep laboratory studies especially since such data on new hypnotics have been regarded as essential by drug regulatory authorities. Quite elaborate protocols have been introduced with some attempt to standardize procedures between laboratories. A short protocol consists of 2 nights without drug to acclimatize the subject to sleeping in the laboratory, 3 nights on placebo, 4 on the active drug and 3 on placebo again. An idealized long protocol would comprise a total of 66 nights, 3 adaptation nights, 7 on placebo, 28 on active drug, 28 on placebo again. Not every night is spent in the laboratory, of course.

Most hypnotics have definite effects on sleep onset, duration, and patterns. At the usual clinical doses, the barbiturates (still used as hypnotics) reduce sleep latency and may increase deep sleep in insomniacs. Rapid-eye-movement sleep, however, is usually markedly reduced. On repeated administration, the reduction in REM sleep gradually wears off, so that after a few weeks, the sleep pattern returns to baseline. On withdrawal of the drug, the REM periods increase in duration and frequency, the so called 'REM rebound'. This in turn wears off after a few weeks, but during that time the patient experiences difficulty in getting off to sleep and his sleep is broken, fitful and punctuated by disturbing dreams (Kales *et al.* 1974).

The benzodiazepines, now more widely used than the barbiturates, also reduce sleep latency and increase total sleep time. Sleep pattern changes come on after a night or two and comprise reductions in both REM and slow wave sleep (Adam *et al.* 1976). Most of the night is spent in stage 2 sleep. Sleep spindles are increased in number. The abnormal patterns tend to persist, and rebound after discontinuation is less than with the barbiturates.

Chloral hydrate in doses of 500–1500 mg produces little distortion of sleep patterns. Sleep latency is definitely decreased and sleep duration modestly prolonged. Glutethimide, methaqualone, and methyprylon resemble the barbiturates in their effects on sleep. The sedative antihistamines such as diphenydramine have some effect on REM time and reduce sleep latency.

All in all, hypnotics do have effects on insomnia, reducing sleep onset and duration. But the more effective the drug, the more sleep patterns are disrupted and the greater the effects on discontinuation. The intensity of rebound insomnia is strongly dose-related (Roehrs *et al.* 1986). The timing is related to the half-life of the hypnotic: the rebound insomnia is prompt, severe, and short-lived with short-acting drugs; delayed, mild and longer with long acting drugs (Lader and Lawson 1987; Bixler *et al.* 1985).

The decision whether or not to take a patient off hypnotics must take account of many factors. The age of the patient is important, many elderly patients actually becoming confused, ataxic, and even incontinent on chronic barbiturate therapy. Physical condition is also crucial, the frail patients being sensitive to quite small doses of hypnotics. The reasons for the initial prescription should be reviewed carefully; often the indication will have resolved itself. An elderly patient who has no signs of drug intoxication but does seem to derive some benefit from hypnotics may be best left alone, at least in the short term. If, however, there is a deterioration in mental functioning, the hypnotic medication must be reviewed immediately.

Barbiturates should be particularly carefully evaluated. Their liver-inducing effects cause interactions with other drugs and the elderly are most likely to be receiving other medication for physical complaints.

The first step in withdrawal of medication is to take the patient into one's confidence telling him frankly of the dangers versus the dubious benefits of continued hypnotic use. The cause of the insomnia in terms of the withdrawal stimulatory effects on the central nervous system must be emphasized. Inevitably, the patient will ask why he was started on such drugs in the first instance, and the doctor should explain frankly the change in attitude towards the prescription of hypnotics now that the drug withdrawal insomnia has been confirmed as a reality by laboratory studies.

Next, one doctor only must assume full responsibility for all prescribing for that patient, lest supplies be given unwittingly by another practitioner. The patient's relatives must understand the need to supervise the drug administration. Prescriptions should be issued on a weekly basis and the patient seen each time. The patient must take the dose as prescribed even if he feels he can sleep without it. Otherwise, withdrawal insomnia may occur.

Thirdly, the drugs are gradually withdrawn. If several drugs are being taken simultaneously (by no means uncommon), one should be withdrawn at a time. About 8 weeks is right for the withdrawal period, so the initial dose should be lowered by 10–12 per cent each week. At each step the patient will experience a worsening of insomnia. If this is too extreme, the withdrawal may need to be decelerated, particularly towards the final steps. Even so, the process should not be prolonged beyond 10 weeks.

The final withdrawal should be without the use of any other psychotropic drugs as 'cover', nor should alcohol be allowed. Some doctors use placebos but this is not generally recommended. After total withdrawal, disturbed sleep may persist for 4–6 weeks. If insomnia persists beyond this time, sleep recordings are invaluable in establishing the extent, if any, of the insomnia, and may give some clues as to an underlying cause.

Stimulant induced insomnia

Several drugs can produce insomnia. The commonest are the methyl xanthines, caffeine and theophylline. Coffee contains caffeine, tea caffeine and theophylline, cola drinks made from the nut of the cola tree, *cola acumniata*, contain caffeine. All stimulate the cerebral cortex and in excess can induce insomnia (Victor *et al*. 1981). Elderly people tend to become less tolerant of caffeine, resulting in an insidiously increasing insomnia.

Other drugs producing insomnia include the amphetamines, ephedrine, some sympathomimetics, and some appetite suppressants. Some psychotropic drugs such as protriptyline and pimozide may induce insomnia.

Specific causes

Nocturnal myoclonus is characterized by difficulty in remaining asleep due to frequent arousals (Guilleminault *et al.* 1975). The patient's muscles jerk, especially in the leg; the tibialis anterior is typically affected, with repetitive contractions lasting a couple of seconds every thirty seconds or so. These jerks are unrelated to the sudden startles which everyone experiences from time to time during the onset of sleep. The EEG during nocturnal myoclonus is normal and the jerks can occur at any stage of sleep, but most frequently in nonREM sleep. The arousal which follows involves the autonomic nervous system, with tachycardia and vasoconstriction.

There is no specific treatment for the condition: some patients obtain relief from diazepam 5–20 mg at bedtime. Sometimes the myoclonic jerks occur only when the patient takes up a particular position in bed. Arranging pillows to prevent that position may help.

The '*restless legs*' syndrome comprises uncomfortable sensations in the legs which lead to an urge to move the limbs (Ekbom 1975). This occurs as the patient prepares to fall asleep but the movements may persist during sleep and be associated with nocturnal myoclonus. In time, the sensations may localize to a glove-and-boot type distribution. A number of treatments have been advocated including quinine, vitamin E and the barbiturates. A controlled study has demonstrated that clonazepam reduces the number of leg movements and the number of arousals when compared with placebo (Peled and Lavie 1987). Carbamazepine and diazepam are sometimes useful.

The third of these syndromes is *central sleep apnea* (Guilleminault *et al.* 1976; Editorial 1985). Patients with this complaint are usually overweight with some upper respiratory airway obstruction. During sleep the obstruction increases, leading to apnea. The patient wakes up struggling for breath. This can happen thirty or more times during the night. The bed partner reports strident snoring in between the apneas, the latter lasting more than 10 seconds. The Pickwick syndrome is a variant. Hypnotics must be avoided as these will depress respiration and may prove fatal. The approach is to ascertain the cause of the respiratory obstruction and to remove it. Dieting is essential to reduce weight.

The use of hypnotics

Many complaints of insomnia are unfounded, the patient having unreal expectations concerning sleep. Elderly people fail to appreciate that it is normal to sleep less as they age. Cat-napping during the day also lessens the need for sleep at night. Some old people cannot afford to heat their rooms for more than a few hours a day, and take to their beds as the warmest place. Not surprisingly their sleep patterns become disrupted.

Other subjects can manage on 5–6 h a night as a normal procedure, and yet worry that this is insufficient. Explanation and reassurance relieves their worries.

In most other cases, the insomnia is either a symptom of psychiatric distress, anxiety, or depression, or it is iatrogenic, caused by the very drugs prescribed to relieve the insomnia. In the first instance, treatment is directed towards the primary condition; in the second, a careful regimen of drug withdrawal or substitution and subsequent withdrawal must be planned, as discussed earlier.

Nevertheless, a residuum of patients will be found not to fit into these categories and yet will complain bitterly of insomnia. Careful evaluation of the symptom may yet reveal some relationship to stresses, transient or persistent. These patients are responding to the pressures of life, the man worrying over possible redundancy, his wife concerned about their delinquent son, their daughter lovelorn, grandfather anxious over his physical decrepitude. Giving drugs may set in train a long term process culminating in drug related insomnia without solving the basic problems (Vela-Bueno and Kales 1986).

Short term symptomatic relief seems appropriate when the stress is undoubtedly severe, but transient (Lader 1986). Even so, the hypnotic should be chosen with care (Nicholson 1986). The elimination half-life is the most important consideration (Table 13.2). Those with half lives over 12 h, such as nitrazepam, are only appropriate where sedation is required during the

Table 13.2. Plasma elimination half-lives of hypnotic benzodiazepines and active metabolites in healthy subjects.

Compound	Elimination half-lives of parent drug (h) (mean + range or SD)	Active metabolite	Elimination half-life of metabolite (h)
Brotizolam	5.0 (3.1–6.1)	1-methylhydroxy-derivative	short
Flunitrazepam	15 (9–25)	7-amino-derivative N-desmethyl-derivative	23 31
Flurazepam	very short	*N*-desalkylflurazepam Hydroxyethyl-derivative	87 (40–144) short
Lormetazepam	9.9±2.4	—	—
Loprazolam	6.3(4–8)	?	?
Midazolam	2.5(1–3)	1-methylhydroxy-derivative	short
Nitrazepam	28(20–34)	—	—
Temazepam	12(8–21)	—	—
Triazolam	2.3(1.4–3.3)	1-methylhydroxy-derivative	short

From Breimer and Jochemsen (1983), with permission.

day as well as sleep induction at night (Bond and Lader 1973). Even here, diazepam, 5–15 mg, one dose at night, may be preferred. For a more selective hypnotic effect, temazepam (Heel *et al.* 1981), or triazolam (Pakes *et al.* 1981) with their shorter half times, will encourage sleep onset without leaving the patient with residual sedative effects the next day. Several other medium- and short-acting compounds have been developed such as lormetazepam (Oswald *et al.* 1982), loprazolam (Clark *et al.* 1986) and brotizolam (Mamelak *et al.* 1983). No other differences in efficacy can be detected among these various drugs.

One problem which has been recently noted with the use of short acting hypnotics such as triazolam is increased anxiety during the day (Kales *et al.* 1983*a*). This is similar to that caused by alcohol and is believed to be due to a rebound effect between each dose (Morgan and Oswald 1982). A related phenomenon is early morning insomnia following use of a short acting hypnotic (Kales *et al.* 1983*b*). The elderly are less tolerant of benzodiazepines than younger people and conservative dosage, at least initially, is essential. It is not clear whether the amino acid, L-tryptophan, has useful hypnotic properties or not (Hartmann and Elion 1977; Adam and Oswald 1979).

Residual effects can be a problem especially when long acting drugs are used repeatedly (Greenblatt *et al.* 1984). It must be emphasized that dosage is important here, a small dose of a long-acting drug having less residual effects than higher doses of a short-acting drug (Greenblatt *et al.* 1989). However, the pharmacokinetic factors are complex (Bond and Lader 1981), and the extrapolation from single doses in normal volunteers to repeated doses in insomniacs is difficult (Johnson and Chernik 1982; Hindmarch 1982). Nevertheless, it should be remembered that hypnotics are the only class of drugs in which the main therapeutic effect (drowsiness) is identical with the main unwanted effect: the two are merely separated by 8 h in time (Fig. 13.4). Thus, a short acting hypnotic compound will be devoid of residual effects the next day, but the patient may wake early. After taking a

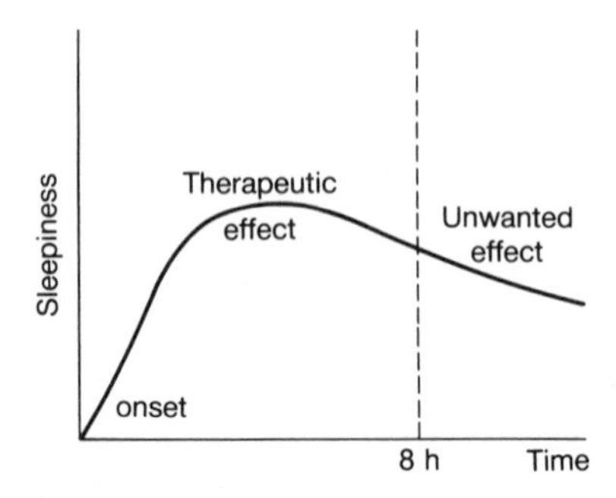

Fig. 13.4. Sleepiness induced by a hypnotic.

longer acting compound, sleep may be prolonged but hangover effects pronounced. It may well be that the ideal treatment will be to administer a hypnotic with a duration of effective hypnotic action of about 8 h, but to 'switch it off' in the morning by administering an antidote. The recent development of a benzodiazepine antagonist (flumazenil) takes this possibility out of the realms of science fiction!

Hypersomnia

This means too much sleep and includes excessive daytime sleepiness. The establishing of the condition is usually easy, especially when observers verify the inappropriateness of the patient's behaviour. Sleep laboratory studies will help confirm the symptom. Care must be taken that the excessive daytime sleepiness is not secondary to insomnia at night. As the objective study of sleep disorders is of recent origin, the hypersomnia syndromes are still being delineated with the narcolepsy group of syndromes being the best documented (Guilleminault and Dement 1977).

Narcolepsy comprises a tetrad of sleep attacks, cataplexy, hypnagogic hallucinations, and sleep paralysis. Frequently, the sleep attacks and only one of the three other features are present. The sleep attack comprises an irresistible urge to sleep during the daytime, often at inappropriate times such as while standing or driving. The patient sleeps for a few minutes or half an hour and awakes feeling refreshed. Cataplexy consists of abrupt attacks of profound muscle weakness which may result in the patient falling helpless to the ground. Emotional states such as laughter or anger may trigger an attack. The sleep onset hallucinations are found in normal people on occasion but are frequent and vivid in narcoleptics. Sleep paralysis is a condition in which the patient lies awake and conscious, but cannot move without an extreme effort of will. Although narcolepsy presumably involves a brain abnormality, nothing definite has been uncovered. The condition typically appears in adolescence or early adulthood, sometimes in association with obesity.

Laboratory recordings reveal a very short latency between sleep onset and the first REM period, sometimes only a few minutes. Similarly, the daytime sleep episodes are characterized by rapid transfer into REM sleep, and cataplexy is accompanied by similar patterns. Consequently, it has been suggested that there is a failure to inhibit REM sleep and that cataplexy represents a dissociated manifestation of the muscular relaxation which accompanies REM sleep.

The treatment of narcolepsy can be divided into the management of the daytime sleepiness and that of the cataplexy. Stimulant drugs such as amphetamine and methylphenidate lessen the incidence of daytime drowsiness but are attended by the usual problems of tolerance, dependence, and rebound hypersomnia and depression on withdrawal. The minimal effective dosage must be sought assiduously; for example, methylphenidate 5–20 mg, three times a day. Part of the problem is the difficulty patients have assessing their own difficulties and a careful observer is invaluable in establishing the extent of any therapeutic effect. As tolerance develops, the stimulant can be withdrawn to allow a 'drug holiday' before re-institution of the drug at a lower dose.

The treatment of the cataplexy is more satisfactory. Antidepressants, both tricyclics and MAOIs, suppress REM episodes and are effective in lessening cataplectic attacks. Clomipramine seems to be currently favoured in the usual antidepressant dosage of 25–50 mg three times a day. The usual unwanted effects are sometimes troublesome. MAO inhibitors have also been used but are less acceptable because of their dietary and drug interactions. They must *never* be combined with clomipramine.

The *Kleine–Levin syndrome* is a rather ill defined condition involving increased sleep and social withdrawal, increased appetite and sometimes heightened libido (Critchley 1962). It is rare and is believed by some to be a depressive variant. The episodes come on mainly in males and in late adolescence, lasting for weeks or months at intervals of a year or longer. There is no treatment and the condition usually remits in time.

Other causes of hypersomnia include lesions of the hypothalamus such as cysts and tumours. In trypanosomiasis ('sleeping sickness'), parasitic infestation occurs in this area of the brain. Encephalitis may be associated with inversion of the sleep rhythm. The torpor of hypothyroidism should also be remembered in the differential diagnosis of excessive sleepiness.

Episodic sleep disorders

This rubric encompasses several conditions which occur episodically during the night. The most frequent occur in children, especially during SWS, and are sometimes called slow-wave sleep dyssomnias. All occur most commonly early in the night, when SWS is most prevalent, usually during a brief arousal from deep sleep. The commonest conditions are sleep-walking, sleep-talking and night terrors. Boys are affected more than girls and there is often a positive family history and twin concordance. Signs of neurological immaturity may be apparent. During the episode the child is unresponsive to the environment, has automatic actions, and retrograde amnesia for the attack. The conditions typically worsen when the child is under emotional strain.

Enforced wakening from SWS is somewhat disturbing for normal people. Many experience disorientation, inco-ordination and confusion, sometimes called 'sleep drunkenness'.

Somnambulism is fairly common, about 15 per cent of children up to the age of 12 having sleep-walked at least once. One or two per cent of the adult population occasionally sleep-walk. The EEG record shows SWS followed by a body movement with arousal. The individual sits up in bed, staring but unseeing. Attempts to walk are clumsy but some people succeed and may endanger themselves. Treatment is usually not required providing the bedroom is made as safe as possible. In severe cases, diazepam at night should help, perhaps by reducing SWS.

Sleep-talking is essentially similar although not related solely to SWS. The child utters gibberish. Parental reassurance is the basis of treatment.

Night terrors (pavor nocturnus) present a more disturbing problem and are quite common in young children. The terrors, being an SWS dyssomnia, occur early in the night. The child (or adult) suddenly sits up and screams. Again, the EEG shows an arousal from stage 3 or 4, together with signs of autonomic arousal. The child often appears to be hallucinating. After a few seconds the attack subsides but in severe cases, it can last 10 or 20 min. The attacks tend to diminish as the child gets older, especially after the age of 5 or 6. Some adults have night terrors after severe traumatic episodes. These attacks, as in concentration camp survivors, tend to persist. Epileptic attacks at night may sometimes resemble night terrors and may need excluding. The treatment is either symptomatic—diazepam to suppress SWS—or, better, psychotherapy in adults and older children to deal with the root cause.

Nocturnal enuresis is also an SWS dyssomnia. It is dealt with in Chapter 14.

Nightmares differ fundamentally from night terrors, being much more common and associated with REM sleep. Like all dreams they occur later in the night, typically towards the end of a long REM period. On awakening from an episode of this sort, the subject reports a vivid and anxiety-provoking dream often culminating in a terrifying threat coupled with helplessness. Nightmares are more common in anxious people and the content is usually related to the daytime worries (Hersen 1971). The treatment, if any is required, is toward the underlying anxieties.

Other disturbances during sleep include bruxism (teeth-grinding) and head-banging, not usually brought to the attention of the psychiatrist. Various medical conditions such as left ventricular failure and asthma may be worse at night and some epileptics only have fits at night, sometimes after an injudicious drinking bout.

References

Adam, K., and Oswald, I. (1979). One gram of L-tryptophan fails to alter the time taken to fall asleep. *Neuropharmacology* **18,** 1025–7.

Adam, K., Adamson, L., Brezinova, V., Hunter, W., and Oswald, I. (1976). Nitrazepam: lastingly effective but trouble on withdrawal. *British Medical Journal* **1,** 1558–60.

Aserinsky, E., and Kleitman, N. (1953). Regularly occurring periods of eye motility and concomitant phenomena during sleep. *Science* **118,** 273–4.

Bixler, E.O., Kales, J.D., Kales, A., Jacoby, J.A., and Soldatos, C.R. (1985). Rebound insomnia and elimination half-life: assessment of individual subject response. *Journal of Clinical Pharmacology* **25,** 115–24.

Bond, A.J., and Lader, M.H. (1973). The residual effects of flurazepam. *Psychopharmacologia* **32,** 223–35.

Bond, A., and Lader, M.H. (1981). After effects of sleeping drugs. In *Psychopharmacology of sleep*. (ed. D. Wheatley) pp. 177-97. Raven, New York.

Breimer, D.D., and Jochemsen, R. (1983). Clinical pharmacokinetics of hypnotic benzodiazepines: a summary. *British Journal of Clinical Pharmacology* **16,** suppl. 2, 277–8.

Clark, B.G., Jue, S.G., Dawson, G.W., and Ward, A. (1986). Loprazolam: a preliminary review of its pharmacodynamic and pharmacokinetic properties and therapeutic efficacy in insomnia. *Drugs* **31,** 500–16.

Cleghorn, J.M., Kaplin, R.D., Bellissimo, A., and Szatmari, P. (1983*a*). Insomnia: I. Classification, assessment and pharmaceutical treatment. *Canadian Journal of Psychiatry* **28,** 339–46.

Cleghorn, J.M., Bellissimo, A., Kaplin, R.D., and Szatmari, P. (1983*b*). Insomnia: II. Assessment and treatment of chronic insomnia. *Canadian Journal of Psychiatry* **28,** 347–53.

Consensus Conference (1984). Drugs and insomnia. The use of medications to promote sleep. *Journal of the American Medical Association* **251,** 2410–14.

Critchley, M. (1962). Periodic hyposomnia and megaphagia in adolescent males. *Brain* **85,** 627–56.

Dement, W., and Kleitman, N. (1955). Cyclic variations in EEG during sleep and their relation to eye movements, body motility and dreaming. *Electroencephalography and Clinical Neurophysiology* **9,** 673–90.

Editorial (1985). Snoring and sleepiness. *Lancet* **2,** 925–6.

Ekbom, K.A. Restless legs. *Acta Medica Scandinavica* 1945, Suppl. 158, 1–123.

Flemenbaum, A. (1976). Pavor nocturnus: a complication of single daily tricyclic or neuroleptic dosage. *American Journal of Psychiatry* **133,** 570–2.

Gerner, R.H., Post, R.M., Gillin, J.C., and Bunney, W.E. (1979). Biological and behavioral effects of one night's sleep deprivation in depressed patients and normals. *Journal of Psychiatric Research* **15,** 21–60.

Greenblatt, D.J., Harmatz, J.S., Engelhardt, N., and Shader, R.I. (1989). Pharmacokinetic determinants of dynamic differences among three benzodiazepine hypnotics. *Archives of General Psychiatry* **46,** 326–32.

Greenblatt, D.J., Shader, R.I., Divoll, M., and Harmatz, J.S. (1984). Adverse reactions to triazolam, flurazepam, and placebo in controlled clinical trials. *Journal of Clinical Psychiatry* **45,** 192–5.

Guilleminault, C., and Dement, W.C. (1977). 235 cases of excessive daytime sleepiness: diagnosis and tentative classification. *Journal of the Neurological Sciences* **31,** 13–27.

Guilleminault, C., Billiard, M., Montplaisir, J., and Dement, W.C. (1975). Altered states of consciousness in disorders of daytime sleepiness. *Journal of the Neurological Sciences* **26,** 377–93.

Guilleminault, C., Tilkian, A., and Dement, W.C. (1976). The sleep apnea syndromes. *Annual Review of Medicine* **27,** 465–84.

Hartmann, E.L. (1980). Sleep and the sleep disorders. In: *Handbook of biological psychiatry* (ed. H.M. van Praag, M. Lader, O. Rafaelsen and E. Sachar) Pt. II. Marcel Dekker, New York.

Hartmann, E., and Elion, R. (1977). The insomnia of 'sleeping in a strange place'. Effects of L-tryptophane. *Psychopharmacology*, **53,** 131–3.

Hauri, P. (1977). *The sleep disorders*. Upjohn, Kalamazoo.

Heel, R.C., Brogden, R.N., Speight, T.M., and Avery, G.S. (1981). Temazepam: a review of its pharmacological properties and therapeutic efficacy as an hypnotic. *Drugs* **21,** 321–40.

Hersen, M. (1971). Personality characteristics of nightmare sufferers. *Journal of Nervous and Mental Disease* **152,** 27–31.

Hindmarch, I. (1982). Hypnotics and residual sequelae. In: *Hypnotics in clinical practice*. (ed. A.N. Nicholson) pp. 7–16. Medical Publishing Foundation: Oxford.

Hobson, J.A. (1984). The cellular basis of sleep cycle control. *Advances in Sleep Research* **1,** 217–50.

Horne, J.A. (1981). The effects of exercise upon sleep: a critical review. *Biological Psychology* **12,** 241–90.

Johnson, L.C., and Chernik, D.A. (1982). Sedative-hypnotics and human performance. *Psychopharmacology* **76,** 101–13.

Kales, A., Bixler, E.O., Tan, T., *et al.* (1974). Chronic hypnotic-drug use. *Journal of the American Medical Association* **227,** 513–17.

Kales, A., Scharf, M.B., Kales, J.D., and Soldatos, C.R. (1979). Rebound insomnia—a potential hazard following withdrawal of certain benzodiazepines. *Journal of the American Medical Association* **241,** 1692–5.

Kales, A., Soldatos, C.R., Bixler, E.O., and Kales, J.D. (1983*a*). Rebound insomnia and rebound anxiety: a review. *Pharmacology* **26,** 121–37.

Kales, A., Soldatos, C.R., Bixler, E.O., and Kales, J.D. (1983*b*). Early morning insomnia with rapidly eliminated benzodiazepines. *Science* **220,** 95–7.

Karacan, I., Blackburn, A.B., Thornby, J.I. *et al.* (1975). The effect of doxepin HCL (Sinequan) on sleep patterns and clinical symptomatology or neurotic depressed patients with sleep disturbance. In *Sinequan (doxepin HCl): A monograph of recent clinical studies* (ed. J. Mendels) pp. 4–22. Excerpta Medica, Amsterdam.

Lader, M.H. (1986). A practical guide to prescribing hypnotic benzodiazepines. *British Medical Journal* **2,** 1048–9.

Lader, M., and Lawson, C. (1987). Sleep studies and rebound insomnia: methodological problems, laboratory findings, and clinical implications. *Clinical Neuropharmacology* **10,** 291-312.

Mamelak, M., Csima, A., and Price, V. (1983). Effects of brotizolam on the sleep of chronic insomniacs. *British Journal of Clinical Pharmacology* **16,** 377S–82S.

McFarland, R.A. (1975). Air travel across time zones. *American Scientist* **63,** 23–30.

Mellinger, G.D., Balter, M.B., and Uhlenhuth, E.H. (1985). Insomnia and its treatment—prevalence and correlates. *Archives of General Psychiatry* **42,** 225–32.

Moldofsky, H., and Scarisbrick, P. (1976). Induction of neurasthenic musculoskeletal pain syndrome by selective sleep stage deprivation. *Psychosomatic Medicine* **38,** 35–44.

Moldofsky, H., Scarisbrick, P., England, R., and Smythe, H. (1975). Musculoskeletal symptoms and non-REM sleep disturbance in patients with 'fibrositis syndrome' and healthy subjects. *Psychosomatic Medicine* **37,** 341–51.

Morgan, K., and Oswald, I. (1982). Anxiety caused by a short-life hypnotic. *British Medical Journal* **284,** 942.

Nicholson, A.N. (1986). Hypnotics—their place in therapeutics. *Drugs*. **31,** 164–76.

Oswald, I. (1984). Symptoms that depress the doctor—insomnia. *British Journal of Hospital Medicine* **27,** 219–24.

Oswald, I., French, C., Adam, K., and Gilham, J. (1982). Benzodiazepine hypnotics remain effective for 24 weeks. *British Medical Journal* **284,** 860–3.

Pakes, G.E., Brogden, R.N., Heel, R.C., Speight, T.M., and Avery, G.S. (1981). Triazolam: a review of its pharmacological properties and therapeutic efficacy in patients with insomnia. *Drugs* **22,** 81–110.

Peled, R., and Lavie, P. (1987). Double-blind evaluation of clonazepam on periodic leg movements in sleep. *Journal of Neurology, Neurosurgery and Psychiatry*. **50,** 1679–81.

Roehrs, T.A., Zorick, F.J., Wittig, R.M., and Roth, T. (1986). Dose determinants of rebound insomnia. *British Journal of Clinical Pharmacology* **22,** 143–7.

Rudolf, G.A.E., and Tolle, R. (1981). Sleep deprivation and circadian rhythm in depression. *Psychiatria Clinica* **11,** 198–212.

Tolle, R. (1981). Sleep deprivation and sleep treatment. In: *Handbook of biological psychiatry*, (eds. H. van Praag, M. Lader, O. Rafaelsen, and E. Sachar) Part VI. Marcel Dekker, New York.

Vela-Bueno, A., and Kales, A. (1986). Benzodiazepine hypnotics in the multidimensional treatment of insomnia. *Drugs of Today*. **22,** 271–81.

Victor, B.S., Lubetsky, M., and Greden, J.F. (1981). Somatic manifestations of caffeinism. *Journal of Clinical Psychiatry* **42,** 185–8.

Vogel, G. (1981). Sleep deprivation. In: *Handbook of biological psychiatry*, (eds. H. van Praag, M. Lader, O. Rafaelsen, and E. Sachar) Part VI. Marcel Dekker, New York.

14. Drug treatment in children

General principles (Werry 1979; Campbell and Cohen 1981)

Child psychiatrists in the UK tend to be conservative in their use of psychotropic drugs. This stems from several factors: the emphasis on social and educational manipulations as forms of treatment; the psychoanalytic background of many child psychiatrists; the realization that many disturbed children are reflecting tensions in the family rather than intrinsic difficulties; the reluctance to use drugs in a developing organism, in particular on a developing brain; and a healthy and often well founded scepticism concerning the efficacy of drug therapy in psychiatrically disturbed children. Also the ready use of drugs in children leads to the erroneous conclusion by child, parents and by other medical attendants that the problem lies within the child and is amenable to drugs so that recourse to drugs in the future becomes too facile. Nevertheless, there are some indications for drug treatment, mainly stimulants in truly hyperkinetic children and antipsychotic drugs in a few severely disturbed psychotic children. However, the selection of such children is complex and time-consuming and ideally should be left to a specialist.

The importance of a careful evaluation need hardly be stressed. An interview and examination of the child is essential. Information from parents, teachers, the family physician, and others enables a full assessment of the child's condition to be made. Standardized ratings by parents, teachers, or nurses are also helpful, and laboratory tests such as the EEG may be needed. Based on all this, the diagnosis and prognosis can be drawn up. Appropriate treatments can be used including drugs where necessary (Blau 1978; Werry 1979).

The particular problems of drug treatment in adolescents have been reviewed by Rifkin and his colleagues (1986) who point out that adolescents are neither adults nor children. The dearth of clinical trials in adolescents is deprecated.

Principles of prescribing

Drug treatment should always be part of a scheme of general management. Children often improve spontaneously; therefore one should never hurry to use drugs. Simple reassurance may be quite effective where anxiety is marked. The lowest effective dose should be used and the dose increased only slowly. Careful monitoring for adverse effects should be carried out by parents and teachers. The long half lives of many psychotropic drugs should be borne in mind when adjusting dosage.

Long term drug administration should be undertaken only when all the risks and benefits have been carefully assessed. The use of medication should be discussed with the child. Frequent review of medication should involve parents and teachers when the child is an out-patient and nursing attendants, teachers, and occupational therapists if the child is in an institution.

Many children for whom drugs are indicated display behaviour disturbances. The drugs used have major effects on cognitive and intellectual performance. Thus, a balance may need to be struck between behavioural improvement and impairment of mental function.

Stimulant drugs

The hyperkinetic syndrome is known by a variety of names including 'minimal brain dysfunction' (MBD) syndrome, 'minimal brain damage', 'attention deficit disorder' and 'hyperactive child syndrome' (Strother 1973). The child is characterized by hyperactivity, excitability, distractibility, impulsiveness, and often by antisocial and aggressive behaviour, emotional lability, and specific learning problems.

The syndrome has excited some controversy (Taylor 1979). Undoubtedly, there are children with definite brain damage who show symptoms of this type. However, the syndrome merges into normality and the criteria for diagnosing the condition remain arbitrary. The definition of normal behaviour in a child is entirely a value judgement. Thus, one observer may dub a child as merely high-spirited and mischievous, whereas another may regard him as suffering from a hyperkinetic syndrome. The apparent prevalence of MBD is much higher in the USA than the UK, reflecting the reluctant use of this label by British child psychiatrists. In the USA as many as 4–10 per cent of children are believed to demonstrate one or more symptoms, boys 3–4 times more frequently than girls.

Central nervous system stimulants are currently the drugs of choice in treating the hyperkinetic syndrome and have been well investigated (Conners and Taylor 1980; Taylor *et al.* 1987). Dextroamphetamine was popular but methylphenidate is currently preferred (Arnold *et al.* 1978). Special arrangements may be needed to obtain it. Both drugs are useful in the short term and most children show some response, occasionally dramatic (Gittelman-Klein and Klein 1976; Butler and Lapierre 1974). A typical treatment using methylphenidate commences with 0.3 mg/kg (5–10 mg/daily), divided into two doses at breakfast and lunch-time. The dose is doubled every week or so but not beyond 2.0 mg/kg/day. High doses carry the risk of anorexia and weight loss: inhibition of growth may become marked and will persist as long as medication is given. The maintenance dose is usually 10–20 mg/daily. Medication should be interrupted whenever possible, for example, at weekends or during vacations. Other side-effects of stimulants include tearfulness, rebound irritability, exacerbation of tics, insomnia, personality change, and even toxic psychosis. Cessation of medication may be followed by a compensatory spurt in growth. If lack of normal weight gain continues during medication, the drug should be changed or stopped. Dependence does not seem to be a problem at the time the drug is given and in later life drug abuse does not seem more likely. Medication is usually not needed after the age of 12 because hyperactivity tends to lessen at about that age. However, personality problems may be noted later in life.

The use of stimulants in hyperactive children should not be embarked on lightly (Millichap 1973). If improvement follows, the pressures from teachers and parents for long term maintenance may become great. Growth inhibition is a worrying side effect but not usually a long-term problem, and there is little evidence that long term benefit to social or personal adjustment or educational achievement follows the use of these drugs. Non pharmacological management should be instituted as the treatment of hyperkinetic syndromes requires a total approach. Remedial educational programmes, counselling of the parents with practical advice on how to structure the child's environment and time-table, and behaviour therapy and psychotherapy as appropriate, should be the mainstay of management. Stimulant drugs should be a short-term adjunct (Quinn and Rapoport 1975; Rifkin *et al.* 1986). Consequently, the management of the truly hyperkinetic child should be under the general guidance of a specialist, a pediatrician or a child psychiatrist.

It is generally argued that the hyperkinetic syndrome be distinguished from conduct disorder but this is not necessarily either easy or valid in adolescents. Stimulant drugs should be avoided in delinquent children, who may be abusing them anyway.

Antipsychotic drugs

Psychotic disturbances in childhood comprise a group of ill-defined disorders characterized by emotional abnormalities, bizarre behaviour disturbances, speech problems, and blunted, uneven, or fragmented intellectual development. 'Pervasive developmental disorder' is often the preferred term nowadays. Infantile autism is the commonest of the childhood psychoses and comprises the development before the age of 2½ of withdrawal, aloofness, isolation, language delays and abnormalities, ritualistic and obsessive activities, dislike of change, and patchy intellectual development. Childhood schizophrenia is uncommon, occurs over the age of 10, and more closely resembles schizophrenia in adults, with disorder of thought processes, delusions, hallucinations, and affective blunting. Psychoses can also occur in the mentally retarded, the brain-damaged and the epileptic.

Antipsychotic drugs are indicated symptomatically in these conditions but should be used sparingly because of the wide range of side effects, in particular, tardive dyskinesia. The antipsychotic drugs exercise a general depressant effect and are consequently most effective against symptoms reflecting overactivity such as aggressive outbursts and explosiveness, irritability, and movement disorders (Jorgensen 1979). In hyperkinetic syndromes without psychosis they are not as effective as the stimulants. The widespread use of these drugs as antianxiety agents in children is not supported by clear data (Rifkin *et al.* 1986).

Each child must be treated individually to arrive at the optimal dosage. The whole range of antipsychotic drugs has been used in children but chlorpromazine, thioridazine, pericyazine, and haloperidol seem most popular. The first three are less likely to lead to acute extrapyramidal effects than haloperidol but oversedation and autonomic effects are more likely. Usually a single bed-time dose will be tried initially but some children do better on divided doses. Fluphenazine or flupenthixol decanoate depot injections should be reserved for very disturbed children who present major problems of compliance.

Extrapyramidal effects can occur, especially acute dystonic reactions with haloperidol; the dosage should therefore be kept conservative. Tardive dyskinesia can supervene and become severe and distressing in children, limb and trunk movements interfering with eating and walking.

One special indication for haloperidol is Gilles de la Tourette syndrome, characterized by widespread tics, involuntary grunting, barking, or coprolalia (Shapiro and Shapiro 1981). The evidence for efficacy is stronger with respect to pimozide (Shapiro *et al.* 1984). Antipsychotic drugs have been advocated in anorexia nervosa but general behavioural management and psychotherapy are more generally used. However, chlorpromazine may be useful to stimulate appetite but must be used carefully in the physically frail anorectic patient.

Antidepressant drugs

Depression is another controversial topic in child psychiatry (Welner 1978; Kashani *et al.* 1981). Children do not generally become sad, withdrawn and retarded but tend to react to adverse circumstances by inappropriate and awkward behaviour, by developing vague physical complaints, dysphoria, sleep difficulties, and anxiety. Although some advocate the use of tricyclic antidepressants in such cases of neurotic depression, most child psychiatrists regard the use of these drugs as unestablished (Schulterbrandt and Raskin 1977), especially as these disorders may remit with psychosocial support.

Manic depressive psychosis is extremely rare before the age of 12 and quite uncommon until the mid teens. Lithium has been tried but reports are few as are those on the use of antidepressants during the depressed phase (Youngerman and Canino 1978). Reports are also unconvincing as to the usefulness of lithium in adolescents with chronic childhood psychoses or conduct disorders with mood swings (Rifkin *et al.* 1986; Jefferson 1982).

Antidepressants can suppress nocturnal enuresis. The mechanism is obscure but probably central. They should only be used in children over the age of 7. Unfortunately, the condition tends to recur when medication is stopped. Behavioural methods such as the pad and alarm are generally more effective (Forsythe and Redmond 1974). Antidepressants (e.g. imipramine 25–50 mg at night) are best reserved for short term use in adverse social circumstances, for example, to relieve the pressure on a harassed mother or when a child is staying away from home when the enuresis would be unacceptably embarrassing.

Antianxiety drugs

Many physicians believe that anxiolytics make hyperkinetic and psychotic children worse and that these drugs have little place in the management of minor disturbances with anxiety and disturbed sleep. Nevertheless, these drugs are widely used in anxious children. Benzodiazepines and antihistamines are the usual drugs prescribed. However, sedation is common in children and it is difficult to attain a dose which lessens symptoms without some impairment of mental functioning. Use of these drugs should be sparing and closely monitored especially as the risk of dependence in children and adolescents is unknown. Panic disorder is best treated with antidepressants.

Conclusions

Only the stimulants such as methylphenidate have been extensively tested in children but their use should be under specialist supervision. Antipsychotic medication may help control the severely disturbed psychotic child but the place of antidepressants, lithium and antianxiety medication is so far unclear. The use of medication in children is attended by the usual side-effects plus ill-documented ones related to the effect of these drugs on the developing brain and body. As well as pharmacological side-effects, the use of drugs in children with behavioural problems has general implications related to the role of drug treatment, relationships with parents and teachers and over-reliance on outside intervention. No childhood psychiatric problems are cured by drugs and relatively few are ameliorated by them to a sufficient degree to outweigh the disadvantages.

References

Arnold, L.E., Christopher, J., Huestis, R., and Smeltzer, D.J. (1978). Methylphenidate vs dextroamphetamine vs caffeine in minimal brain dysfunction. *Archives of General Psychiatry* **35,** 463–73.

Blau, S. (1978). A guide to the use of psychotropic medication in children and adolescents. *Journal of Clinical Psychiatry* **39,** 766–72.

Butler, H.J., and Lapierre, Y.D. (1974). The effect of methylphenidate on sensory perception and integration in hyperactive children. *International Pharmacopsychiatry* **9,** 235–44.

Campbell, M., and Cohen, I.L. (1981). Psychotropic drugs in child psychiatry. In *Handbook of Biological Psychiatry, Part VI.* (ed. H.M. van Praag, M.H. Lader, O.J. Rafaelsen, and E.J. Sachar) pp. 215–41. Marcel Dekker, New York.

Conners, C,K, and Taylor, E. (1980). Pemoline, methylphenidate and placebo in children with minimal brain dysfunction. *Archives of General Psychiatry* **37,** 922–30.

Forsythe, W.I., and Redmond, A. (1974). Enuresis and spontaneous cure rate. *Archives of Disease in Children* **49,** 259–63.

Gittelman-Klein, R., and Klein, D.F. (1976). Methylphenidate effects in learning disabilities. Psychometric changes. *Archives of General Psychiatry* **33,** 655–64.

Jefferson, J.W. (1982). The use of lithium in childhood and adolescence: an overview. *Journal of Clinical Psychiatry* **43,** 174–7.

Jorgensen, O.S. (1979). Psychopharmacological treatment of psychotic children: a survey. *Acta Psychiatrica Scandinavica* **59,** 229–38.

Kashani, J.H., Husain, A., Shekim, W.O., Hodges, K.K., Cytryn, L., and McKnew, D.H. (1981). Current perspectives on childhood depression: an overview. *American Journal of Psychiatry* **138,** 143–53.

Millichap, J. (1973). Drugs in management of minimal brain dysfunction. *Annals of the New York Academy of Sciences* **205,** 321–34.

Rifkin, A., Wortman, R., Reardon, G., and Siris, S.G. (1986). Psychotropic medication in adolescents: a review. *Journal of Clinical Psychiatry* **47,** 400–8.

Quinn, P.O., and Rapoport, J.L. (1975). One-year follow-up of hyperactive boys treated with imipramine or methylphenidate. *American Journal of Psychiatry* **132,** 241–5.

Schulterbrandt, J.G., and Raskin, A. (eds.) (1977). Depression in childhood. Diagnosis, treatment and conceptual models. Department of Health, Education and Welfare Publication No (ADM), Washington, D.C.

Shapiro, A.K., and Shapiro, E. (1981). The treatment and etiology of tics and Tourette syndrome. *Comprehensive Psychiatry* **22,** 193–205.

Shapiro, A.K., Shapiro, E., and Flyer, P.A. (1984). Controlled study of pimozide vs. placebo in Tourette syndrome. *Journal of the American Academy of Child Psychiatry* **23,** 161–73.

Strother, C. (1973). Minimal cerebral dysfunction: a historical overview. *Annals of the New York Academy of Sciences* **205,** 6–17.

Taylor, E. (1979). The use of drugs in hyperkinetic states: clinical issues. *Neuropharmacology* 951–8.

Taylor, E., Schachar, R., Thorley, G., Wieselberg, H.M., Everitt, B., and Rutter, M. (1987). Which boys respond to stimulant medication? A controlled trial of methylphenidate in boys with disruptive behaviour. *Psychological Medicine* **17,** 121–43.

Welner, Z. (1978). Childhood depression: an overview. *Journal of Nervous and Mental Disease* **166,** 588–93.

Werry, J.S. (1979). Principles of use of psychotropic drugs in children. *Drugs* **18,** 392–7.

Youngerman, J., and Canino, I. (1978). Lithium carbonate use in children and adolescents. *Archives of General Psychiatry* **35,** 216–24.

15. Drug treatment in the elderly

Mental illness in the elderly

The proportion of the aged in developed countries will increase three- to four-fold from 1950 to the end of the century. This will place an increasing burden on health services especially psychiatric facilities.

Psychopathology increases with age and at least 10 per cent of the elderly are mentally disturbed. Organic disturbances such as dementia become increasingly common with age to constitute a formidable problem in the over-80s. But functional psychoses such as paranoid states and affective disorders also increase in frequency. Suicide rates rise sharply with age. Neurotic reactions are also a problem as the old person's adaptability wanes so that minor stresses precipitate depressions and anxiety states (Turnbull and Turnbull 1985). Thus, age alone does not mean that a patient's emotional disorder is due to a dementing (and hence, almost by definition) irreversible process. Depression, paranoid reactions and anxiety states should be as vigorously treated in the old as in the young.

Treatment of these conditions by drugs or other physical methods does not differ in principle from that in younger patients (Eisdorfer and Fann 1973; Sathananthan *et al.* 1977; Jenike, 1985). It must form part of a general strategy combining these approaches with psychotherapy, family counselling, and use of social resources. In addition, physical conditions which often aggravate or even precipitate the mental condition must be rectified. Age, however, does modify the choice and use of psychotropic medication because drug actions are altered in the elderly (Lader 1982; Small 1988). Both pharmacokinetic and pharmacodynamic aspects of drug action may be modified in old people but individual variation can be very great.

Pharmacokinetics

All four main aspects of pharmacokinetics are altered in old age (Crooks *et al.* 1976; Friedel 1978). As gastric secretion declines, absorption may be impaired, especially if the drug is optimally absorbed from an acid medium.

The disintegration of tablets and solution of capsules is sometimes slower or less complete in the elderly. Absorption may thus be delayed which is not in itself a disadvantage as drug levels may be less variable and peaked. However, absorption may be delayed to the point that it is incomplete.

Distribution is altered in the elderly. Plasma protein concentration lessens with age so the amount of drug bound to protein diminishes. This leaves more drug in the plasma water and hence tissue concentrations will also tend to be higher. Body mass is less in the elderly than in younger people. Consequently, a standard dose in absolute terms will be a high dose in the elderly in terms of dose per kilogram of body weight.

Metabolism of drugs is mainly carried out by the liver microsomal enzymes. The different enzymes metabolizing drugs change in different ways with age. Hydroxylation and demethylation are common metabolic processes and are usually slower in the elderly, sometimes markedly so. By contrast, conjugating processes (for example, with glucuronic acid) are little changed.

Finally, renal capacity declines steadily with age, resulting in diminished renal clearance of drugs. The kidney also seems more susceptible to toxic effects.

Overall, ageing is associated with a definite prolongation of the action of most, but not all, psychotropic drugs. As a general rule, therefore, the action of a dose of a drug will be longer, sometimes several times longer, in an aged person than in a young or middle-aged adult.

Pharmacodynamics

Much less is known of the mechanisms whereby elderly people respond more than younger people to the same tissue concentration of drug (Bender 1974). Whether this is related to a change in the number of receptors, in their affinity for the drug, or in the coupling between surface receptor and intracellular processes is unclear. Perhaps, several mechanisms operate.

Practical implications

Thus, as a general rule, the elderly are more sensitive than young to drugs, by a factor of up to about three. The dose of drug, as well as having a more pronounced effect also acts longer. Consequently, less drug is needed, less often (Cole and Stotsky 1974). The prudent initiate treatment with between a third and a half of the normal adult dose and increase it gradually. Frail, thin, physically ill patients may respond to even lower proportional doses (Davis *et al.* 1973). Some elderly patients, however, need and tolerate full doses. Clinical judgement is needed to arrive at the therapeutic dose without pushing the dose too rapidly and risking toxicity or raising the dose too slowly and postponing the therapeutic response unduly.

The half-lives of many psychotropic compounds are so prolonged in the elderly that smaller doses at less frequent intervals are justifiable. Once the body levels have built up, the increase following each dose is not proportionately large. In addition, compliance is better, the simpler the regimen. Sustained release preparations are the logical answer to providing a smooth, low profile absorption curve, thereby avoiding toxicity in the elderly. However, such preparations require sophisticated formulation such as plastic matrices, and the change in characteristics of these vehicles in the elderly has not been much studied.

Because of possible impaired disintegration and absorption of tabletted drugs, liquid preparations such as elixirs are often to be preferred. Care should be taken in switching from one formulation to another lest the bioavailabilities differ significantly.

Drug interactions

Psychotropic drugs have many pharmacological actions, as best instanced by the antipsychotic drugs, the antidepressants and lithium. They therefore interact with many other drugs, psychotropic and non-psychotropic. Elderly people tend to have a multiple pathology, both physical and psychiatric, and are commonly being treated with several powerful drugs simultaneously. The whole topic of drug interactions is uncertain. Although many interactions, both pharmacokinetic and pharmacodynamic, can be demonstrated in animal preparations, it is much less clear which are important in clinical practice. The general rule must be, not withstanding, that the fewer the drugs, the better. There is no rationale for combining several drugs of the same class.

Questions about concomitant medication are particularly essential in the elderly. If possible, close relatives or friends, acting as informants should be asked about drugs being taken. Over-the-counter, patent medicines should be also enquired for. Where several drugs are being taken, hospital admission may be needed to rationalize the treatment or to withdraw the patient from say, a barbiturate. Confusion in the elderly may be due to over-medication with psychotropic drugs and unsuspected drug interactions may elevate body concentrations of drug. The general metabolic state such as salt depletion or thyroid insufficiency may also alter drug effects and such metabolic alterations are commonest in the elderly.

Antidepressant drugs

Depression is the most common psychiatric disorder of old age (Blazer 1980). Both recurrences of depression and first episodes occur frequently in the elderly. In this, the last period of life, psychosocial factors become increasingly important in precipitating, contributing to, or perpetuating affective disturbances. In particular, life events of loss, known to be often associated with the onset of depression, are distressingly frequent for the elderly. Physical and mental vigour wanes; retirement has occurred; income drops; friends and relatives die, and spouse, too, perhaps. From leading a full life, the elderly person can become enfeebled and isolated. It is hardly surprising that depressive reactions commonly ensue. Nevertheless, the presence of adverse personal and social circumstances should not lead to half-hearted attempts to alleviate symptoms of depression in an elderly individual. What seems hopeless to a person when depressed may seem tolerable or even trivial when the mood reverts to normal. Response to medication can be gratifying and rapid in the elderly (Post 1972), but the overall prognosis is poor (Murphy 1983).

Drug therapy, as always, must be part of a coherent and flexible treatment schedule. Physical illness must be carefully sought as this may have led to the depressed state, or the symptoms of depression may mimic physical complaints. The social and personal background of the patient should be assessed with respect to assets and drawbacks. Thus, the outlook is much better for a depressed old man cared for by his wife than for the isolated widower. Compliance is particularly poor in the elderly, probably because side effects are more troublesome.

The symptoms of depression in the elderly are generally similar to those in younger patients but bodily complaints and intellectual impairment are more noticeable because elderly people tend to have physical problems and lessened mental vigour anyway, and the depressive illness decompensates them. Severe depression in the elderly may include symptoms such as psychomotor retardation or agitation, anorexia and weight loss, sleep disturbance, constipation, fatigue, social withdrawal, delusions and hallucinations. Intellectual capacity may be so impaired as to constitute a pseudodementia and some patients are mistakenly regarded as senile dements. Social isolation may increase and this in turn increases the risk of suicide, which is already appreciable, especially in males living alone.

Prior to initiation of treatment, a thorough physical examination is advisable, together with a laboratory test battery including hepatic, renal, and thyroid function tests (Gerner 1985). An ECG should be recorded and blood pressure and pulse taken with the patient lying and standing. These clinical measures should be repeated until the patient is on a stable dose of medication. The ECG should also be repeated, with greater frequency in patients with a history of cardiovascular disease.

Tricyclic antidepressants with sedative effects are generally preferred in the elderly because the clinical picture is typically coloured with anxiety or agitation (Kantor and Glassman 1980). Amitriptyline is still very popular but produces marked anticholinergic effects, hypotension, and sedation and some suspicion of cardiotoxicity (Grossberg and Nakra 1986). Imipramine is somewhat less sedative. Doxepin is also recommended for the elderly. Of the newer drugs, mianserin (available in the UK and many other European countries) is almost devoid of anticholinergic effects, is usefully sedative, and is much less cardiotoxic than its predecessors. However, blood dyscrasias are more likely in the elderly. Lofepramine is also worth considering as it has fewer anticholinergic side-effects than other tricyclic compounds.

Because elderly people are generally sensitive to these drugs, one should start with a third or half of the usual dosage. Thus, for a frail old lady, 10 mg three times a day of amitriptyline or imipramine, is appropriate. The dosage can then be increased cautiously in some cases to full dosage: smaller dosage requirements are not inevitable in all elderly people. The rate of increase is 25–30 mg per week for an out-patient; a faster rate of increase is possible in in-patients under close supervision. Dosage should be divided. The single dose at night which is appropriate in some younger patients is not advisable in the elderly because side effects may be troublesome in the morning, and if the patient wakes at night the side-effects, such as blurred vision, difficulty in micturition, and dry mouth may be excessive, hypotension may result in a fall, or confusion may also occur. Elderly patients find it difficult to remember to take thrice-daily dosage so the best compromise is to administer the drug night and morning in roughly equal proportions.

If the patient does not improve by the end of three weeks or if side-effects prove intolerable, the tricyclic antidepressant should be withdrawn over the course of a week and alternative treatment substituted. The MAO inhibitors have a particular propensity for producing side-effects in the elderly and postural hypotension may preclude attainment of adequate dosages for MAO inhibition. L-tryptophan is worth considering in doses of 3–6 g/day either alone or with a tricyclic antidepressant. This amino acid is marketed as a drug in the UK and is sometimes available from health food stores elsewhere. Its only appreciable side-effect is drowsiness, so it is also useful when side effects to the tricyclic drug are too great. Evidence to date suggests that L-tryptophan is fairly effective in mildly and moderately depressed patients but should not be used in the severely depressed where ECT remains the treatment of choice.

Drug therapy is generally maintained for several months after response has occurred. As the depression lifts appropriate social measures may be instituted. In particular, social isolation must be reversed by day hospital or day centre attendance, or membership of clubs. It is worth trying to persuade an elderly person to join an interest group which caters for all ages rather than an old age group. Side effects with the tricyclic drugs are more marked in the elderly. Constipation may be particularly troublesome in the elderly and acute retention of urine may occur. The patient should be questioned about bowel habits and elderly males about existing symptoms of urinary hesitancy. Glaucoma is usually exacerbated by tricyclic antidepressants which are thus contraindicated. Mianserin is probably safe in this indication, but cautious dosage should be used with careful monitoring.

Cardiovascular changes include ECG and myocardial changes. A pretreatment ECG is a wise precaution to exclude arrhythmias which often worsen with tricyclic antidepressants. Either hypotension or hypertension may be induced. Hypotensive episodes can be quite severe and should be treated by reducing medication and by bed rest. The antihypertensive effects of such drugs as guanethidine, bethanidine, debrisoquine, and clonidine are attenuated by most tricyclic antidepressants. A diuretic or a beta-adrenoceptor blocking agent should be substituted as these do not interact with tricyclic antidepressants. Alternatively, or in addition the patient's depression can be treated with mianserin or L-tryptophan, neither of which interact significantly with antihypertensive therapy.

Other treatments include antipsychotic medication combined with antidepressants, to reduce severe agitation. Sedatives and hypnotics may lessen anxiety or induce sleep but should be used sparingly. Barbiturates should never be instituted in the elderly. Stimulant drugs such as amphetamine have no place in antidepressant therapy in the elderly.

Lithium

Lithium has not been used extensively in the aged, but as the population maintained on lithium ages, experience of its use is increasing. Manic episodes are not common in the elderly but can occur even for the first time. The prognosis for the elderly used to be poor, with symptoms sometimes persisting and necessitating institutionalization.

The half-life of lithium is prolonged 50–100 per cent in the elderly mainly due to reduced renal clearance. Also, elderly patients seem more sensitive to lithium than are younger patients. Lithium should be started at a low dose (say 300 mg/day in divided doses) and gradually increased. For the treatment of mania, serum concentrations of 0.8–1 mmol/litre are usually sufficient. For the prevention of recurrent affective episodes, much lower concentrations may suffice.

The side-effects of lithium are many and in general the pattern in the elderly resembles that in younger patients (Thompson *et al.* 1983*b*). The elderly are prone to develop memory disturbance and even confusion as a toxic effect of lithium which is thus another cause of pseudosenile dementia. Polyuria and polydipsia are particular problems in the elderly, who may complain of intolerable nocturia with many wakenings in the night to urinate. Another side-effect is hypothyroidism which may precipitate an elderly person with marginal thyroid function into frank myxoedema.

Electrolyte imbalance may result in lithium toxicity. The use of diuretics in the elderly must be very careful as must be any attempt to alter the diet of someone maintained on lithium. Renal disease, acute or of insidious onset, may also lead to lithium toxicity.

Antipsychotic drugs

The aged suffer commonly from psychotic illnesses. Schizophrenic disorders may occur as prolongations of earlier breakdowns or as paranoid states of late onset. Affective disorders may be severe and psychotic in intensity. Organic brain disorders may also result in a psychosis. In all these instances, antipsychotic drugs are indicated for symptomatic relief of the condition. Response, however, may be incomplete (Birkett and Boltuch 1972).

The choice of antipsychotic medication depends on whether sedation is required and on the pattern of side-effects tolerated by the patient. Many antipsychotic drugs such as chlorpromazine and thioridazine are markedly sedative. This may be useful in an agitated patient but unnecessary or even unwanted in other patients, especially those characterized by inertia. In these cases the patient may spend his day dozing and quickly loses touch.

The extrapyramidal effects are similar to those in younger individuals but dystonias are uncommon and akathisia infrequent. However, as agitation is frequent in the elderly, it is important to distinguish akathisia from it lest the dose of antipsychotic drug be mistakenly increased. The patient usually retains insight into akathisia, regarding it as foreign to himself whereas he typically regards his agitation as justified by his predicament. Akinetic parkinsonism is the commonest extrapyramidal effect in the elderly, coming on within a few weeks of starting treatment but usually fading away after a few months. Unless the patient begins to relapse, it is best to treat the symptoms by lowering the dose of antipsychotic drug rather than by adding an antiparkinsonian agent. The latter course is liable, especially in the elderly, to lead to excessive anticholinergic effects with severe constipation, retention of urine or toxic psychosis. Under no circumstances should an antiparkinsonian drug be prescribed routinely with an antipsychotic drug.

The most worrying extrapyramidal effect is tardive dyskinesia which is commonest in the elderly, partly because they have inevitably been longest on antipsychotic medication if they are chronically ill and partly because brain damage and degeneration may predispose to the disorder (Greenblatt *et al.* 1968). There is a spontaneous prevalence of tardive dyskinesia in non-antipsychotic drug-treated elderly people of 1 or 2 per cent.

The anticholinergic activity of antipsychotic drugs produces a range of symptoms, especially in the elderly, including dry mouth, blurring of vision, raised intraocular pressure, constipation, and urinary hesitancy. A central anticholinergic syndrome has been described comprising memory impairment, disorientation, anxiety and restlessness, and perceptual disturbances such as visual illusions and hallucinations. The danger of misdiagnosing this condition is greater in the elderly where psychotic conditions tend to be more pleiomorphic than in younger patients. Treatment comprises lowering the dose of antipsychotic medication and withdrawing any antiparkinsonian medication.

Severe orthostatic hypotension can be a particular problem in the elderly. It may manifest itself as recurrent ischaemic attacks, cerebral or cardiac, or as confusion. Fainting can occur, leading to falls and fractured limbs. Taking the blood pressure with the patient recumbent and then standing may suggest the degree of alpha adrenergic block which underlies the condition and allow the clinician to warn the patient of possible problems. Treatment of the established condition comprises bed rest. Sympathomimetic drugs are not indicated. In less severe states, the dose of antipsychotic medication can be lowered somewhat.

As with other drugs used in the elderly, dosage of antipsychotics should initially be modest and dosage increments gradual. Oral medication is generally preferred to injections because of the reduced muscle mass in the elderly. Thioridazine is popular as it has few extrapyramidal effects. For patients with mild psychotic symptoms, agitation, and restlessness, promazine is often effective, and is almost devoid of extrapyramidal effects.

Antianxiety and hypnotic drugs

The barbiturates were most used until the benzodiazepines ousted them a decade or two ago. The barbiturates are poorly tolerated by the elderly who may become sleepy and over-sedated, or even ataxic, stumbling and confused (Gershon 1973). Toxic delirious states have been reported. An insidious impairment of intellectual performance may occur, leading to admission to hospital under the mistaken idea that a dementing process is present. Despite these major drawbacks, barbiturates are still used and prescribing figures suggest that their usage is appreciable in the elderly. In most cases, the use of barbiturates has continued for many years but careful review should be made and gradual withdrawal of the barbiturate considered (Shader and Greenblatt 1982).

The benzodiazepines have largely replaced the barbiturates, but their widespread use in the elderly cannot be advocated (Hall 1973). Many of the side effects of the barbiturates are produced by benzodiazepines as well, ataxia and confusion being most notable. Thus, the use of benzodiazepines in the elderly should be restricted to short-term relief in patients with marked primary anxiety (Nakra and Grossberg 1986). Warnings must be given about day-time sedation (Fancourt and Castleden 1986).

Benzodiazepines have complex metabolic patterns but can be roughly divided into (a) chlordiazepoxide, diazepam, medazepam, clorazepate, clobazam, and prazepam, with active metabolites and metabolic pathways of oxidation and demethylation, and (b) lorazepam and oxazepam, which have no active metabolites and are inactivated by conjugation with glucuronic acid. In general, glucuronic acid conjugation capacity is maintained in the elderly whereas the ability to oxidize and demethylate drugs wanes. Thus, the half-life of diazepam is on average at least twice as long in the elderly as in younger people, whereas that of oxazepam is almost unchanged. Thus, if a benzodiazepine is used it is preferable to try oxazepam as unduly prolonged half-lives are unlikely (Salzman *et al.* 1983). Even so, elderly people are more sensitive to benzodiazepines than younger patients even allowing for pharmacokinetic differences, so dosage should be conservative (Reidenberg 1980).

With hypnotic drugs similar considerations apply as with antianxiety drugs. The continued administration of hypnotic drugs is common in the elderly. Sleep requirements wane with age and further problems can arise if the old person spends some time napping during the day (Roehrs *et al.* 1984). Some indigent elderly spend a lot of time in bed because it is the only place they feel warm. Older people take longer to fall asleep than younger people, have more frequent awakenings, and have little and sometimes no deep (slow-wave) sleep.

Chronic administration of hypnotics to induce sleep can itself lead to insomnia. Whenever attempts are made to discontinue or merely to reduce the dose of hypnotic, rebound insomnia may ensue with disturbing effects on the old person. Thus, the use of hypnotics in the elderly for sleeping disorders should be minimal. After long-term use withdrawal may be less severe in the elderly than in younger subjects, but a tapering schedule is essential (Schweizer *et al.* 1989). If the insomnia is associated with depression or anxiety, treatment should be of the primary affective disorder, with perhaps the bulk of the dose of the antidepressant or anxiolytic at night to induce sedation and sleep. If a hypnotic is required, temazepam or triazolam seem most appropriate (Quan *et al.* 1984). Many other compounds have been used as hypnotics in the elderly. Chloral hydrate may be useful but may interact with other medication by displacing drugs such as warfarin and phenytoin from plasma proteins (Thompson *et al.* 1983*a*). It may thus induce a sudden increase in the concentrations of the free (unbound) drug and increase their effects, perhaps to the point of side-effects. Alcohol is a favourite self-administered nostrum and may help induce sleep (Mishara and Kastenbaum 1974). However, sleep later in the night may be more broken after alcohol and its diuretic effect is particularly troublesome in the elderly. Chlormethiazole, with its short duration of action, has achieved popularity in some countries as an hypnotic for the elderly. Its dependence potential even in the modest dosages used is poorly documented so cautious short-term prescribing is essential.

Apart from morning sedation and forgetfulness, hypnotics carry the danger of producing confusion and unsteadiness of gait in the night if the patient wakes up to go to the toilet. General measures such as subdued lighting and clear signs lessen this problem but even so the use of hypnotics in the elderly is not a measure to be embarked on lightly.

Drugs affecting mental functioning

This is a contentious topic with problems in assessing mental functioning and a range of drugs whose actions and rationale are often unclear (Reisberg *et al.* 1981; Gurski 1981; Coper and Herrmann 1988).

Central nervous system stimulants

Caffeine is a mild cerebral stimulant and widely used as a 'pick-me-up'. Excessive use of coffee can produce symptoms of anxiety, especially in the elderly.

More powerful stimulants include pentylenetetrazol, magnesium pemoline, methylphenidate, and amphetamine. Pentylenetetrazol is an analeptic agent which is sometimes used in elderly patients to increase their alertness and thereby enhance motivation and ability to learn. Methylphenidate and amphetamine are sympathomimetic stimulants. The former has been extensively used to treat the elderly in the United States. The possible value of these drugs remains controversial (Crook 1979). Against the reports of enhancement of new learning must be set the drawbacks: increased sympathomimetic activity with some of the drugs, decreased appetite, increase in irritability, and perhaps psychotic manifestations. In most patients the drawbacks outweigh the advantages but occasionally a patient with cognitive deficits does well on a stimulant drug such as methylphenidate or magnesium pemoline.

Vasodilators

Vasodilator drugs have been advocated in the treatment of arteriosclerotic dementia but the arteriosclerotic blood vessels are incapable of dilating. The general bodily vasodilation results in a lowering of blood-pressure and hence a diminution, not an increase, in cerebral perfusion.

The three drugs most widely used as vasodilators in the treatment of dementia are papaverine, isoxsuprine, and cyclandelate. The results with papaverine suggest some improvement in mental functioning but it is doubtful whether this justifies the side-effects, postural hypotension, flushing, dizziness, headaches, and sweating. Cyclandelate has been available for over 25 years and many studies have examined its effects. In those studies which reach adequate criteria of design, execution and interpretation (Yesavage *et al.* 1979), several show some positive effects of the drug on mental functioning but only a few report practical benefit (Hall 1976; Judge *et al.* 1973). This problem bedevils much of the work in the area of dementia (Spagnoli and Tognoni 1983). Although test results may improve or mood may lighten or stabilise, the practical consequences both in the day-to-day management of the patient and in longer term prognosis are nugatory. Isoxsuprine has been evaluated in even fewer trials and there is little firm evidence that it has beneficial effects, let alone that these are of practical value.

Hyperbaric oxygen has been used extensively to improve cerebral oxygenation in patients with multi-infarct dementia. Despite early encouraging uncontrolled studies, controlled evaluations have failed to establish any therapeutic utility.

Mixed vasodilator/cerebral 'activators'

These drugs have complex actions producing some vasodilatation but in addition altering cerebral metabolism in an ill-understood way. It is believed that they improve the utilization of glucose and oxygen, thereby improving dementia especially of the vascular type. Naftidrofuryl improves the oxidative capacity of animal brains and alters the metabolism of glucose. It protects against the metabolic effects of hypoxia. In controlled trials in a variety of patients, mainly elderly people with mental deterioration and confusion, naftidrofuryl proved superior to placebo, improving such variables as ability to concentrate, memory, social adaptation, alertness, and intellect. However, not all the studies showed the same pattern of change, and improvement in test function or in general condition was not always translated into useful clinical response.

Co-dergocrine mesylate is a mixture of three hydrogenated alkaloids of ergot. It has complex neuronal effects perhaps related to its actions on enzyme systems in the brain together with improved cerebral circulation. A wide variety of functions have been assessed and in general drug effects are scanty and rather inconsistent from trial to trial. Generally some improvement occurs in social skills and general activity but cognitive function is not generally augmented (Hollister and Yesavage 1984). Improvement in dementia is only marginally clinically significant (Hughes *et al.* 1976).

Cerebral 'activators'

Meclofenoxate is a drug which modifies cerebral neuronal metabolism without producing vasodilatation. It reduces the need of the brain for oxygen and is claimed to improve memory function. Evidence for its efficacy in improving test functions is not compelling and its clinical effectiveness is unestablished.

Piracetam and its analogues, deanol, propranolol, procaine amide (Gerovital) and various vitamins have all been advocated in the treatment of cerebral deterioration in the elderly. The piracetam-type compounds ('nootropics') alter brain metabolism, facilitate memory in animals and enhance cognitive performance in normal human subjects. However, efficacy in treating dementing patients remains poorly established (Crook 1985).

Future developments

The area of intellectual deterioration in old age was relatively poorly researched until quite recently. A very full account of recent work is available in Roth and Iversen (1986). However, interest is now focused on Alzheimer's disease, a progressive and insidious form of dementia associated with characteristic microscopic changes; namely, neurofibrillary tangles and senile plaques. These neuropathological changes are associated with a deficit in choline acetyltransferase, the enzyme which synthesizes acetylcholine (Davies and Maloney 1976; Perry *et al.* 1977). The postsynaptic muscarinic receptors remain intact suggesting a presynaptic neuronal degeneration (Davies and Verth 1978). Other neurotransmitters are also involved (Adolfsson *et al.* 1979; Rossor *et al.* 1984). The aetiology of the degeneration is unclear but may be related to abnormalities in microtubular protein (Glenner 1989).

Senile dementia of Alzheimer's type is much more common than Alzheimer's disease, comes on at a later age, and is associated with few biochemical abnormalities. It is unclear whether the two are separate conditions (Gottfries 1985). It is also unclear whether these conditions are an extreme of normal ageing or a separate disease (Editorial 1989).

Acetylcholine is important in memory functions, anticholinergic drugs such as atropine and scopolamine impairing memory, cholinomimetic drugs enhancing it. Thus, compounds increasing brain acetylcholine levels have been suggested in the treatment of Alzheimer's dementia, as L-dopa is used in parkinsonism. Choline availability governs the synthesis of acetylcholine and the neuronal uptake of choline may be impaired in Alzheimer's disease. However, increasing choline concentrations in the body does seem to result in increased acetylcholine turnover in the brain. Another way of increasing acetylcholine concentrations is to administer lecithin.

The early results administering choline or lecithin to patients with Alzheimer's disease have not been encouraging. In patients with the well-established disease, little change has been noted. In earlier, mild cases, some improvement in test functioning and in some behavioural measures were noted. Thus, the utilization of the increased choline supplies may be deficient, either because uptake is a limiting factor or because the neurones are unable to synthesize acetylcholine in any significantly increased amount. However, dosages have been modest and short-term and further studies are certainly warranted.

An alternative approach is to block the breakdown of acetylcholine with a cholinesterase inhibitor. Unfortunately, there is no long acting compound capable of crossing the blood–brain barrier. Physostigmine (eserine) is short-acting and has to be injected. Some improvements in memory have been reported in patients with Alzheimer's disease given physostigmine or the direct muscarinic agonist, arecholine. The latter approach is potentially the most rewarding as it does not depend on acetylcholine synthesis for its therapeutic mode of action. Tetrahydroaminoacridine (THA) is a centrally acting anticholinesterase and cerebral stimulant and has been claimed to have major therapeutic effects in Alzheimer's disease. Further studies have shown only modest albeit worthwhile improvements and hepatotoxicity is common (Byrne and Arie 1989). Nicotine is a cholinergic receptor agonist and produced marked improvements in some psychological test functions in patients with Alzheimer-type dementia (Sahakian *et al.* 1989). Further developments of cholinomimetic drugs are awaited with interest. Indeed, this area is the focus of intense activity by many drug companies (Hershenson and Moos 1986).

Meanwhile, treatment of Alzheimer's disease remains unsatisfactory. Many clinicians regard all drug therapy as useless, or even worse than useless because of the side-effects, and will not use them outside a research setting (Byrne and Arie 1985; Castleden 1984). Others recommend a trial of treatment with co-dergocrine mesylate or a cerebral activator (Hollister 1985; Lehmann 1983).

References

Adolfsson, R., Gottfries, C.G., Roos, B.E., and Winblad, B. (1979). Changes in the brain catecholamines in patients with dementia of Alzheimer type. *British Journal of Psychiatry* **135,** 216–23.

Bender, A.D. (1974). Pharmacodynamic principles of drug therapy in the aged. *Journal of the American Geriatric Society* **22,** 296-303.

Birkett, D.P., and Boltuch, B. (1972). Chlorpromazine in geriatric psychiatry. *Journal of the American Geriatric Society* **20,** 403–6.

Blazer, D. (1980). The diagnosis of depression in the elderly. *Journal of the American Geriatric Society* **28,** 52–8.

Byrne, J., and Arie, T. (1985). Rational drug treatment of dementia? *British Medical Journal* **290,** 1845–6.

Byrne, J., and Arie, T. (1989). Tetrahydroaminoacridine (THA in Alzheimer's disease. *British Medical Journal* **298,** 845–6.

Castleden, C.M. (1984). Therapeutic possibilities in patients with senile dementia. *Journal of the Royal College Physicians of London* **18,** 28–31.

Cole, J.O., and Stotsky, B.A. (1974). Improving psychiatric drug therapy. A matter of dosage and choice. *Geriatrics* **29,** 74–8.

Coper, H., and Herrmann, W.M. (1988). Psychostimulants, analeptics, nootropics: an attempt to differentiate and assess drugs designed for the treatment of impaired brain functions. *Pharmacopsychiatrica* **21,** 211–217.

Crook, T. (1979). Central nervous system stimulants: appraisal of use in geropsychiatric patients. *Journal of the American Geriatric Society* **27,** 476–7.

Crook, T. (1985). Geriatric psychopathology: An overview of the ailments and current therapies. *Drug development research* **5,** 5–23.

Crooks, J., O'Malley, K., and Stevenson, I.H. (1976). Pharmacokinetics in the elderly. *Clinical Pharmacokinetics* **1,** 280–96.

Davies, P., and Maloney, A.J.F. (1976). Selective loss of central cholinergic neurons in Alzheimer's disease. *Lancet* **2,** 1403.

Davies, P., and Verth, A.H. (1978). Regional distribution of muscarinic acetylcholine receptor in normal and Alzheimer's type dementia brains. *Brain Research* **138,** 385–92.

Davis, J.M., Fann, W.E., El-Yousef, M.K., and Janowsky, D.S. (1973). Clinical problems in treating the aged with psychotropic drugs. *Advances in Behavioural Biology* **6,** 111–25.

Editorial, (1989). Senile dementia of Alzheimer's type—normal ageing or disease? *Lancet* 476–7.

Eisdorfer, C., and Fann, W.E. (1973). *Psychopharmacology and aging*. Plenum Press, New York.

Fancourt, G., and Castleden, M. (1986). The use of benzodiazepines with particular reference to the elderly. *British Journal of Hospital Medicine* **35,** 321–6.

Friedel, R.O. (1978). Pharmacokinetics in the geropsychiatric patient. In *Psychopharmacology: A generation of progress* (eds. M.A. Lipton, A. DiMascio, and K.F. Killam) pp. 1149–505. Raven Press, New York.

Gerner, R.H. (1985). Present status of drug therapy of depression in late life. *Journal of Affective Disorders* (Suppl.) **1,** S23–S31.

Gershon, S. (1973). Antianxiety agents. *Advances in Behavioural Biology* **6,** 183–7.

Glenner, G.G. (1989). The pathobiology of Alzheimer's disease. *Annual Review of Medicine* **40,** 45–51.

Gottfries, C.G. (1985). Alzheimer's disease and senile dementia: biochemical characteristics and aspects of treatment. *Psychopharmacology* **86,** 245–52.

Gottfries, C.G. (1987). Pharmacology of mental aging and dementia disorders. *Clinical Neuropharmacology* **10,** 313–29.

Greenblatt, D.L., Dominick, J.R., Stotsky, B.A., and DiMascio, A. (1968). Phenothiazine-induced dyskinesia in nursing home patients. *Journal of the American Geriatric Society* **16,** 27–34.

Grossberg, G.T., and Nakra, B.R.S. (1986). Treatment of depression in the elderly. *Comprehensive Psychiatry* **12,** 16–22.

Gurski, G.E. (1981). Evaluation of geriatric patients with special reference to clinical trials of so called nootropic drugs. I. General considerations and screening. *Pharmacopsychiatrica* **14,** 51–60.

Hall, M.R.P. (1973). Drug therapy in the elderly. *British Medical Journal* **3,** 582–4.

Hall, P. (1976). Cyclandelate in the treatment of cerebral arteriosclerosis. *Journal of the American Geriatric Society* **24,** 41–5.

Hershenson, F.M., and Moos, W.H. (1986). Drug development for senile cognitive decline. *Journal of Medicinal Chemistry* **28,** 1125–30.

Hollister, L.E. (1985). Alzheimer's disease. Is it worth treating? *Drugs* **29,** 483–8.

Hollister, L.E., and Yesavage, J. (1984). Ergoloid mesylates for senile dementias: unanswered questions. *Annals of Internal Medicine* **100,** 894–8.

Hughes, J.R., Williams, J.G., and Currier, R.D. (1976). An ergot alkaloid preparation (hydergine) in the treatment of dementia. Critical review of the clinical literature. *Journal of the American Geriatric Society* **24,** 490–7.

Jenike, M.A. (1985). Handbook of geriatric psychopharmacology. PSG Publishing Company, Littleton, Mass.

Judge, T.G., Urquhart, A., and Blakemore, C.B. (1973). Cyclandelate and mental functions: a double-blind cross-over trial in normal elderly subjects. *Age Ageing* **2,** 121–4.

Kantor, S.J., and Glassman, A.H. (1980). The use of tricyclic antidepressant drugs in geriatric patients. In *Psychopharmacology of aging* (eds. C. Eisdorfer, and W.E. Fann) pp. 99–118. MTP Press, Lancaster.

Lader, M. (1982). Psychopharmacology of old age. In *The psychiatry of late life* (eds. R. Levy and F. Post) pp. 143–62. Blackwell, Oxford.

Lehmann, H.E. (1983). Psychopharmacological approaches to the organic brain syndrome. *Comprehensive Psychiatry* **24,** 412–30.

Mishara, B.L., and Kastenbaum, R. (1974). Wine in the treatment of long-term geriatric patients in mental institutions. *Journal of the American Geriatric Society* **22,** 88–94.

Murphy, E. (1983). The prognosis of depression in old age. *British Journal of Psychiatry* **142,** 111–19.

Nakra, B.R.S., and Grossberg, G.T. (1986). Management of anxiety in the elderly. *Comprehensive Therapy* **12,** 53–62.

Perry, E.K., Perry, R.H., Blessed, G., and Tomlinson, B.E. (1977). Necropsy evidence of central cholinergic deficits in senile dementia. *Lancet* **1,** 189.

Post, F. (1972). The management and nature of depressive illnesses in late life: a follow-through study. *British Journal of Psychiatry* **121,** 393–404.

Quan, S.F., Bamford, C.R., and Beutler, L.E. (1984). Sleep disturbances in the elderly. *Geriatrics* **39,** 42–7.

Reidenberg, M.M. (1980). Drugs in the elderly. *Bulletin of the New York Academy of Medicine* **56,** 703–14.

Reisberg, B., Ferris, S.H., and Gershon, S. (1981). An overview of pharmacologic treatment of cognitive decline in the aged. *American Journal of Psychiatry* **138,** 593–600.

Roehrs, T., Zorick, F., and Roth, T. (1984). Sleep disorders in the elderly. *Geriatric Medicine Today* **3,** 76–86.

Rossor, M.N., Iversen, L.L., Reynolds, G.P., Mountjoy, C.Q., and Roth, M. (1984). Neurochemical characteristics of early and late onset types of Alzheimer's disease.

Roth, M., and Iversen, L.L. (1986). Alzheimer's disease and related disorders. *British Medical Bulletin* **42**(1), 1–116.

Sahakian, B., Jones, G., Levy, R., Gray, J., and Warburton, D. (1989). The effects of nicotine on attention, information processing and short-term memory in patients with dementia of the Alzheimer type. *British Journal of Psychiatry* **154,** 797–800.

Salzman, C., Shader, R.I., Greenblatt, D.J., and Harmatz, J.S. (1983). Long v short half-life benzodiazepines in the elderly. Kinetics and clinical effects of diazepam and oxazepam. *Archives of General Psychiatry* **40,** 293–7.

Sathananthan, G.L., Ferris, S., and Gershon, S. (1977). Psychopharmacology of aging: current trends. *Current Developments in Psychopharmacology* **4,** 250–64.

Schweizer, E., Case, G., and Rickels, K. (1989). Benzodiazepine dependence and withdrawal in elderly patients. *American Journal of Psychiatry* **146,** 529–31.

Shader, R.I., and Greenblatt, D.J. (1982). Management of anxiety in the elderly: the balance between therapeutic and adverse effects. *Journal of Clinical Psychiatry* **43,** Sec. 2, 8–18.

Small, G.W. (1988). Psychopharmacological treatment of elderly demented patients. *Journal of Clinical Psychiatry* **49,** (5, Suppl), 8–13).

Spagnoli, A., and Tognoni, G. (1983). 'Cerebroactive' drugs. Clinical pharmacology and therapeutic role in cerebrovascular disorders. *Drugs* **26,** 44–69.

Thompson, T.L., Moran, M.G., and Nies, A.S. (1983*a*). Psychotropic drug use in the elderly. *New England Journal of Medicine* **308,** 134–8.

Thompson, T.L., Moran, M.G., and Nies, A.S. (1983*b*). Psychotropic use in the elderly. *New England Journal of Medicine* **308,** 194–9.

Turnbull, J.M., and Turnbull, S.K. (1985). Management of specific anxiety disorders in the elderly. *Geriatrics* **40,** 75–82.

Yesavage, J.A., Tinklenberg, J.R., Hollister, L.E., and Berger, P.A. (1979). Vasodilators in cerebral dementias. A review of the literature. *Archives of General Psychiatry* **36,** 220–3.

16. Electroconvulsive Therapy

Introduction

In the 1930s several physical treatments were introduced including insulin shock, sleep narcosis, leucotomy and camphor, metrazol and shock-induced electroconvulsive therapy. Chemically-induced convulsions were initially used, based on the mistaken premise that epilepsy and schizophrenia were mutually incompatible in the same person, and, *ergo*, fits would ameliorate schizophrenic illnesses (Meduna 1938). Electrically produced convulsions were found to be more easily controlled and more acceptable to the patient (Cerletti and Bini 1938), and soon it was recognized that depressed patients often showed the most gratifying responses to electroconvulsive therapy (ECT). Schizophrenic patients are still sometimes given ECT, as are a few manic patients, but its use in conditions such as general paresis, delirium tremens, and even epilepsy is now of historical interest only.

Like other physical treatments, ECT has been severely criticized both from within and without the psychiatric profession (Friedberg 1977; Crowe 1984). Undoubtedly, abuses have occurred and vigilance is needed to protect patients from the over-enthusiastic and uncritical, but it is no longer true that strictly controlled comparative trials of ECT are lacking (Kendell 1981). Several trials now corroborate the mass of clinical experience that ECT has worthwhile and sometimes dramatic effects in accelerating recovery in patients suffering from moderate and especially severe depression. Such benefits far outweigh the minor risks and troublesome side-effects of the treatment (Fink 1977; Ottosson 1981).

An authoritative publication covering the practical administration of ECT was produced by the Royal College of Psychiatrists in 1989 (ECT Sub-committee 1989). This excellent document should be consulted for a detailed account of the topic.

Effectiveness in depression

A survey of all studies of antidepressant treatment in in-patients published between 1958 and 1963 in American, Canadian and British journals listed

153 studies totalling 5864 patients (Wechsler *et al.* 1965). The mean improvement with placebo was 23 per cent, with MAO inhibitors 50 per cent, tricyclic antidepressives 65 per cent and with ECT 72 per cent. For depressive illnesses of recent onset the effectiveness of ECT was more apparent—86 per cent improvement as compared with 24 per cent with placebo and 62 per cent with drugs. The active treatments were less effective in chronic depressions, ECT 37 per cent, drugs 32 per cent and placebo 21 per cent. Many of these trials were uncontrolled and exaggeration of drug/ECT differences may have occurred. Even later controlled trials comparing ECT with tricyclic antidepressants have often been methodologically deficient.

Two large multicentre trials were carried out in the early 1960s. In the USA, ECT, imipramine, phenelzine, isocarboxazid, and placebo were compared in 281 severely depressed patients. Of these 76 were manic depressive, depressed; 50 were involutional melancholics; 60 depressed schizophrenics; and 44 had miscellaneous diagnoses. Treatment was assessed over 8 weeks during which time at least 9 ECTs were given. With ECT 76 per cent of patients showed marked improvement, with imipramine or phenelzine 50 per cent, isocarboxazid only 28 per cent and placebo 48 per cent (Greenblatt *et al.* 1962 1964).

In the UK, the Medical Research Council (1965) carried out a multicentre trial involving 259 patients aged between 40 and 65 with primary depressive illnesses. Admission and outcome criteria were clearly defined and symptoms were evaluated at 4 and 20 weeks. At 4 weeks, patients showing no or slight symptoms comprised 71 per cent of the ECT group, 52 per cent on imipramine, 30 per cent on phenelzine and 39 per cent on placebo. By 20 weeks, despite the complications of treatment changes after the first 4 weeks, ECT maintained its advantage over phenelzine and placebo but was about equal in effectiveness to imipramine. Women did particularly well with ECT.

An open evaluation compared the charts of 1495 patients admitted over a 12-year period (Black *et al.* 1987*a*). Of those receiving ECT, 70 per cent improved compared with only half of those given antidepressant drugs.

Thus, in the treatment of depression, ECT is better than placebo (Barton 1977) and more rapidly acting and at least as effective as tricyclic antidepressants (Turek and Hanlon 1977; Royal College of Psychiatrists 1977; Kendell 1978).

Which depressed patients respond to ECT?

One approach has been to define clinical features indicative of ECT response. Three scales have been produced (Hobson 1953; Mendels 1965;

Carney *et al.* 1965) but only two features are common to all three scales: hypochondriasis and hysterical attitude to illness were unfavourable prognosticators. In general, favourable features approximate to the stereotype of endogenous depression: early waking, somatic and paranoid delusions, retardation and absence of neurotic traits and emotional lability. However, these prognostic factors were not found useful by Abrams *et al.* (1973), although outcome in this study was assessed rather prematurely. Also, these features tend to predict response to imipramine (Kiloh *et al.* 1962) and may merely be associated with a good outcome whatever the treatment.

Studies using diagnostic labels suggest that ECT is most effective in psychotic depressives and depressed bipolar patients (Greenblatt *et al.* 1964; Perris and d'Elia 1966; Minter and Mandel 1979). Biological indicators such as DST status are not helpful in predicting responders (Scott 1989).

Failure to respond occurs in 15–25 per cent of depressed patients. It is more common in patients who have been ill the longest and tend to have longer illnesses. It has been suggested that ECT may be effective only when it is given within 6 months of the time when spontaneous remission would have occurred anyway (Kukopulos *et al.* 1977).

In summary, the main indications for ECT in depressive illness are generally regarded as: an illness of endogenous type which has failed to respond to a course of tricyclic antidepressants given at adequate dosage for at least 4 weeks; recurrent depression in a patient who has responded well to ECT in previous episodes; depression of such severity with high suicidal risk or profound retardation that rapid response is essential; depression characterized by major mood-congruent delusions and hallucinations (Gill and Lambourn 1979; Black *et al.* 1987*a*).

Effectiveness in other conditions

Mania

Although there are no controlled studies of ECT in mania, 60 per cent of psychiatric centres in the New York area believe that it is indicated as a treatment, although only one centre uses it as treatment of choice. McCabe (1976) retrospectively compared groups of patients treated in the same institution before and after the introduction of ECT. Manics treated with ECT spent less time in hospital, had fewer symptoms on discharge and made a better social recovery than those treated by other means. Similar results were obtained in an Iowa study (Black *et al.* 1987*b*). Electroconvulsive therapy is worth considering in manic patients who are severely disturbed and refusing medication (McCabe and Norris 1977). One or two applications are usually sufficient to quieten the patient enough for drug treatment to be tried again. A comparison of ECT and lithium found that ECT may effect a more rapid improvement than lithium (Small *et al.* 1988).

Puerperal psychosis

About two-thirds of these psychoses are primarily affective so the use of ECT is reasonable, especially as the clinical state is often florid.

Schizophrenia

The view of many psychiatrists especially in the USA that ECT is of value in some schizophrenics is not supported by firm evidence (Salzman 1980). May (1968) compared ECT with drugs alone, drugs plus psychotherapy, milieu therapy and psychotherapy alone in 228 schizophrenic patients. On a number of outcome variables, ECT was consistently less effective that either drugs or drugs plus psychotherapy although more effective than milieu therapy or psychotherapy alone. In a British trial any benefits of ECT were short-lived (Taylor and Fleminger 1980).

Depressed schizophrenic patients respond less to ECT than do depressed patients. Catatonia is generally believed to be a definite indication for ECT, but one study failed to distinguish between pentothal anaesthesia and ECT in such patients (Miller *et al.* 1953).

There is thus little evidence that ECT is of any value in schizophrenic patients (Ottosson 1985), although it will undoubtedly continue to be used by some psychiatrists in patients with catatonia, affective symptoms, or drug-resistant states (Greenblatt 1977; Van Vakenburg and Clayton 1985).

Types of ECT

Bilateral

The electrical current is passed across both hemispheres via electrodes placed over both fronto-temporal regions. More anterior placements have been advocated but no particular advantages have been demonstrated.

Unilateral

It has been suggested that the unwanted side-effects of ECT such as confusion and memory loss might be minimized without affecting the therapeutic efficacy. The current is passed through the non-dominant hemisphere by means of electrodes on one side of the head only. One electrode is usually over the frontotemporal region but there is no agreement as to the optimum position for the other one—frontal, parietal, and occipital have all been used.

Unilateral vs. bilateral

The memory disturbance and the therapeutic effects of ECT are mediated via different mechanisms (Ottosson 1960). The memory impairment is mainly determined by the amount of electrical energy used to induce the fit and the length of the fit, whereas the effectiveness seems mainly dependent on the length of the induced seizure. Unilateral non-dominant ECT causes less memory impairment than bilateral ECT (d'Elia 1970) partly because less electricity is used and partly because the current does not traverse the dominant hemisphere. However, a review of 29 comparative studies (d'Elia and Raotma 1975) disclosed that in two unilateral ECT was superior to the bilateral procedure, in 14 it was equal, but in 12 studies it was somewhat inferior. In the final study unilateral ECT was definitely less effective.

Multiple ECT

The administration of several ECTs within one session does not lead to increased effectiveness and the side effects are greater (Abrams 1974). It would appear that a finite interval between seizures is necessary.

Maintenance ECT

Chronically relapsing depressives have been treated with one ECT every 2–4 weeks. The effectiveness of this procedure is unestablished.

Fluoroethyl-induced seizures

Fluoroethyl (Indoklon) is a convulsant gas which produced comparable results to ECT with perhaps less memory disturbance (Small 1974). It is no longer available.

Mortality

Electroconvulsive therapy is associated with a small but distinct risk of death. Maclay (1953) ascribed 62 deaths to ECT in England and Wales between 1947 and 1952. Perrin (1961) estimated from American studies that the risk of death was 1 in 12 500 treatments and 1 in 950 patients. In the UK, Barker and Baker (1959) calculated the risk, based on a questionnaire survey of a quarter of a million treatments, to be 1 in 28 000 treatments. Other studies confirm that the risk is quite low, especially when set against the risk of suicide in untreated or drug-treated patients. Avery and Winokur (1976) in their 3-year follow-up of 579 depressed patients reported a significantly lower mortality rate in those given ECT than in those treated by other means.

Fatalities usually occur during or just after the ECT, the commonest cause being cardiac arrest due to excessive vagal inhibition. Other causes include myocardial infarction, cerebral haemorrhage, pulmonary embolism, and, later, pneumonia. Adequate atropinization should prevent vagally-mediated cardiac arrest (Barron and Sullivan 1967). Less than half the deaths follow the first treatment so survival of one ECT is no guarantee that the patient will survive the course. As expected, the elderly and the physically ill are more at risk.

Morbidity

Major non-fatal complications of ECT are rare. Cardiac morbidity includes myocardial infarction, arrhythmias, congestive cardiac failure and angina; they affect about 1 patient in 500. Respiratory problems comprise aspiration pneumonia, pulmonary embolism, prolonged apnea, and exacerbation of tuberculosis. Cerebrovascular accidents, nasal or subconjuctival haemorrhage, and bleeding from a peptic ulcer have also been reported. Status epilepticus has been described but persisting epilepsy is very rare.

Orthopaedic complications such as spinal and long bone fractures, fat embolism, and dislocation of the jaw have been almost eliminated by the use of muscle relaxants. Muscle aches and pains are complained of by less than 10 per cent of patients and headaches by 2–3 per cent. Muscle pains generally affect neck, shoulders and masseters and tend to subside after the first treatment.

Greenblatt *et al.* (1964) provide data for side effects from their comparative trial. Table 16.1 shows that some complaints are actually more common in the placebo-treated patients.

Contraindications

There are no absolute contraindications to ECT but the depression must be very severe before one administers ECT within 3 months of a myocardial infarct or stroke, or in patients with acute respiratory infections or raised intracranial pressure. Conditions requiring particular caution include congestive cardiac failure, cardiac arrhythmias especially with a pacemaker, aneurysm, peptic ulceration, severe osteoporosis, major bone fracture, and an intracranial space-occupying lesion. Pregnant women should be very thoroughly relaxed to protect the fetus.

Table 16.1. 'Side-effects' of ECT and placebo

	ECT %	Placebo %
Headaches	29	15
Hypotension	16	26
Confusion	16	Not reported
Drowsiness	16	15
Anorexia	13	Not reported
Palpitations	10	Not reported
Weakness	10	15

From Greenblatt *et al.* 1964).

It must be remembered that other antidepressive therapies and the depression itself carry an appreciable risk, e.g. cardiac problems with some tricyclic antidepressants. Each patient must be evaluated in conjunction with the anaesthetist, the patient and his relatives, balancing the severity and type of depression against the risks of ECT.

Memory impairment

The memory impairment associated with ECT has been extensively studied (Harper and Wiens 1975). Nevertheless, depressive illnesses themselves are associated with poor memory so that it is difficult to disentangle the two factors. Memory impairment might be attributable to persistence of the depression rather than to ECT itself. Indeed, patients who improved most after ECT complained least about memory impairment (Cronholm and Ottosson 1963). Electroconvulsive therapy may impair retention whereas acquisition is deficient as a consequence of the depression.

The duration of the memory impairment following ECT is unclear. One study reported that test performance had returned to normal after 30 days, whereas another detected deficits persisting at 3 months. Memory impairment is probably related to the number of shocks given. It is much less marked after brief-pulse than sinusoidal wave ECT. Ability to learn new material recovers in the 24 h after each shock but is more impaired after the fourth than the first shock.

The memory loss is of several types:

Retrograde amnesia for distant events

Some patients complain of pockets of memory loss relating to events in the distant past, and impairment which is not easy to confirm. Squire (1977) asked patients to recognize the names of television programmes screened nationally for one season only during the previous 15 years. Bilateral ECT was associated with an inability to recall programmes broadcast in the 3 years before ECT with no impairment for programmes broadcast 4 years or more earlier. This deficit disappeared 2 weeks after the ECT. Patients also mixed up the order of events and this defect was more persistent (Squire *et al.* 1981). Unilateral ECT was not associated with impairment of memory for recent events.

Retrograde amnesia for recent events

Although many patients recall events right up to the anaesthetic induction, others have a total amnesia for anything up to a few hours. The magnitude and persistence of this side effect is not known.

Anterograde amnesia

As the patient recovers from the fit, he passes through a confused phase for which there is amnesia (Daniel and Crovitz 1982). As mentioned above, the learning of new material, verbal and non-verbal, is affected. Bilateral ECT produces more problems than unilateral ECT (Squire and Slater 1978). The memory impairment lasts only a few weeks.

Long-term impairment

Some patients are adamant that ECT has resulted in persisting memory impairment and many studies have been addressed to this problem (Taylor *et al.* 1982). These patients complain that they cannot remember names, faces, shopping lists, or important dates as well as they could before ECT. Such complaints, of course, are also made by normal people as they age and are common in depressed and anxious patients, especially those treated with psychotropic drugs. It is thus difficult to attribute long-term memory disturbances unequivocally to ECT because many patients with such complaints have some residual affective disturbance and are receiving medication. Nevertheless, subjective complaints about memory 6–9 months after ECT are made by 67 per cent of patients after bilateral ECT and only 27 per cent after non-dominant unilateral ECT suggesting some involvement of bilateral ECT (Squire and Chace 1975). Objective impairment could not be demonstrated but the numbers were small. It is likely that ECT does not produce prolonged memory defects but may induce some subtle deficiencies in the recall of autobiographical material (Taylor *et al.* 1982).

Mechanism of action (Bolwig and Rafaelsen 1981)

Animal experiments

Mice were more active 3 and 6 days after the last in a series of 7 daily electroconvulsive shocks but not after a single shock. Mice receiving shocks showed greater locomotor activity after reserpine pretreatment and the dopamine agonist apomorphine or the noradrenalin agonist clonidine than did non-shocked mice. This suggests that the shocks sensitize catecholamine mechanisms in some way, perhaps the receptors directly. Similarly, the stimulating effects of tranylcypromine and L-dopa were potentiated by shocks, as were the effects of tranylcypromine and L-tryptophan, presumed to act on serotoninergic mechanisms (Evans *et al.* 1976). That a postsynaptic site of action is involved was implied by enhanced responses also following the use of catecholamine and serotonin agonists (Green *et al.* 1977; Costain *et al.* 1979). Growth hormone responses to apomorphine and clonidine are also altered.

Longer-term changes have been described: noradrenalin but not serotonin turnover is enhanced.

Human studies

The role of the convulsion in the effectiveness of ECT is somewhat unclear. Electroconvulsive therapy is an elaborate procedure with induction of anaesthesia and muscle relaxation which themselves could have non-specific therapeutic effects. Some studies have directly compared ECT with pseudo-ECT; namely, every aspect of ECT except the actual switching on of the current and induction of a seizure. Miller *et al.* (1953) compared anaesthesia and ECT with anaesthesia and subconvulsive shock in 40 patients with chronic schizophrenia and observed no difference in therapeutic outcome. Another study using mainly schizophrenics was that of Brill *et al.* (1959).

Much more important are the trials comparing real and simulated ECT in depressed patients. In one study, a course of bilaterally applied ECT which began with two simulated ECTs was associated with significantly slower improvement than a course which included real ECTs from the start (Freeman *et al.* 1978). By contrast, Lambourn and Gill (1978) reported improvement to be as rapid with 6 sessions of simulated ECT as with 6 real ECTs. However, they used unilateral ECT.

The largest trial was that carried out at Northwick Park involving 70 patients with primary depressive illnesses selected for features favourable to an ECT response (Johnstone *et al.* 1980). They were allocated randomly either to a course of 8 real ECT or 8 simulated ECT. The improvement was significantly greater in those given real ECT but the absolute differences were small in relation to the considerable improvements over time in both groups. No differences were found between the two groups at 1 month and 6-month follow-up. It was concluded that 'the therapeutic benefits of electrically induced convulsions in depressions were of lesser magnitude and were more transient than has sometimes been claimed'. However, examination of the data reveal a rapid and major improvement in the patients treated with simulated ECT, leaving little scope for any active treatment to be proved effective. It may be that the selection criteria were predictive of improvement in general rather than to ECT in particular.

The fourth trial involved only 22 patients with primary depressive illness but yielded very clear advantages of a course of 6 ECT as compared with 6 simulated ECT (West 1981). When those patients who had received simulated ECT were later switched to real ECT, they too were significantly improved.

The Nottingham ECT study compared the effects of bilateral, unilateral and simulated ECT in 69 depressed patients (Gregory *et al.* 1985). Both bilateral and unilateral ECT were significantly superior to simulated ECT. In this study, in contrast to the Northwick Park investigation, simulated ECT was associated with little change.

Biochemical changes following ECT have not been established. No changes in serotonin or dopamine metabolites have been detected. Noradrenaline turnover has not been estimated.

Physiological changes during ECT have been studied in detail (Perrin 1961). An initial bradycardia is followed by a rapid rise in heart rate and a subsequent fall. This bradycardia is abolished by atropine. Blood-pressure changes are similar to heart-rate changes, and again the hypotension is abolished by atropine. Blood pressure rises still occur, and systolic levels may reach 200 mmHg. Cerebral blood flow about doubles and peripheral blood flow falls. Transient arrhythmias are common, especially at the end of the seizure, and may be mediated by either division of the autonomic nervous system. Vagal arrhythmias can be lessened by atropine, especially in high dose. The arrhythmias are almost always evanescent.

The electroencephalogram shows increased voltage, slow-wave activity and a decrease in fast-wave activity. The delta activity is related to the number of seizures and disappears 8–12 weeks after the last ECT. The total sleep time is reduced whereas the number of REM periods increases.

Administration of ECT (Freeman 1979)

Unilateral vs. bilateral

This is an unresolved controversy and no categorical advice can be given. Unilateral ECT to the nondominant hemisphere is associated with less verbal memory disturbance but evidence regarding non-verbal memory disturbances is less clear-cut (Daniel and Crovitz 1983*b*). However, brief-pulse bilateral ECT is associated with less side-effects than the older machines so the possible advantages of unilateral ECT are much less apparent. Furthermore, some misgivings have been expressed over the efficacy of unilateral ECT and one trial cited earlier showed that patients receiving bilateral ECT recovered more quickly than those given unilateral applications (Gregory *et al.* 1985). However, if the ECT is monitored by EEG recordings and the current reapplied if the seizure lasts less than 25 s, unilateral ECT is as good as bilateral, with less memory disturbance (Horne *et al.* 1985). Thus, unilateral ECT seems less effective because it may not always induce the necessary fit.

As the memory impairment is usually temporary, it would appear, on balance, that there is insufficient evidence to warrant the routine use of unilateral ECT where brief-pulse ECT machines are in use. However, it should be considered in patients who have been upset by memory loss after previous courses of brief-pulse ECT, who have previously needed more than average numbers of ECT in a session, who have previously had several courses of ECT, or who complain of persisting memory loss from their previous course. As giving unilateral ECT to the dominant hemisphere by mistake is likely to produce increased side-effects, it is important to establish the dominant side.

Establishing cerebral dominance

Asking about handedness is not adequate. In addition the patient should be observed writing (Levy and Reid 1976). Most people write normally with the thumb and forefinger pointing away from them. This indicates that the contralateral hemisphere is dominant (Table 16.2) and unilateral ECT can be given to the same side as the preferred writing hand. People who curl their hands round so the thumb and forefinger are directed towards them ('inverted writers') probably have either ipsilateral or mixed dominance. Bilateral ECT is indicated. In cases of doubt, especially in left-handed females, side-effects should be assessed after the first ECT.

Need for an anaesthetist

Anaesthesia is a complex procedure which requires an expert. Psychiatrists are not experts in anaesthesia and, although they may be competent to deal with routine procedures, they are not competent to cope with the unexpected and with emergencies. An anaesthetist should always administer the anaesthetic and remain until the patient has regained consciousness.

Premedication

Atropine 0.6 mg by intramuscular injection produces oral dryness and inhibition of bronchial secretions within 15 min. However, this dose is insufficient to prevent vagally-induced cardiovascular effects such as bradycardia and hypotension. It is better to give a dose of 0.6 mg intravenously at the same time as the anaesthetic. It is also less painful. Some centres no longer administer atropine routinely.

Table 16.2. Handedness and ECT

Sex	Handedness	Writing position	Dominant hemisphere	Type of ECT
Male	Right	Normal	Left	Right
	Right	Inverted (rare)	Right or mixed	Bilateral
	Left	Normal	Right	Left
	Left	Inverted	Left or mixed	Bilateral
Female	Right	Normal	Left	Right
	Right	Inverted	Mixed	Bilateral
	Left	Normal	Right (sometimes mixed)	Left
	Left	Inverted	Mixed	Bilateral

Muscle relaxation

A muscle relaxant should always be used to modify the fit and prevent orthopaedic complications. Suxamethonium chloride 30–60 mg intravenously is the drug of choice given through the same needle as the anaesthetic but from a different syringe. The aim is as full a relaxation as possible without obscuring the fit entirely. As suxamethonium is a depolarizing agent, it produces muscle twitching which must be allowed to subside before the seizure is induced. The dose used should be recorded together with degree of modification of the seizure so the anaesthetist can alter the dose next time if necessary. The dose of suxamethonium varies appreciably from patient to patient.

Rarely, a patient manifests prolonged apnea after suxamethonium. Most such patients have an atypical plasma cholinesterase or a deficiency of the enzyme, due to a genetic factor, a nutritional disturbance or hepatic disease (Marco and Randels 1979). In some, however, enzyme type and level are normal. In prolonged apnea, the patient must be ventilated mechanically and another relaxant used in future.

Anaesthetic

False teeth, earrings, and other jewellery and hairpins should be removed before ECT. Oxygen should be given before the induction of the seizure as this prevents oxygen saturation dropping below 90 per cent during the fit. Thiopentone sodium is the traditional anaesthetic but tends to persist into the post-ictal phase. Methohexitone has been shown to produce quicker induction and recovery with fewer cardiac abnormalities; it is now the drug of choice.

After induction of anaesthesia, a bite-block should be placed between the teeth and the seizure induced. An airway should be substituted when the seizure has abated and additional oxygen given.

Electrode placement

The usual bilateral electrode placement is fronto-temporal with the electrodes 4 cm above the midpoint of a line joining the angle of the orbit and the external auditory meatus, just on or above the hairline. The most common placements for unilateral ECT, that of Lancaster *et al.* (1958), uses the same frontotemporal site as with bilateral ECT, with the second electrode 9 cm above and behind.

The hair should be moistened at the electrode sites but left dry in between to prevent the current short-circuiting. The electrodes should be held, one in each hand, and firmly applied and the current switched on. The patient should be carefully observed for evidence of both the tonic and clonic phases of the seizure. Typically, the feet plantar-flex slightly and the arms and fingers flex. Then, muscle twitching occurs most easily seen in the lips and face. Although most patients go into a fit within a few seconds, a delay of up to 30 seconds can occur. If no fit ensues, no more than one more attempt should be made, perhaps at a higher pulse frequency. The anaesthetist must be apprised of any difficulty in inducing the fit.

Types of electrical current

The object is to induce a seizure as reliably as possible and yet to minimize side-effects by keeping the electrical current as low as possible. Little research has been carried out on this aspect of ECT (Daniel and Crovitz 1983*a*). Several machines are available in the U.K., differing in many technical respects (Mikhail *et al.* 1984). Newer machines deliver brief DC pulses which are greatly preferable to the sinusoidal wave forms given by older machines.

Length of course

Six treatments seem to be the norm in the UK although enthusiasts for ECT give up to 12 applications. Some patients respond to 3 or even 2. Older patients and men typically require more applications. Patients who are going to respond to the course typically show an ephemeral improvement after the second, third or fourth application. After one or two more ECTs, the improvement is more substantial and more prolonged. Once recovery has taken place an additional ECT does not reduce the chances of relapse. Treatment should be 2 or 3 times per week but not daily.

If a patient shows no response at all to a course of 6 ECTs the treatment should be abandoned. It is best to wait 3 months or more before ECT is reinstituted to increase the chances that the patient has entered a treatment-responsive phase.

Consent to treatment

The need for ECT should be fully explained to the patient and his relatives and the slight risks spelt out. Many misconceptions envelope ECT and the procedure should be described in detail. Unfortunately, even with careful explanations, few patients seem to fully understand the nature of their treatment (Malcolm 1989). Most patients are not distressed by the experience (Hughes *et al.* 1981). The use of anaesthetics and muscle relaxants should be emphasized. The inadvisability of discontinuing the course prematurely should be pointed out but the freedom of the patient to withdraw consent at any point must be acknowledged. It is best to give these explanations in the presence of other members of the therapeutic team.

It is customary for the patient to sign a consent form, the wording of which must take account of the law of the land and of local custom. Both doctor, patient, and another member of the therapeutic team should sign this document. In the UK, a special form must be completed by the consultant if the patient is detained under the Mental Health Act 1983.

If the detained patient does not or cannot consent, then local legal practices must be strictly observed. In the UK, the Mental Health Act Commission must be contacted. They then send a doctor who consults with the responsible consultant and two other professionals involved in the patient's care. One must be a nurse, the other neither a nurse nor a doctor. If the Commission doctor concludes that ECT is likely to alleviate or prevent a deterioration in the patient's condition and that the patient is not capable of understanding the nature, purpose, and effect of the treatment, or will not consent, he will authorize the ECT after completing the appropriate form. The whole plan of treatment is considered and not just each individual ECT.

In an emergency when ECT is considered necessary to save the patient's life or to prevent serious deterioration, it can be given on the consultant's responsibility and the position regularized as soon as possible.

Ethical considerations

Although ECT has been used for over 40 years, its role in the management of psychiatric conditions remains controversial, its use is empirical and its mode of action is unknown. Opposition to its use has increased, especially in the USA, on the grounds that it produces brain damage. Numerous instances are known of patients receiving many courses of ECT, totalling over 100 applications, and claims have been made that the indications for its use have not been clear-cut. It has even been alleged that it has been given to control the behaviour of unruly institutional inmates. Some restrictions on its use have been introduced in some states in the USA, and questions have been asked about it in the British Parliament.

Many psychiatrists regard it as an indispensable treatment for the severely depressed patient and are concerned lest its use be banned. More research is needed on the indications for ECT and favourable prognostic features identified. Further evaluation of possible long-term memory defects using sensitive tests are essential.

It is the responsibility of every psychiatrist to use ECT sparingly and carefully, and never as a treatment of desperation or as a quasi-punishment for a patient's disturbed behaviour (Salzman 1977). He should also seek to curb the untrammelled enthusiasm of any colleague who is using ECT excessively for inappropriate or minor indications. In the long run, if abuses of ECT occur or are believed to occur, the psychiatric profession will only have itself to blame if ill-informed but well-intentioned pressure groups succeed in their aim of having ECT totally banned and not merely professionally regulated.

Other physical treatments for affective disorders

Seasonal patterns have long been known in affective disorders. Recently, syndromes of Seasonal Affective Disorder (SAD) have been described (Lam *et al.* 1989). The most typical pattern is autumn/winter depressions followed by spring/summer remissions. The syndrome often contains atypical elements such as hypersomnia and weight gain. No definite biochemical abnormalities have been established although several hypotheses have been suggested involving melatonin, lack of light, or shifts in circadian rhythm.

Many cases of SAD respond satisfactorily or even dramatically to 'phototherapy'—exposure to white light of at least 2000 lux. (Indoor lighting ranges from 30–300 lux, outdoors on a dull day 1000–5000 lux, and a bright sunny day up to 10 000 lux.) About 2 h per day is usually sufficient, and morning exposure seems more effective than other times of the day. Using strict improvement criteria, Terman (1988) estimated that about half of SAD patients responded to morning light, 38 per cent to evening light and only 11 per cent to dim light conditions. There is little evidence to support the use of phototherapy in non-seasonal disorders.

Sleep deprivation has received attention as a treatment for depression, particularly where there is a marked diurnal fluctuation in mood. However, improvements are usually ephemeral (Gillin 1983).

References

Abrams, R. (1974). Multiple ECT—what have we learned? In *Psychobiology of convulsive therapy*. (eds. M. Fink., S.S. Kety., J.L. McGaugh, and T.A. Williams) pp. 79–84. John Wiley, New York.

Abrams, R., Fink, M., and Feldstein, S. (1973). Predicton of clinical response to ECT. *British Journal of Psychiatry* **122,** 457–60.

Avery, D., and Winokur, G. (1977). The efficacy of electroconvulsive therapy and antidepressants in depression. *Biological Psychiatry* **12,** 507–23.

Barker, J.C., and Baker, A.A. (1959). Deaths associated with electroplexy. *Journal of Mental Science* **105,** 339–48.

Barron, S.P., and Sullivan, T.M. (1967). The use of the cardiac pacemaker in an ECT-induced cardiac arrest. *American Journal of Psychiatry* **124,** 395–6.

Barton, J.L. (1977). ECT in depression: The evidence of controlled studies. *Biological Psychiatry* **12,** 687–95.

Black, D.W., Winokur, G., and Nasrallah, A. (1987*a*). The treatment of depression: electroconvulsive therapy v antidepressants: a naturalistic evaluation of 1495 patients. *Comprehensive Psychiatry* **28,** 169–82.

Black, D.W., Winokur, G., and Nasrullah, A. (1987*b*). Treatment of mania: a naturalistic study of electroconvulsive therapy versus lithium in 438 patients. *Journal of Clinical Psychiatry* **48,** 132–9.

Bolwig, T.G., and Rafaelsen, O.J. (1981). Working action of electroconvulsive therapy. In *Handbook of biological psychiatry*, Part VI. (eds. H.M. van Praag., M.H. Lader., O.J. Rafaelsen, and E.J. Sachar). pp. 405–18, Marcel Dekker, New York.

Brill, N.Q., Crumpton, E., Eiduson, S. *et al.* (1959). Relative effectiveness of various components of electroconvulsive therapy. *Archives of Neurology and Psychiatry* **81,** 627–35.

Carney, M.W.P., Roth, M., and Garside, R.F. (1965). The diagnosis of depressive syndromes and the prediction of ECT response. *British Journal of Psychiatry* **111,** 659–74.

Cerletti, U., and Bini, L. (1938). Un nuovo metodi di shock terapia. *Bollettino della Academia di Medica di Roma* **64,** 136–8.

Costain, D.W., Green, A.R., and Grahame-Smith, D.G. (1979). Enhanced 5-hydroxytryptamine-mediated behavioral responses in rats following repeated electroconvulsive shock: relevance to the mechanism of the antidepressive effect of electroconvulsive therapy. *Psychopharmacology* **61,** 167–70.

Cronholm, B., and Ottosson, J.O. (1963). The experience of memory function after electroconvulsive therapy. *British Journal of Psychiatry* **109,** 251–8.

Crowe, R.R. (1984). Electroconvulsive therapy—a current perspective. *New England Journal of Medicine* **311,** 163–7.

Daniel, W.F., and Crovitz, H.F. (1982). Recovery of orientation after electroconvulsive therapy. *Acta Psychiatrica Scandinavica* **66,** 421–8.

Daniel, W.F., and Crovitz, H.F. (1983*a*). Acute memory impairment following electroconvulsive therapy. 1. Effects of electrical stimulus waveform and number of treatment. *Acta Psychiatrica Scandinavica* **67,** 1–7.

Daniel, W.F., and Crovitz, H.F. (1983*b*). Acute memory impairment following electroconvulsive therapy. 2. Effects of electrode placement. *Acta Psychiatrica Scandinavica* **67,** 57–68.

d'Elia, G. (1970). Unilateral electroconvulsive therapy. *Acta Psychiatrica Scandinavica* **46,** (Suppl. 215), 1–98.

d'Elia, G., and Raotma, H. (1975). Is unilateral ECT less effective than bilateral ECT? *British Journal of Psychiatry* **126,** 83–9.

ECT Sub-Committee of the Research Committee (1989). *The practical administration of electroconvulsive therapy (ECT)*, Gaskell, London.

Evans, J., Grahame-Smith, D.G., Green, A.R., and Tordoff, A.F.C. (1976). Electroconvulsive shock increases the behavioural responses of rats to brain 5-hydroxytryptamine accumulation and central nervous system stimulant drugs. *British Journal of Pharmacology* **56,** 193–9.

Fink, M. (1977). Myths of 'shock therapy'. *American Journal of Psychiatry* **134,** 991–6.

Fink, M., and Feldstein, S. (1973). Prediction of clinical response to ECT. *British Journal of Psychiatry* **122,** 457.

Freeman, C.P. (1982). *Electroconvulsive therapy: a practical guide*. SK and F Publications, Welwyn Garden City.

Freeman, C.P.L., Basson, J.V., and Creighton, A. (1978). Double blind controlled trial of electroconvulsive therapy (ECT) and simulated ECT in depressive illness. *Lancet* **1,** 738–40.

Friedberg, J. (1977). Shock treatment, brain damage, and memory loss: a neurological perspective. *American Journal of Psychiatry* **134,** 1010–14.

Gill, D., and Lambourn, J. (1979). Indications for electric convulsion therapy and its use by senior psychiatrists. *British Medical Journal* **1,** 1169–71.

Gillin, J.C. (1983). The sleep therapies of depression. *Progress in Neuropsychopharmacology and Biological Psychiatry* **7,** 351–64.

Green, A.R., Heal, D.J., and Grahame-Smith, D.G. (1977). Further observations on the effect of repeated electroconvulsive shock on the behavioral responses of rats produced by increases in the functional activity of brain 5-hydroxytryptamine and dopamine. *Psychopharmacology* **52,** 195–200.

Greenblatt, M. (1977). Efficacy of ECT in affective and schizophrenic illness. *American Journal of Psychiatry* **134,** 1001–5.

Greenblatt, M., Grosser, G.H., and Wechsler, H. (1962). A comparative study of selected antidepressant medications and EST. *American Journal of Psychiatry* **119,** 144–53.

Greenblatt, M., Grosser, G.H., and Wechsler, H. (1964). Differential response of hospitalized depressed patients to somatic therapy. *American Journal of Psychiatry* **120,** 935–43.

Gregory, S., Shawcross, C.R., and Gill, D. (1985). The Nottingham ECT study. A double-blind comparison of bilateral, unilateral and simulated ECT in depressive illness. *British Journal of Psychiatry* **146,** 520–4.

Harper, R.G., and Wiens, A.N. (1975). Electroconvulsive therapy and memory. *Journal of Nervous and Mental Disease* **161,** 245–54.

Hobson, R.F. (1953). Prognostic factors in electric convulsive therapy. *Journal of Neurology, Neurosurgery and Psychiatry* **16,** 275–81.

Horne, R.L., Pettinati, H.M., Sugerman, A., and Varga, E. (1985). Comparing bilateral to unilateral electroconvulsive therapy in a randomized study with EEG monitoring. *Archives of General Psychiatry* **42,** 1087–92.

Hughes, J., Barraclough, B.M., and Reeve, W. (1981). Are patients shocked by ECT? *Journal of the Royal Society of Medicine* **74,** 283–5.

Johnstone, E., Deakin, J.F.W., Lawler, P., Frith, C.D., Stevens, M., McPherson, K., and Crow, T.J. (1980). The Northwick Park electroconvulsive therapy trial. *Lancet* **2,** 1317–20.

Kendell, R.E. (1978). Electroconvulsive therapy. *Journal of the Royal Society of Medicine* **71,** 319–21.

Kendell, R.E. (1981). The present status of electroconvulsive therapy. *British Journal of Psychiatry* **139,** 265–83.

Kiloh, L.G., Ball, J.R.B., and Garside, R.F. (1962). Prognostic factors in the treatment of depressive states with imipramine. *British Medical Journal* **i,** 1225–27.

Kukopulos, A., Reginaldi, D., Tondo, L. *et al.* (1977). Spontaneous length of depression and response to ECT. *Psychological Medicine* **7,** 625–9.

Lam, R.W., Kripke, D.F., and Gillin, J.C. (1989). Phototherapy for depressive disorders: a review. *Canadian Journal of Psychiatry* **34,** 140–7.

Lambourn, J., and Gill, D. (1978). A controlled comparison of simulated and real ECT. *British Journal of Psychiatry* **133,** 514–19.

Lancaster, N., Steinert, R., and Frost, I. (1958). Unilateral electroconvulsive therapy. *Journal of Mental Science* **104,** 221–7.

Levy, J., and Reid, M. (1976). Variations in writing posture and cerebral organization. *Science* **194,** 337–9.

McCabe, M.S. (1976). ECT in the treatment of mania: a controlled study. *American Journal of Psychiatry* **133,** 688–91.

McCabe, M.S., and Norris, B. (1977). ECT versus chlorpromazine in mania. *Biological Psychiatry* **12,** 245–56.

Maclay, W.S. (1953). Death due to treatment. *Proceedings of the Royal Society of Medicine* **46,** 13–20.

Malcolm, K. (1989). Patients' perceptions and knowledge of electroconvulsive therapy. *Psychiatric Bulletin* **13,** 161–5.

Marco, L.A., and Randels, P.M. (1979). Succinylcholine drug interactions during electroconvulsive therapy. *Biological Psychiatry* **14,** 433–45.

May, P.R.A. (1968). *Treatment of schizophrenia: a comparative study of five treatment methods*. Science House, New York.

Medical Research Council (1965). Report by Clinical Psychiatry Committee. Clinical trial in the treatment of depressive illness. *British Medical Journal* **i,** 881–6.

Meduna, L. (1938). General discussion of the cardiazol therapy. *American Journal of Psychiatry* **94,** (Suppl), 40–50.

Mendels, J. (1965). Electroconvulsive therapy and depression. II. Significance of endogenous and reactive syndromes. *British Journal of Psychiatry* **3,** 682–6.

Mikhail, W.I., Perinpanayagam, M.S., and Sivakumar, K. (1984). ECT machines. *British Journal of Hospital Medicine* **31,** 369–73.

Miller, D.H., Clancy, J., and Cumming, E. (1953). A comparison between unidirectional current nonconvulsive electrical stumulation given with Reiter's machine, standard alternating current electroshock (Cerletti method), and pentothal in chronic schizophrenia. *American Journal of Psychiatry* **109,** 617–20.

Minter, R.E., and Mandel, M.R. (1979). The treatment of psychotic major depressive disorder with drugs and electroconvulsive therapy. *Journal of Nervous and Mental Disease* **167,** 726–33.

Ottosson, J.O. (ed). (1960). Experimental studies of the mode of action of electroconvulsive therapy. *Acta Psychiatrica Scandinavica*, Suppl. 145.

Ottosson, J.O. (1981). Convulsive therapy. In *Handbook of biological psychiatry*, Part VI (eds. H.M. van Praag, M.H. Lader, O.J. Rafaelsen and E.J. Sachar) pp. 419–54, Marcel Dekker, New York.

Ottosson, J.O. (1985). Use and misuse of electroconvulsive treatment. *Biological Psychiatry* **20,** 933–46.

Perrin, G.M. (1961). Cardiovascular aspects of electric shock therapy. *Acta Psychiatrica Neurologica Scandinavica*, Suppl. 152.

Perris, C., and d'Elia, G. (1966). A study of bipolar (manic-depressive) and unipolar recurrent depressive psychoses. *Acta Psychiatriac Scandinavica* **42** (Suppl.) **194,** 153–63.

Royal College of Psychiatrists (1977). *Memorandum on the use of electroconvulsive therapy* **131,** 261–72.

Salzman, C. (1977). ECT and ethical psychiatry. *American Journal of Psychiatry* **134,** 1006–9.

Salzman, C. (1980). The use of ECT in the treatment of schizophrenia. *American Journal of Psychiatry* **137,** 1032–41.

Scott, A.I.F. (1989). Which depressed patients will respond to electroconvulsive therapy? *British Journal of Psychiatry* **154,** 8–17.

Small, I.F. (1974). Inhalant convulsive therapy. In *Psychobiology of convulsive therapy* (eds. M. Fink, S.S. Kety, J.L. McGaugh, and T.A. Williams) pp. 65–7. John Wiley, New York.

Small, J.G., Klapper, M.H., Kellams, J.J., Miller, M.J., Milstein, V., Sharpley, P.H., and Small, I.V. (1988). Electroconvulsive treatment compared with lithium in the management of manic states. *Archives of General Psychiatry* **45,** 727–32.

Squire, L.R. (1977). ECT and memory loss. *American Journal of Psychiatry* **134,** 997–1001.

Squire, L.R., and Chace, P.M. (1975). Memory functions six to nine months after electroconvulsive therapy. *Archives of General Psychiatry* **32,** 1557–64.

Squire, L.R., and Slater, P.C. (1978). Bilateral and unilateral ECT: effects on verbal and nonverbal memory. *American Journal of Psychiatry* **135,** 1316–20.

Squire, L.R., Slater, P.C., and Miller, P.L. (1981). Retrograde amnesia and bilateral electroconvulsive therapy. Long-term follow-up. *Archives of General Psychiatry* **38,** 89–95.

Taylor, J.R., Tompkins, R., Demers, R., and Anderson, D. (1982). Electroconvulsive therapy and memory dysfunction: is there evidence for prolonged defects? *Biological Psychiatry* **17,** 1169–93.

Taylor, P.J., and Fleminger, J.J. (1980). ECT for schizophrenia. *Lancet* **1,** 1380–2.

Terman, M. (1988). On the question of mechanism in phototherapy for seasonal affective disorder: considerations of clinical efficacy and epidemiology. *Journal of Biological Rhythms* **3,** 155–72.

Turek, I.S., and Hanlon, T.E. (1977). The effectiveness and safety of electroconvulsive therapy ((ECT). *Journal of Nervous and Mental Diseases* **164,** 419–31.

Van Valkenburg, C., and Clayton, P.J. (1985). Electroconvulsive therapy and schizophrenia. *Biological Psychiatry* **20,** 699–700.

Wechsler, H., Grosser, G.H., and Greenblatt, M. (1965). Research evaluating antidepressant medications on hospitalized mental patients: a survey of published reports during a five-year period. *Journal of Nervous and Mental Disease* **141,** 231–9.

West, E.D. (1981). Electric convulsion therapy in depression: a double-blind controlled trial. *British Medical Journal* **282,** 355–7.

17. Brain surgery for psychiatric disorders

History

Operations on the brain are the most controversial physical treatments in psychiatry today. In no other area, not even electroconvulsive therapy, is opinion so diverse and even polarized. Brain surgery, misleadingly and euphemistically termed 'psychosurgery', is enthusiastically advocated by a few practitioners who between them are responsible for the bulk of the operations in the U K and U S A. In opposition are lay people and professionals who with vigour and articulateness regard these operations, 'leucotomies', as an unwarranted insult to the brain of hapless patients who are cajoled into accepting professional advice to have the operation. This state of affairs has risen largely because for the first 25 years, crude operations were performed on the wrong patients. The more recent anatomically-refined operations are attended by better results with few untoward effects, providing that patients are carefully selected and that the operation is part of a wider treatment and rehabilitation programme. Some historical background is essential to judge the present state of affairs and this will be outlined.

Damage to the frontal lobes has long known to be associated with personality changes. A well-documented example is that of Phineas P. Gage who was employed building a railway in 1848. While tamping explosive with an iron bar, a detonation occurred driving the iron bar through Gage's frontal lobes. Consciousness was lost for only a few minutes and Gage miraculously survived. However, from being an efficient and capable foreman before his accident, he became fitful, profane, impatient, capricious, and vacillating at one time, stubborn and intractable at others. His intellectual capacities reverted to those of a child. He started having epileptic fits 12 years after the accident and died in status epilepticus three months later.

The first brain operations to attempt to transform a 'disturbed to a quiet dement' were carried out by Dr Gottlieb Burckhardt, Superintendent of the Insane Asylum at Prefargier in Switzerland. In several operations, reported in 1891, he removed a few grams of cerebral cortex from six psychotic patients. Results were not encouraging and were attended by an ominous harbinger of what would happen in 50 years time: one patient made a social recovery but one died and two developed fits.

Psychosurgery really stems from the International Neurological Congress in London in 1935 when Fulton and Jacobsen described the effects of removing the frontal association areas in two chimpanzees. After the operation the animals seemed devoid of emotional expression and no longer reacted to frustrating choice situations. Doctor Egas Moniz of Lisbon was in the audience and asked Fulton if it would be possible to alleviate anxiety states in man by surgical means. Fulton thought this would be a formidable undertaking. Moniz was a remarkable man—historian, musician, literary critic and politician. With his neurosurgical colleague, Almeida Lima, Moniz carried out the first leucotomy on 12 November, 1935 by injecting alcohol. Soon Moniz designed a special leucotome but carried out less than 100 operations as he wished to assess the long-term effects before embarking on large numbers of operations. Tragically Moniz was shot and rendered paraplegic by a leucotomized psychotic patient. Moniz reported that results were better in non-schizophrenics (depression, anxiety, and obsessional neurosis) than in schizophrenics. It is a pity that this careful clinical observation was ignored.

The neurologist Walter Freeman and the neurosurgeon James Watts modified Moniz' operation and became the most enthusiastic advocates of this approach to major mental illness. In their operation, a blunt knife was introduced from a lateral or a temporal aspect and swept in a coronal plane through the frontal lobes. Because of anatomical variation, there were major differences in the site of lesion, some being too far caudal with pronounced adverse effects. These included major personality change with disinhibition or inert states, prolonged incontinence, and convulsions. Over 10 000 modified leucotomies were carried out in the UK in the 1940s and 1950s, perhaps 4–5 times this number in the USA. Several surveys demonstrated the uselessness and negative effects of leucotomy in psychotic patients. For example, Tooth and Newton (1961) examined the records of the 10 365 patients operated on in the UK from 1942–51. Two-thirds were schizophrenics, and one-quarter suffered from affective illnesses. Less than a fifth (18 per cent) of the schizophrenic patients had a good outcome, as compared with half of the depressives. Three per cent of the patients had personality changes severe enough to require continued stay in hospital. Fits persisted in 1.3 per cent of those operated on; the mortality rate was 0.3 per cent.

Such results were obviously not appreciated at the time the operations were being carried out wholesale as enthusiasm mounted rather than waned. Indeed, Watts dissociated himself from Freeman when the latter proposed to do leucotomies through the roof of the orbit, the patient having been rendered insensate by two rapidly applied unmodified electroconvulsive shocks.

With hindsight it may be difficult to appreciate why so many operations were carried out on schizophrenic patients when the results were so unrewarding. However, it must be remembered that the modern antipsychotic drugs became established only in the mid-1950s and the outlook and conditions for chronic schizophrenic patients before that time were grim. The 19 per cent figure above should be set against that background rather than the present optimism, drug therapy, and social rehabilitation.

The surgical procedures were also being further modified. It was established early on that bilateral operations of the frontal lobes were the most strategic therapeutic target. Bimedial leucotomy was developed, the approach being from the vertex with the lesion restricted to the medial 2 cm. This divided the frontothalamic pathways from above. This operation was shown to be superior to the standard leucotomy (Greenblatt and Solomon 1952). About half of depressives and three-quarters of obsessionals did well but at the cost of up to 20 per cent adverse effects. About 6 per cent suffered disabling personality changes.

Another adaptation was orbital undercutting with an anterior entry and a horizontal sweep on each side of the midline (Scoville 1949). Knight carried out over 300 of these operations. Results were similar to those of the bimedial operation, good results in the majority of carefully-selected patients but a high incidence of side effects.

A more rational approach was advocated by Crow (1973) who introduced a large number of wire electrodes into the frontal lobes. The sheaf of electrodes remained implanted for up to 6 months while highly selective electrocoagulation was gradually built up. Over 100 patients were treated in this way, but the disadvantages of infection risk and the need for 6 months' detailed evaluation militated against the widespread use of this technique.

Modern operations

It can be seen that the crude slashes in deteriorated schizophrenics were attended by such poor results and major adverse effects as to bring the operation into disrepute with many psychiatrists and to engender lay opposition to psychosurgery in general. Indeed, psychosurgical operations of all types are banned in the USSR, and there are many places in the world where such operations are not performed. At present less than 100 operations are carried out per year in the UK (Barraclough and Mitchell-Heggs 1978). Four specialized units did two-thirds of those operations. In the USA, with 4 times the population the figure is less than 200 operations per year (Donnelly 1978). Before describing the operations currently used it is necessary to outline the anatomical features and neuronal circuits involved.

Anatomy

The frontal lobe has a wealth of connexions to the limbic system. From the dorsal convexity of the frontal lobe, pathways run to the cingulate gyrus and hippocampus; a similar pathway runs down to the hypothalamus and tegmental area of the midbrain. The orbital surface of the frontal lobe projects to the septal area and also the hypothalamus.

The limbic system comprises the hippocampus, amygdalum, hippocampal and cingulate gyri, limen insulae, and the posterior part of the orbital regions of the frontal lobe. Organization of these structures results in two parallel circuits in the frontolimbic–hypothalamic–midbrain axis. First, is a medial frontal, cingulate, hippocampal axis; second, an orbital frontal, temporal, amygdala circuit. Both influence the hypothalamus, altering autonomic and endocrine functions and also the brainstem reticular formation. The first circuit connects via the fornix, mamillary bodies, mamillothalamic tract, and thalamofrontal fibres; the second runs between the amygdala, dorsomedian thalamic nuclei, and into the thalamofrontal bundle. Both axes connect together in the septal region, pre-optic area, hypothalamus and midbrain. This establishment of the anatomy of frontal lobe connexions led to the understanding of the close relationship between overt emotional behaviour and covert physiological changes accompanying that behaviour.

The 'standard lobotomy' resulted in massive division of fronto-limbic structures and the adverse effects produced can be appreciated with hindsight as due to the extent of the impairment of frontal lobe function. Operations on the anterior cingulate gyrus and thalamofrontal bundle (modified bimedial leucotomy) divide different parts of the same main circuit, the latter in particular affecting more of the frontolimbic connexions (Fig. 17.1).

Orbital undercutting effectively severs the fibre tracts running from the posterior orbital cortex to the limbic system.

Current operations

Four operations are currently favoured (Fig. 17.1).

1. *Lower medial quadrant leucotomy:* (LMQ; Fig. 20.1). This is essentially a development of the modified leucotomy mentioned in the historical introduction. It is, however, still carried out in the UK by a third of units, although the numbers operated on are less than 3 patients per unit per year. A superior frontal approach is usually used and the white matter is cut for a width of about 20 mm above grey matter medially and inferiorly. The lesion is just in front of the fourth ventricle and transects the thalamofrontal radiation (Schurr 1973). In a series of Maudsley Hospital patients, 69 per

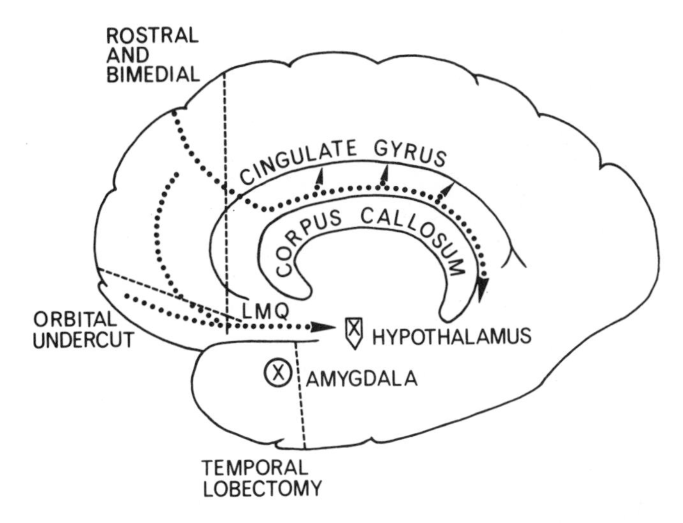

Fig. 17.1. Diagrammatic representation of some operations on the brain.

cent were relieved of their most severe symptoms but there were 'lasting and troublesome' or 'severely disabling' effects in about 20 per cent (Post *et al.* 1968). Depressed patients responded better to anteriorly placed than to more caudal lesions (Newcombe 1975). The incidence of side-effects is higher than with prefrontal leucotomies (Birley 1964), operations which are still carried out by some units.

2. *Stereotactic subcaudate tractotomy* comprises the use of a stereotaxic device which is a metal rectangular frame which fits around the head. Radiographs are taken of the head to establish the anatomy. At subsequent operation the insertion of an electrode or probe can be carried out to an accuracy of 1 mm, the stereotaxic device being replaced in the identical position.

The lesion can be produced by severing the tract or by introducing an array of small ceramic rods, each 7 mm long and 1 mm in diameter, containing radioactive yttrium (90Y) which has a half-life of 62 h. A lesion 25 mm × 15 mm × 5 mm is produced. The posterior half of such lesions lie in the subcaudate area, the anterior part lies beneath the central segment of frontal white matter.

A review of the first 210 patients operated on by this technique was followed by a survey of the next 209 (Strom-Olsen and Carlisle 1971; Goktepe *et al.* 1975). The results are shown in Table 17.1. Over half of patients show a favourable response and the incidence of untoward effects is fairly low. Knight (1973), the main protagonist of this operation, reported that the subcaudate lesion helps obsessional patients with depression more than purely obsessional cases. Some depressed patients recover dramatically

Table 17.1. Rough comparisons of the wanted and unwanted effects of brain surgery

	Standard prefrontal	Bimedial	Orbital undercut	Stereotactic tractotomy		Limbic leucotomy
	Tooth and Newton (1961)	Birley (1964)	Sykes and Tredgold (1964)	Strom-Olsen and Carlisle (1971)	Goktepe *et al.* (1975)	Mitchell, Heggs *et al.* (1976)
Good response for:						
Depression	50%	50%	69%	56%	68%	56%
Anxiety			44%	41%	63%	27%
Obsessional states		75%	30%	50%	50%	67%
Adverse events:						
Schizophrenia	18%		4/13			4/7
Death	0.3%	0	1.5%	0	0.5%	0
Fits	1.3% (persisting)	1%	16%	1%	2%	1.5%
Severe adverse effects on personality	3.1%	6%	5%	2.6%	Less than 7%	1.5%
N =	10365	92	350	210	208	66

after their operation with few, if any, affective episodes. It is unclear which factors are associated with this particularly good prognosis.

3. *Cingulectomy*: Operations on the anterior cingulate gyrus have been carried out since 1948, the first being performed in Oxford by Cairns. In the 'open' operation, the anterior 40 mm of cingulate gyrus, extending up to 10 mm into the white matter, is removed bilaterally. Lewin (1961) reported that this approach was particularly beneficial for obsessional symptoms but that orbital cortex operations were more appropriate for anxious and depressive symptoms. Occasional operations have been performed on the posterior cingulate gyrus.

4. *Stereotactic limbic leucotomy*: This operation was suggested by Kelly *et al.* (1973), as a rational development of rostral leucotomy. In limbic leucotomy two pairs of sites are routinely operated on by electrocoagulation or by cryogenic techniques (freezing). Lesions are placed stereotactically in the subcaudate area of the lower medial quadrant of the frontal lobe and, in addition, via entry from above, lesions are made in the anterior cingulate gyrus (Richardson 1973). These are designed to interrupt frontolimbic pathways.

Although stereotactic techniques are used, the precise localization of the lesion is aided by introducing an electrode at the proposed site of operation. Stimulation via this electrode should result in a diminution of respiration and cardiovascular alterations. If not, the electrode is moved a few millimetres and stimulation tried again. Responses are very similar from both the cingulate and lower medial quadrant areas.

Kelly (1976) has reported on 66 patients followed up for a mean interval of 16 months. Of the 27 patients with obsessional neurosis, 89 per cent improved. The improvement rate was a little less in the 9 depressives (78 per cent) and only 66 per cent of 15 anxiety states improved. Six out of 7 chronic schizophrenics improved, but Kelly states that symptoms of severe anxiety, depression or obsessional rituals or ruminations must be present before limbic leucotomy should be envisaged in such patients. The remaining 8 patients were of various diagnoses including anorexia nervosa and personality disorder with affective symptoms. Overall, ratings of neuroticism, anxiety and depression dropped by about a third within 2 months of the operation, with some slight further improvement in the ensuing months. Obsessional symptoms were ameliorated to a greater extent. Adverse effects were uncommon. Some patients became more outspoken, some became mildly lethargic. One patient developed a memory disturbance.

Other operations

Many other parts of the brain have been operated on in attempts to lessen symptoms of anxiety, depression and obsessions. More controversially, some operations have been designed to diminish aggressive behaviour whether or not this was in the context of epilepsy.

Stereotactic techniques have been used to place lesions in the amygdala, the hypothalamus and the stria terminalis. Amygdalectomy has been reported as decreasing aggressiveness and maladaptive behaviour in 18 patients of whom 16 were epileptic (Hitchock and Cairns 1973). Marked calming effects are claimed to follow medial or posteromedial hypothalamotomy (Sano *et al.* 1972; Kim and Umbach 1973). Another site claimed to be important is the stria terminalis, linking the hypothalamus and amygdala; lesions here are reported to lessen violently aggressive behaviour (Burzaco 1973).

Indications for brain surgery

As brain surgery involves irreversible changes in brain function, it should never be recommended to a patient without the greatest care and most detailed review. In both the UK and the USA, such operations are advised infrequently.

The indications for brain surgery refer more to symptoms than to diagnostic categories. In particular, the chronicity of symptoms should be carefully assessed, 10 years or so of intractable symptoms being a typical history. Most important, the entire range of non-operative treatments should have been tried first. These treatments must have been applied vigorously and sensibly before it can be concluded that the condition is refractory. A few weeks' drug treatment at low dosage or a few sessions of half-hearted behaviour therapy with an inexperienced practitioner do not constitute an adequate trial. Most patients being considered for leucotomy will have had one or more courses of ECT especially as chronic risk of suicide is a strong indication to consider surgery. Excessive use of ECT is often associated with a persisting memory disturbance. As leucotomies can on occasion affect memory this must be taken into account. Often, patients previously refractory to other treatments become more responsive after surgery, any residual symptoms being controlled by drugs, behaviour therapy or supportive psychotherapy.

Severity of symptoms is an important factor. Many patients considered for leucotomy are totally incapacitated by the symptoms, unable to work or carry out their household duties. They are a great burden to their families and friends.

Chronic, severe depression, especially of the endogenous type, is the best indication for psychosurgery. Patients with recurrent depressive illnesses are also suitable, especially if there is a risk of suicide at the onset and offset of each episode. The premorbid personality is important, a balanced, integrated personality with family support and a stable environment being associated with a better outcome than a manipulative, dependent, histrionic, immature person.

Anxiety states, especially those with previously calm personalities, also generally respond well. Patients with previously anxious personalities, timid, fearful and easily dismayed, have a less certain outcome. A history of drug or alcohol abuse is not uncommon and a wide variety of drugs will have been tried over the years. Occupational, familial and social handicap is usually severe.

Obsessional symptoms, as mentioned before, have a good prognosis when limbic leucotomy is used. Schizophrenic patients usually respond poorly to leucotomy except a very few with marked anxiety and tension and some preservation of personality and insight.

Among other conditions, intractable pain has been associated with disappointing results as has depersonalization. Anorexia nervosa has improved in a few instances but most personality disorders are not helped. Aggression and antisocial behaviour, especially in an epileptic, are claimed to respond to amygdalectomy, but this remains a controversial research procedure. Temporal lobectomy is not strictly a psychosurgical procedure as the excised brain tissue is anatomically abnormal.

Patients with dementia or organic pathology, including cerebrovascular disease, should not be considered for brain surgery, but old age by itself is not a contraindication. Hypertension and blood dyscrasias and bleeding tendencies are usually contraindications. Patients with psychopathy, drug abuse and alcoholism are not suitable for operation.

An agreed statement on indications for psychosurgery was published by surgeons and psychiatrists from three major U.K. centres (Bartlett *et al.* 1981). Their suggestions are marginally wider than the indications given above.

Assessment and rehabilitation

Careful and detailed assessment of the patient's symptoms, handicaps and problems should be carried out in every case. Formal rating scales are very useful in establishing a preoperative baseline. The premorbid personality must be carefully assessed by perusal of school reports, work records and by obtaining the history from one or more informants. The previous treatments should be listed and efforts made to verify dose regimes, the intensity of psychotherapy and the frequency and length of behaviour therapy.

The current symptoms should be meticulously elicited especially with respect to depression, anxiety and compulsive phenomena. Suicidal thoughts and intent must be sought. Psychological capacities should be routinely tested including careful assessment of memory functions. An EEG is useful to exclude focal or diffuse epileptic foci.

Following operative procedures, improvement is usually slow with symptoms resolving slowly. This is particularly true of stereotactic procedures, and the patient and his relatives must be warned of this lest premature disappointment ensue. With freehand leucotomies, improvement is often more rapid but laziness and apathy may also supervene and need careful handling.

Depressive symptoms usually resolve fairly steadily but mood swings can occur especially during the first two months and may be sufficiently marked as to require symptomatic drug therapy. Obsessional symptoms wane more gradually and retraining is necessary in order to maximize benefit from the operation. Thus, a programme of distraction from carrying out compulsive rituals or ruminating excessively must be instituted. The patient can be treated by any of the behaviourally-based techniques such as modelling. Anxiety symptoms usually diminish after the operation but again behaviour therapy may be necessary for situational, social, and specific fears. Such manoeuvres have a greater chance of success than before operation.

As well as these specific symptomatic treatments, a carefully constructed programme of social rehabilitation is essential. Patients must be warned that the operation is not a panacea which will restore them to normality but that the expected lessening of symptoms will provide an opportunity for adjustments in the occupational, marital, and social spheres of functioning. For example, help is needed in finding a job after years of unemployability. The spouse must be encouraged to actively help in the rehabilitation, in taking up those threads of life severed by the illness.

Ethics

The understandable controversy concerning the ethics of psychosurgery stems partly from the disastrous effects of some of the early extensive freehand operations. The tidal wave of over-enthusiasm for leucotomy in the 1940s and 1950s has left signs of its detritus in the form of patients in grossly withdrawn or disinhibited states in the chronic wards of our mental hospitals. Unfortunately, all operations have been tarred with the same brush and, more recently, the introduction of procedures designed to control aggressive and antisocial behaviour has only complicated the issues. Also, in the United States, the psychodynamic views which prevailed until recently implied that even major psychiatric illnesses could be controlled and perhaps cured by psychotherapy and social readjustment. By corollary, physical treatments, drugs, ECT, and especially psychosurgery became regarded as unwarranted assaults on mental functioning. However, the National Commission for the Protection of Human Subjects of Biomedical and Behavioral Research investigated psychosurgery and concluded that the newer forms of operation should not be banned but should be studied further (Culliton 1976).

Nevertheless, it cannot be denied that surgical procedures, even the modern ones, have not been subject to the controlled evaluations which are now not only routine but essential before the introduction of a new drug therapy. All the assessments have been in the absence of a control group, before and after comparisons having to suffice. In view of the magnitude of the operative procedure together with all its attendant diagnostic and assessment routines, as carried out in the major centres, the possibility of a major placebo effect cannot be discounted. In addition, the postoperative rehabilitation procedures are intensively carried out by expert, experienced and dedicated teams. On the other hand, these teams are convinced from their assessment and follow-up data that the selective modern operations are effective in carefully selected patients with an acceptably low rate of complications. These results must be set against the natural history of chronic psychiatric syndromes with indefinite invalidism and possible suicide.

Certain ethical points can be suggested. First, no patient who is compulsorily detained should be subjected to operation nor should release from an institution be made conditional on undergoing an operation. Second, fully informed consent must be obtained from the patient and from the caring relatives. To ensure that consent is obtained fairly, the benefits and risks should be explained at a ward round attended by all involved in the care of the patient, including people from outside the operative team.

We would recommend that should surgery be considered in a patient who is chronically ill and has failed to respond to all other therapeutic procedures. The patient should be referred to a specialized unit rather than to the local neurosurgeon who carries out only a few operations per year. These units are generally in teaching centres and many medical and paramedical people and trainees have the opportunity to see for themselves the type of patients selected for operation. The detailed evaluations and assessments before and after operation are carried out by a multidisciplinary team. In this way public disquiet that such operations are clandestine is likely to be allayed.

References

Barraclough, B.M., and Mitchell-Heggs, N.A. (1978). Use of neurosurgery for psychological disorder in British Isles during 1974–6. *British Medical Journal* **2,** 1591–3.

Bartlett, J., Bridges, P., and Kelly, D. (1981). Contemporary indications for psychosurgery. *British Journal of Psychiatry* **138,** 507–11.

Birley, J.L.T. (1964). Modified frontal leucotomy: a review of 106 cases. *British Journal of Psychiatry* **110,** 211–21.

Bridges, P.K. (1978). A contemporary view of psychosurgery. In *Current Themes in Psychiatry* (eds. R.J. Gaind and B.L. Hudson), pp. 307–32. Macmillan, London.

Burzaco, J.A. (1973). Fundus striae terminalis, an optimal target in sedative stereotactic surgery. In *Surgical Approaches in Psychiatry* (eds. L.V. Laitinen and K.E. Livingston), pp. 135–7. Medical and Technical Publishing, Lancaster.

Crow, H.J. (1973). Intracerebral polarisation and multifocal leucocoagulation in some psychiatric illnesses. *Psychiatrica, Neurologia and Neurochirugia (Amsterdam)* **76,** 365–81.

Culliton, B.J. (1976). Psychosurgery: National Commission issues surprisingly favorable report. *Science* **194,** 299–301.

Donnelly, J. (1978). The incidence of psychosurgery in the United States 1971–1973. *American Journal of Psychiatry* **135,** 1476–80.

Goktepe, E.O., Young, L.B., and Bridges, P.K. (1975). A further review of the results of stereotactic subcaudate tractotomy. *British Journal of Psychiatry* **126,** 270–80.

Greenblatt, M., and Solomon, H.C. (1952). Survey of nine years of lobotomy investigations. *American Journal of Psychiatry* **109,** 262–5.

Hitchcock, E., and Cairns, V. (1973). Amygdalotomy. *Postgraduate Medical Journal* **49,** 894–904.

Kelly, D. (1976). Neurosurgical treatment of psychiatric disorders. In *Recent advances in clinical Psychiatry* No. 2. (ed. K. Granville-Grossman) pp. 227–61. Churchill Livingstone, Edinburgh.

Kelly, D. (1981). Psychosurgery. In *Handbook of biological psychiatry*, Part VI (eds. H.M. van Praag, M.H. Lader, O.J. Rafaelsen, and E.J. Sachar) pp. 455–72. Marcel Dekker, New York.

Kelly, D., Richardson, A., and Mitchell-Heggs, N. (1973). Stereotactic limbic leucotomy: neurophysiological aspects and operative technique. *British Journal of Psychiatry* **123,** 133–40.

Kim, Y.K., and Umbach, W. (1973). Combined stereotactic lesions for treatment of behaviour disorders and severe pain. In *Surgical approaches in psychiatry* (eds. L.V. Laitinen and K.E. Livingston) pp. 182–8. Medical and Technical Publishing, Lancaster.

Knight, G. (1973). Further observations from an experience of 660 cases of stereotactic tractotomy. *Postgraduate Medical Journal* **49,** 845–54.

Lewin, W. (1961). Observations on selective leucotomy. *Journal of Neurology, Neurosurgery and Psychiatry* **24,** 37–44.

Mitchell-Heggs, N., Kelly, D., and Richardson, A. (1976). Stereotactic limbic leucotomy: A follow-up at 16 months. *British Journal of Psychiatry* **128,** 226–31.

Newcombe, R. (1975). The lesion in stereotactic subcaudate tractotomy. *British Journal of Psychiatry* **126,** 478–81.

Post, F., Linford Rees, W., and Schurr, P.H. (1968). An evaluation of bimedial leucotomy. *British Journal of Psychiatry* **114,** 1223–46.

Richardson, A. (1973). Stereotactic limbic leucotomy. Surgical technique. *Postgraduate Medical Journal* **49,** 860–4.

Sano, K., Sekino, H., and Mayanagi, Y. (1972). Results of stimulation and destruction of the posterior hypothalamus in cases with violent, aggressive and restless behaviors. In *Psychosurgery* (eds. E. Hitchock, L. Laitinen, and K. Vaernet), p. 57. Thomas, Springfield, Illinois.

Schurr, P. (1973). Psychosurgery. *British Journal of Hospital Medicine* **10,** 53–60.

Scoville, W.B. (1949). Selective cortical undercutting as a means of modifying and studying frontal lobe function in man. *Journal of Neurosurgery* **6,** 65–73.

Strom-Olsen, R., and Carlisle, S. (1971). Bifrontal stereotactic tractotomy. *British Journal of Psychiatry* **118,** 141–54.

Sykes, M., and Tredgold, R. (1964). Restricted orbital undercutting. A study of its effects on 350 patients over the ten years 1951–60. *British Journal of Psychiatry* **110,** 609–20.

Tooth, G.C., and Newton, M.P. (1961). *Reports on public health and medical subjects*, No. 104, Ministry of Health. HMSO London.

18. Miscellaneous disorders and drugs

In this chapter we deal briefly with a variety of conditions which the general psychiatrist may be called on to treat or about which his advice may be sought. The many interfaces between psychiatry and neurology, internal medicine and clinical psychology are ever-changing and the psychiatrist has to be adept at adjusting his role, being aware of changing views and techniques, keeping himself informed and participating in management when called upon to do so.

Alcoholism and other addictions

Addictive behaviours, whether they involve the use of chemical substances, as in alcoholism, or not, as in bulimia, have much in common including a rather poor prognosis. The behavioural disturbance is therefore more than a simple pharmacological adaptation to a particular chemical agent and treatment of the latter is, in consequence, a minor component of management.

In the assessment and treatment of these problems a number of general matters should always be kept in mind. Patients tend to minimize the extent of their problem or even to deny it, and it is always wise to obtain evidence from an acquaintance of the patient who will probably give a more accurate history. Also, there are often multiple core problems such as other addictions or coexisting psychiatric illness. For example, alcoholics tend to be heavy smokers, they commonly abuse benzodiazepines (Ciraulo *et al*. 1988) or other drugs (Norton and Colliver 1988) and they gamble. Depression, anxiety or personality disorder may be present and withdrawal of the addictive agent may expose depression (Penick *et al* 1988), phobias (Smail *et al* 1984), and insomnia (Wagman and Allen 1977) which may be long-lasting and predispose to a return to drugs and alcohol. The social aspects of the addiction such as the community ambience of the habit, financial loss, family disruption, and physical complications affect the prognosis and they, too, require attention. Management therefore has to be concerned with a number of aspects, and drug treatments currently play a minor role, mainly in easing withdrawal and in treating coexisting psychiatric illness. Patients frequently break contact with treatment; they both want to stop and to continue their habit. The motivational nexus is undoubtedly complex and significant advances in treatment probably depend on understanding it. Whether chemotherapy will find a place here remains to be seen.

Alcohol-related problems

The consumption of alcohol is a widespread habit and the weekly consumption which is considered safe is set at progressively lower levels as knowledge accumulates. Twenty-one units for a man, 14 for a woman are now considered the safe upper levels of consumption. About 6 per cent of men and 1 per cent of women have serious problems with alcohol in any given year in the UK. Clearly, where treatment methods are of very limited efficacy, prevention is the best course. However, the diverse paths leading to alcohol addiction and the different patterns of alcohol abuse make targeted prevention difficult; the spontaneous improvement after drinking is established and the marked differences in the vulnerability to the physical and social complications obscure the changes wrought by any intervention in the long term. Former certainties about the management of alcoholism have therefore faded and in the present state of knowledge treatment consists of simple support and counselling of the patient and his family, calling upon any additional stratagem which will interrupt, delay and lessen the amount of alcohol consumed (Edwards and Grant 1980; Heather and Robertson 1985). Treatment should be offered whenever there is evidence that alcohol intake is above safe levels, when adverse consequences show themselves, and certainly if there is evidence of the dependence syndrome (escalating intake, withdrawal symptoms, a life-style centring increasingly around alcohol).

The use of drugs falls into two main situations, facilitation of alcohol withdrawal and prevention of alcohol dependence and abuse.

Acute alcohol withdrawal, in its most severe form, delirium tremens, can be controlled by substituting a drug which is cross tolerant with alcohol, and then tapering off that drug. Barbiturates were used for this indication, and although largely supplanted by the benzodiazepines and chlormethiazole, are probably more effective than their successors (Kramp and Rafaelsen 1978). Most alcoholics, however, can withdraw from alcohol with general supportive care only and do not need routine drug substitution (Peachey and Naranjo 1984). If a benzodiazepine is deemed necessary, chlordiazepoxide 10 mg three times daily or diazepam 5 mg three times daily, tapering the dose over 5–10 days should lessen apprehension and physical symptoms such as tension, tremor, sweating, and nausea. Should these be especially severe and delirium emerge, a higher dose, such as 20 mg of diazepam orally every hour until the patient is sedated, is both rapid and effective. Lorazepam is equally effective (Miller and McCurdy 1984) but gives a less smooth control of symptoms (Ritson and Chick 1986). It may be preferable in patients with liver impairment because of its simpler metabolism.

In the UK, chlormethiazole is popular in the management of alcohol withdrawal (McInnes 1987). It is given in tapering doses over 6 days. However, there is a very real risk of transferring dependence to it if it is given long-term. Furthermore, the combination of alcohol and chlormethiazole can lead to fatal respiratory depression. Thus, it should not be used in alcoholics who continue to drink, or as a treatment of 'alcoholism' itself. In the management of alcohol withdrawal chlormethiazole should only be given in hospital or under very close out-patient supervision (Committee on Safety of Medicines 1987).

Other drugs used in withdrawal include propranolol for patients with severe tremor and phenytoin for those with a history of fits. Paraldehyde, chloral hydrate and barbiturates (with the possible exception of phenobarbitone) are now obsolete. Bromocriptine, a dopamine agonist, has been tried with some encouraging results (Borg and Weinholdt 1982). Vitamins are probably essential in most patients because alcoholics commonly have a poor diet, and malabsorption and increased requirement of vitamins have been demonstrated. Thiamine is especially necessary but it is usual to give multiple vitamins, intramuscularly or orally depending on the nutritional status of the patient and the severity of the addiction. The degree of vitamin deficiency and response to treatment is highly variable (Brown *et al* 1983).

Alcohol-sensitizing drugs to reduce alcohol consumption have been used for many years, but opinion is divided concerning their efficacy and usefulness. The only one available in the UK is disulfiram. When taken before alcohol, disulfiram produces a strong and unpleasant reaction with tachycardia, hypotension, flushing, dyspnoea, headache, nausea, and vomiting (Peachey *et al.* 1981). Disulfiram produces irreversible inhibition of aldehyde dehydrogenase, thus causing an accumulation of acetaldehyde. This inhibition builds up over 12 h and slowly wears off as new enzyme is synthesized. However, repeated small doses of alcohol can accelerate this waning effect.

Marked interactions can follow the accidental or intentional ingestion of alcohol, with tachycardia, severe hypotension and cardiac arrhythmias. Patients already on alpha- and beta-adrenoceptor agents, tricyclic antidepressants, antipsychotic drugs, or some forms of chemotherapy, e.g. metronidazole, are particularly at risk.

Disulfiram itself has a range of side-effects. Commonly, drowsiness, fatigue, and lethargy occur; more rarely psychosis and acute encephalopathy have been reported. More rare still are peripheral neuropathy, increased plasma cholesterol, and hepatotoxicity.

Co-administration of phenytoin may result in phenytoin toxicity due to inhibition of the microsomal mixed-function enzymes which metabolize it.

Disulfiram should only be given to alcoholics who clearly wish to be abstinent, agree to take the drug regularly and have no history or presence of major psychiatric disorder. The dosage is 250 mg once at night by mouth. It is no panacea but when used thoughtfully can make a useful contribution to treatment. Controlled studies demonstrate that disulfiram reduces the number of days in which alcohol is taken (Fuller *et al* 1986; Fuller and Roth 1979), though in one study a pharmacologically inactive dose was effective, suggesting that it may operate as much through psychological rather than pharmacological mechanisms. These can be productively construed in terms of learning theory in which disulfiram alters the reinforcements operating in drinking behaviour. Importantly disulfiram replaces the delayed with the immediate negative consequences of alcohol intake and therefore makes it less likely that drinking will occur again. Patterns of reinforcement can be further altered by punishing non-compliance (e.g. by loss of a monetary deposit), a task aided by a sensitive measurement of compliance such as detecting the metabolic products of disulfiram (Fuller and Neiderhiser 1981). Compliance is likely to improve if the patient knows it is being checked and can be further improved by building in some form of supervision by, perhaps, a relative and improved again by some form of contract between the patient and his supervisor (Azrin *et al.* 1982). The effectiveness of disulfiram is therefore enhanced when drug treatment is incorporated within a programme in which psychological and social forces are carefully analysed. Reliance on technical ingenuity alone is less impressive: disulfiram implants are available (Wilson *et al.* 1984), but have doubtful efficacy.

The benzodiazepines are widely used in the management of patients with alcohol problems. They lessen anxiety and help sleep but are very likely to be abused, with the substitution, or even addition of one drug problem for another. Their use may be justified when they promote abstinence, but this must be carefully monitored. Other drugs evaluated as 'abstinence-promoters' include bromocriptine (Borg 1983) and selective 5-HT uptake inhibitor antidepressants.

Drug dependence

Although the psychosocial aspects of dependence to various drugs also have common threads running through them, major pharmacological differences exist (see Table 18.1). The opioids are the best studied class of drugs of dependence (Martin 1984). Attempts to develop analgesics that do not have the side-effects of respiratory depression, vomiting, constipation, tolerance and physical dependence have been boosted by the recent major advances in

Table 18.1. Estimated relative tolerance, psychological and physical dependence, and withdrawal in humans of different addictive drugs.

Drug	Tolerance	Psychological dependence	Physical dependence	Withdrawal
Psychomotor stimulants				
Amphetamines	+++	++++	++	+
Cocaine	+++	++++	+	?
Caffeine	+/−	+	+/−	+/−
Nicotine	+	+++	++	++
Hallucinogens				
LSD	++	+	0	0
Mescaline	+	+	0	0
PCP	+	+	+	0
^{9}-THC	+	+++	+	0
Narcotics				
Morphine	+++	++++	++	++
CNS depressants				
Barbiturates	++	+	+++	+++
Benzodiazepines	+	++	++	++
Ethanol	++	++	+++	+++

Key: + = observed; 0 = usually not observed; +/− = observation only in some studies; ? = not enough information available.
Abbreviations: LSD = lysergic acid diethylamide; PCP = phencyclidine; ^{9}-THC = 1- ^{9}-tetrahydrocannabinol.

our understanding of the basic pharmacology of these substances (Henderson and McFadzean 1985).

As with alcohol-related problems, the use of drugs in the management of opioid dependence can be roughly divided into two areas, withdrawal and prevention of relapse. Withdrawal from opioids is very uncomfortable for the addict but it is not life-threatening as withdrawal from alcohol or barbiturates can be. Tapering off the dose over a few days under heavy sedation is the usual management. The antihypertensive agent clonidine has been found effective presumably because it dampens down noradrenergic overactivity which is believed to underlie the withdrawal syndrome (Charney *et al.* 1984). Rapid detoxification can be induced by administration of an opioid antagonist such as naltrexone, and the clonidine–naltrexone combination has been found effective (Charney *et al.* 1982).

A range of drugs has been used to attempt to lessen the risk of relapse. Apart from symptomatic remedies such as antidepressants and anxiolytics, opioid antagonists have been tried. They work by breaking down the euphoriant, reinforcing effects of the opioid so that 'fixes' of heroin, say, have no effect. Naltrexone has been evaluated but has so far not established itself in practice (Gonzalez and Brogden 1988).

Cocaine dependence has become commoner in some countries in recent years (Kleber 1988). In particular there has been a several fold increase in abuse in North America over the past decade (Pollack *et al.* 1989). Cocaine can be taken by injection, it may be inhaled from snuff or as the freebase from cigarettes (known as 'crack'). The latter is absorbed especially rapidly with almost immediate effect and is therefore particularly addictive. Delirium, convulsions, stereotyped behaviour, and psychosis have been described in cocaine abusers (Murray 1986). Diazepam is the usual treatment if convulsions are present or threatened. Initial cocaine abstinence can be facilitated by the use of noradrenalin re-uptake inhibitors such as desipramine (Gawin *et al.* 1989) and bromocriptine. Longer-term studies are in progress. As with other drug addictions, drug treatments have a more enduring effect if integrated into a behavioural programme (O'Brien *et al.* 1988). Adverse reactions to psychedelic drugs such as LSD are common and comprise acute panic reactions, LSD 'psychoses' and flashbacks (Strassman 1984). Treatment is symptomatic. Cannabis abuse can also produce these phenomena but less commonly and less severely (Hollister 1986).

The most serious dependence syndrome, at least in respect of long-term consequences for physical health, is that to nicotine. Nicotine chewing gum has been introduced as an aid to stopping smoking but its status is uncertain (Raw 1985). Efficacy data suggests that it has a useful effect, alleviating nicotine withdrawal symptoms and improving abstinence success rates significantly but modestly (Lam *et al.* 1987). However, it is unpleasant to use for some people, and can be irritant. Other ways of administering nicotine as a substitute for tobacco smoking are being assessed.

Epilepsy and anticonvulsant drugs

The management of epilepsy is a very large topic in its own right which, in the UK at least, is mostly dealt with by neurologists. Consequently, the following brief account will concentrate on the therapy of epileptic patients with psychological disorders (Reynolds 1982).

The management of epilepsy has, perhaps inevitably, been heavily influenced by the treatment of chronic epilepsy with the consequent danger that treatment is often too complex and given for too long to many patients. Much more knowledge is needed of the natural history of unselected populations with prospective studies beginning early in the disorder so that a more balanced appraisal of epilepsy, its treatment and complications is obtained. Studies of this kind have recently begun (Goodridge and Shorvon 1983). The nature of epilepsy and the processes involved in its progression are not really known but there is the possibility, first suggested by Gowers that, 'the effect of a convulsion on the nerve centres is such as to render the occurrence of another more easy, to intensify the predisposition that already exists' and, if this is so, the adequacy of early treatment may have important long-term consequences (Shorvon and Reynolds 1982). The life-time prevalence of epilepsy is about 6.5 per thousand in Europe and the USA. Some patients have only a single seizure or single attacks at widely spaced intervals whilst others have frequent attacks of varying type, the pattern of epilepsy changing over the years. Some of the factors predisposing to a more entrenched disorder have been identified: they include the presence of a neurological lesion, abnormalities in the EEG and psycho-social difficulties and, when these are present, the institution and supervision of treatment are especially important. Perhaps a third of epileptics have psychological disorders due to brain damage, seizure activity and anticonvulsant drug treatment, especially where several drugs are used. Inevitably the consequences for interpersonal and social life pose difficulties for psychological adjustment.

Anticonvulsant Drugs

A large number of drugs are used to treat epilepsy and comprise the hydantoins, barbiturates, succinimides, benzodiazepines, carbamazepine, and sodium valproate. Several interesting compounds are in the process of development. Phenobarbitone, phenytoin and primidone are indicated in the treatment of tonic–clonic (*grand mal*) epilepsy, carbamazepine in partial seizures (including temporal lobe epilepsy), ethosuximide in *petit mal* and clonazepam and sodium valproate in all types. The indications for particular anticonvulsants have been determined by clinical experience hardened by dogmatic tradition rather than scientific evidence, partly perhaps because some of the drugs in present use were introduced long before the era of controlled trials. Treatment decisions must necessarily be guided by the natural history of the disease, knowledge of which has been biased by the study of those patients with more severe and chronic epilepsy. This is now being corrected (Goodridge and Shorvon 1983) and it is clear that remission occurs in a substantial number of epileptics. The mode of action of anticonvulsant drugs is unknown: they may simply suppress seizures but it is possible that they slowly correct the basic disorder. Clearly, careful consideration should be given to the starting and stopping of medication and, in between these major decisions, treatment should be regularly monitored optimizing the balance between seizure suppression and untoward effects (Chadwick and Reynolds 1985). The initiation of treatment is not indicated by a single natural seizure, by seizures occurring during the withdrawal of alcohol, benzodiazepines, or drugs of abuse, and probably not even when there is a high prospective risk of seizures following head injury or craniotomy. Where seizures recur after an interval of less than a year the institution of anticonvulsant treatment is probably of advantage to the patient. The choice of drug, apart from the rough guidelines given above, is dictated more by freedom from side-effects rather than differences in efficacy. Indeed, few studies have addressed the problem of comparative efficacy. The potentialities of one drug should be fully explored before resorting to another and certainly before trying combinations of drugs. For example, sodium valproate will control generalized tonic–clonic convulsions in 70 per cent of patients and in 80 per cent of general absences in children. Plasma drug concentration estimations are valuable in optimizing efficacy and minimizing toxicity. Appropriate values are set out in Table 18.2.

Once treatment is established the patient should be seen regularly to monitor the adequacy and toxicity of treatment, to improve compliance and to allow counselling on matters such as social stress, alcohol use, and drug interactions. Clearly, a drug which is well-tolerated is more likely to be taken regularly: carbamazepine is often preferred because its incidence of adverse effects is lower than with phenytoin or phenobarbitone and it may have positive psychotropic effects such as the combating of depressed mood. Newer compounds are not necessarily less toxic: clonazepam and sodium valproate have appreciable side-effects. The epileptic process waxes and wanes and doses may need to be altered. There is, of course, a tendency for drug regimens to become more complex and doses to remain high. It is difficult to know when the dose can be lowered again although, very occasionally, the epilepsy has a clear pattern as, for example, premenstrual incidence: in such cases treatment can be intermittent (Feely and Gibson 1985). After a period without seizures (generally considered a minimum of two years but longer where epilepsy has been severe or difficult to control) anticonvulsants should be slowly withdrawn over at least a 6-month period. During this time, and for some months afterwards, there is a risk of increased seizure frequency due to withdrawal rather than the return of

Table 18.2. Seizures and drugs of choice

Type of seizure	Drug	Optimal plasma concentration (μg/ml)
Tonic-clonic	Phenobarbitone	15–40
	Phenytoin	10–20
	Primidone	15–40
	Clonazepam	?usefulness
	Sodium valproate	50–100
Partial	Carbamazepine	4–10
Petit mal	Ethosuximide	40–80
	Clonazepam	?usefulness
	Sodium valproate	50–100

natural epilepsy. Withdrawal reactions other than seizures, including anxiety and insomnia, are found with phenobarbitone and the benzodiazepines but are not seen with phenytoin, carbamazepine and valproate (Duncan *et al.* 1988).

Management of status epilepticus

Status epilepticus is a seizure lasting more than 10 min or several distinct episodes without consciousness being regained. It is a highly dangerous condition and permanent brain damage may result if the patient survives. The longer the fits proceed the more difficult it is to control the condition. The patient must be turned to the lateral semi-prone position, false teeth removed if possible but nothing placed in the mouth. The standard treatment is 10 mg of diazepam intravenously with a further 10 mg in 2 mg boluses over the ensuing 30 seconds. Clonazepam and lorazepam are also very effective. Benzodiazepines need to be given with great care because they are irritant to vessel walls and may cause thrombophlebitis. Care must be taken not to cause respiratory depression, and differences in the kinetics of these drugs should be borne in mind with repeated doses. Admission to hospital is essential.

If fits continue, further diazepam (20 mg) can be given. When control has been obtained, phenytoin, 15 mg/kg in normal saline, should be infused at a rate not greater than 50 mg/minute. If control is not obtained after diazepam by bolus injection and phenytoin, chlormethiazole or paraldehyde or an infusion of diazepam can be tried (Brodie 1989). Intensive care management techniques will be needed.

Chronic patients with psychological disorders

High doses and polypharmacy can undoubtedly result in unacceptable levels of toxicity including behavioural problems (Reynolds 1975). Minor side-effects include drowsiness, dysarthria, ataxia and nausea, and phenytoin commonly causes hirsutism and gum hypertrophy. More serious effects include cerebellar degeneration, peripheral neuropathy, Dupuytren's contracture, benign lymphadenopathy, disseminated lupus erythematosus, osteomalacia, and megaloblastic anaemia.

The anticonvulsants interact with many other drugs. Phenytoin is highly bound to plasma albumin and can displace drugs such as tricyclic antidepressants. Most anticonvulsants are powerful inducers of hepatic microsomal enzymes and accelerate the metabolism of many substances including steroid hormones, oral anticoagulants and many psychotropic drugs. Metabolic interactions among the anticonvulsants are complex. Usually induction results in low levels of all the agents administered, but occasionally competition can produce high concentrations and toxicity.

For all these and many other reasons, the management of seizures and of psychological complications in epileptic patients can be a complex and difficult undertaking. Polypharmacy should be rationalized and minimized but this should be done slowly lest seizure frequency increases or even that status epilepticus is precipitated. In such patients, carbamazepine may prove to be the most useful single agent. Such rationalization should be combined with psychosocial measures aimed at establishing a sensible life-style with regular habits. Simple psychological support can sometimes have a dramatic effect on seizure frequency and allow reduced anticonvulsant dosage: this in turn sometimes produces a considerable change in personality, a mature, rational individual emerging from a mass of hypochondriacal complaints, irritability, dependence, and histrionic behaviour.

Anticonvulsants and Behaviour Disorder

The relationships between seizures, emotional disorder and personality are complex and it is often difficult to determine the source of any change. Whilst drugs sometimes cause emotional and personality problems, they may alleviate them. It is not too surprising that drugs with sedative actions ease anxiety and any depression and irritability arising from it, but some drugs, used primarily as anticonvulsants, have other psychotropic effects which have found clinical use in non-epileptic patients. For example, carbamazepine and sodium valproate are established in the treatment and prophylaxis of manic depressive psychosis (see Stromgren and Boller 1985 for review of controlled trials, and Chapter 10). Other anticonvulsants have been studied in psychiatric illness. For example, phenytoin has some beneficial effect on psychoneurotic symptoms (Stephens and Schaffer 1970) but it is ineffective in chronic schizophrenia (Simopoulos *et al.* 1974). Anticonvulsants are sometimes effective in patients, both epileptic and non-epileptic, where irritability and aggression are the major problem, especially where this is explosive or stands out against the customary behaviour of the individual (e.g. intermittent explosive disorder: DSM III). Phenytoin, carbamazepine and primidone have been reported to reduce such episodes, sometimes dramatically (see review by Mattes 1986). Anticonvulsants can also alleviate disturbed behaviour, especially aggression, in mentally subnormal people (Al-Kaisi and McGuire 1974; Reid *et al.* 1981). The psychotropic effects of anticonvulsants require further study. Such studies would be especially valuable if they found a therapeutic niche not covered by established drugs or helped behaviour problems outside the classical syndromes, as seems possible (Blumer *et al.* 1988). Aggressiveness arising within a well recognized psychiatric disorder, particularly a psychosis, is, of course, treated by the drugs mainly indicated for that disorder. It may be noted here that a number of drugs have been found helpful in managing aggression in the individual case: propranolol and lithium salts have received some attention. Aggression secondary to sexual arousal can in some cases be eased by oestrogens or antiandrogens.

The female reproductive role and psychotropic drugs

Premenstrual tension

Many women report the occurrence of a number of physical and psychological symptoms at certain phases of the menstrual cycle. Typically they occur in the luteal phase, 7–10 days before the start of menstruation, though many other patterns are seen and the range and the intensity of symptoms may vary in the same woman over time. Typical somatic symptoms include breast pain, increase in weight, abdominal distension, and headache. Psychological symptoms comprise tension, depression, anxiety, aggression and inability to concentrate. The incidence in women of childbearing age has been variously estimated as between 5 and 95 per cent, but the usually accepted figure is 40 per cent. The wide variation in incidence at least partly reflects the differences in definition and methods of elicitation of symptoms. To note some examples: at least 150 symptoms have been described in this syndrome, their periodicity tends to be exaggerated by women reporting retrospectively (Clare 1983) and the frequency of premenstrual symptoms is reduced considerably when the purpose of enquiry is disguised (Slade 1984). Studies of aetiology and treatment response are necessarily impeded by such problems of definition and detection and inevitably the subject is frequently reviewed (e.g. O'Brien 1987; Reid 1985; Rubinow and Roy-Byrne 1988), some being attempts at rational therapy based on hypothesized pathophysiology. Most have been poorly evaluated, mainly due to the absence of controls, a major defect in a condition with high placebo response rates. Psychotropic drugs which have been tried include the benzodiazepines, monoamine oxidase inhibitors, tricyclic antidepressants, and lithium carbonate: controlled trials, where available, show no consistent effects. Controlled studies do not support the effectiveness of progesterone but there is some, not uncontested, support for synthetic progestogens such as dydrogesterone. Pyridoxine probably has some effect, especially where depression is marked and some evidence supports its use in a dosage of 40 mg twice daily from day 14 of the cycle until menstruation (see Chapter 16). Bromocriptine, because of its effects on prolactin disposition, may be helpful in patients who complain of breast symptoms. In patients with weight gain and water retention diuretics may help, spironolactone being most appropriate, given in a dose of 100 mg commencing 3 days before the expected onset of symptoms. 'Loop' and thiazide diuretics are less desirable because of the problem of secondary aldosteronism and idiopathic oedema. There is no cure-all for premenstrual tension. Treatment should be tailored to the individual woman, her symptoms and their timing preferably documented prospectively by a diary started before treatment is instituted.

Postmenstrual oestrogen deficiency state

Physical and mental symptoms of middle and late life have, in both sexes, been attributed to endocrine changes, especially in women after the cessation of menstruation (Greenblatt *et al.* 1979). Much of the literature examining these matters suffers from the methodological deficiencies found in studies of premenstrual tension. Rigorous studies of symptomatology and treatment response indicate that few symptoms are truly menopausal and that only these respond to hormonal replacement. Hot flushes and night sweats are more common at the time of the menopause or shortly after it, minor psychological symptoms such as impaired concentration, anxiety, and lack of confidence occur a little earlier and some complaints, such as irritability, aching breasts and low back pain steadily decline in the years following the cessation of menstruation (Bungay *et al.* 1980). Treatment with oestrogens reduces flushes and sweating but has little effect on the other symptoms (Coope *et al.* 1975). Treatment with oestrogen reduces osteoporosis and loss of collagen from the skin, has some protective effect against cardiovascular disease, but may predispose to breast and endometrial cancer, although the latter can be reduced by the addition of sequential progestogen. The use of hormone replacement therapy is therefore controversial (Young and Goldzieher 1987) although women find it helpful and are likely to demand it (Hunt 1988). Psychological symptoms require other forms of management. Psychological support, such as may be provided at a menopause clinic, may be very effective; depressive symptoms may require treatment with antidepressant drugs. If hormonal preparations are not acceptable, the severity of flushes may be reduced by clonidine, propranolol or both.

Pregnancy and puerperium

This topic has been touched on in the various chapters on individual classes of drugs but is brought here under one heading because of its importance. The use of psychotropic drugs may be complicated by pregnancy in several different ways including the following:

(1) a woman maintained on prophylactic or maintenance treatment may wish to become pregnant;

(2) a woman previously well may develop a psychiatric illness during pregnancy;

(3) psychotropic drugs may be administered to a woman during labour;

(4) a nursing mother may develop a psychiatric illness and need medication.

At least 10 per cent of women attending antenatal classes will experience appreciable psychological distress, mainly anxiety. During the puerperium 0.2 per cent of mothers develop a psychotic illness, at least 10 per cent a depressive illness, and a further 16 per cent a self limiting depressive reaction which lasts upto a month and is qualitatively different from the 'birth time blues' (Loudon 1987).

Safety of psychotropic drugs and practical implications.

Antidepressants

Although occasional reports are received of congenital abnormalities associated with the use of tricyclic and MAOI antidepressants during pregnancy, no firm evidence is available to prove or disprove any teratogenic risk (Thiels 1987). Nevertheless, caution is advisable during the first trimester, i.e. the fact that the patient is pregnant should make the practitioner less ready to use drug treatments. Towards the end of the pregnancy, attempts should be made to lower the dose of antidepressant to lessen the likelihood of withdrawal reactions in the baby. Opinion is divided as to whether antidepressants reach the mother's milk in appreciable amounts. However, so little is known about the long-term effects of even small amounts of psychotropic drugs on the developing brain that it is wisest for women on psychotropic medication not to breast-feed (Robinson *et al.* 1986).

Lithium

This drug has excited the greatest concern. A register of all pregnant women exposed to lithium in at least the first trimester was set up: of 225 such pregnancies, 25 resulted in congenitally malformed babies (Weinstein 1980). Cardiovascular disorders, especially Epstein's anomaly (tricuspid valve malformation) are particularly common. A recent study has confirmed the risk at about 7 per cent (Kallen and Tandberg 1983).

Lithium concentrations fall during pregnancy due to increased renal clearance. After delivery, the clearance falls back to normal which may result in toxicity if the previous dose is not reduced. Lithium enters breast milk freely.

If a woman maintained on lithium wishes to become pregnant, and assuming no psychiatric contraindications, the lithium should be gradually withdrawn over 2–3 months and the patient monitored for signs of relapse. A patient who conceives while on lithium should stop the drug immediately. Any pregnancy which has continued for some time with the mother on lithium should be examined using ultrasound to exclude cardiac abnormalities. If lithium is essential, as in a severe manic-depressive illness, the dosage should be adjusted to maintain the serum concentration between 0.5 and 0.7 mmol/litre at 12 h after ingestion of the dose. When labour starts lithium should be stopped and reinstituted during the puerperium. Diuretics should be avoided. The mother should not breastfeed.

Antipsychotic drugs

There is no evidence that any of the subclasses of the antipsychotic drugs are teratogenic. Intoxication and withdrawal in the neonate are possible if high doses are given towards the end of pregnancy. Antipsychotic drugs do not usually pass into the breast milk in clinically important quantities.

In practical terms, antipsychotic drugs should be used in the minimally effective doses in pregnancy, especially towards the end. Breast feeding is best avoided.

Anxiolytics and hypnotics

The teratogenic potential of the benzodiazepines is unclear. Earlier, reports of greater use of benzodiazepines by the mothers of babies with defects of the palate were not confirmed. However, the report of abnormalities (see Chapter 12) must give rise to concern. Barbiturates may have similar properties.

Benzodiazepines accumulate in the fetus which can result in the 'floppy infant syndrome' on birth, characterized by hypotonia, hypothermia, depressed respiration, and poor suckling. A withdrawal syndrome may supervene. Benzodiazepines, being mainly highly lipophilic, are readily transferred into the maternal milk, so that accumulation can occur in the baby. This is possibly less of a problem with lorazepam and oxazepam which undergo conjugation rather than metabolism.

Benzodiazepines are best avoided in pregnancy so they should be withdrawn if a long term user wishes to become pregnant. However, the severely anxious woman may need continuing medication and the risks will have to be discussed. Lowering of dose should be attempted in late pregnancy but full withdrawal may be too upsetting a procedure psychologically and physiologically, to be attempted. Women taking benzodiazepines should not breast-feed.

Disorders of appetite

Many psychotropic drugs affect appetite (Silverstone 1983). Some antipsychotic drugs such as chlorpromazine or fluphenazine make patients feel very hungry and over a third of patients in one survey receiving regular depot injections were clinically obese. Antidepressant drugs increase appetite, over and above the improvement in mood. The exception is the group of selective 5-HT uptake inhibitor drugs such as fluvoxamine and fluoxetine, which are associated with decreased appetite and even loss of weight despite elevation of mood.

The amphetamines and related compounds lessen appetite and have been used extensively to help reduce weight. However, dependence is a real danger, the efficacy of these drugs tends to wane due to tolerance, and side effects of anxiety, tension and palpitations can be troublesome. Consequently, their use as appetite suppressants is not encouraged. Fenfluramine differs in not being stimulant. Dependence is rare, but abrupt withdrawal may be followed by depression.

A range of drugs has been used to treat patients with anorexia nervosa (Garfinkel and Garner 1987). Antidepressants are appropriate for the mood disorder which is a common problem, but lithium poses all sorts of toxicity problems in patients who severely restrict food and fluid intake, self-induce vomiting, and abuse laxatives or diuretics (Johnson *et al.* 1983). Antipsychotic drugs, especially chlorpromazine, have been advocated in treatment but controlled studies are lacking. Cyproheptadine, a serotonin antagonist, has been evaluated as a promoter of weight gain, but seems ineffective.

Drugs have also been used in bulimia nervosa. Antidepressants have been tried because many bulimics are depressed; indeed the depression may antedate the eating disorder, although in many cases the reverse obtains (Huon and Brown 1984). Most studies have found a favourable effect of tricyclic or MAOI antidepressants on bingeing behaviour. Selective 5-HT uptake inhibitors are particularly promising. It is not clear whether this is a direct therapeutic effect or whether it is secondary to the treatment of depression (Griffiths *et al.* 1987).

Drugs have a very limited role in the treatment of anorexia and bulimia nervosa which are helped more by psychological techniques, notably behavioural methods. Drugs may help at certain phases of these treatment programmes to sedate an overactive anorexic or to lessen intense craving in a bulimic but they can also impede treatment. For example, an anorexic patient resisting hunger in order to avoid exacerbating her perceived obesity will not be helped by a drug which increases appetite, causes carbohydrate craving, increases weight, and promotes water retention!

Anaesthesia and psychotropic drugs

An extensive review of this topic was presented by Janowsky and her colleagues (1981). As both anaesthetics and most drugs used in psychiatry act on the brain, interactions both additive and subtractive are to be expected. These interactions will be briefly listed with respect to each major class of psychotropic drug.

Antidepressants

The uptake-inhibiting and the anticholinergic properties of the tricyclic antidepressants (TCAs) are those most germane to interactions with anaesthetic agents. The pressor responses to directly acting sympathomimetic agents such as adrenalin, noradrenalin and phenylephrine are potentiated twofold to tenfold. Hyperthermia, sweating and hypertensive crises with severe headache and rupture of cerebral vessels can result. Adrenalin's arrhythmic effect on the heart may be markedly potentiated. Pre-operative administration of centrally active anticholinergic drugs may be additive with the TCA and cause postoperative confusion and delirium. Accordingly, it is advisable to stop all TCAs 2 weeks prior to surgery. If this is impossible, or surgery needed in an emergency, avoidance of directly-acting sympathomimetics is advisable. Treatment of hypertensive crises comprises sodium nitroprusside or an alpha-adrenoceptor antagonist. Severe anticholinergic effects can be treated with physostigmine.

The MAOIs produce a different pattern of interactions. Indirectly acting sympathomimetics like the amphetamines, methylphenidate, ephedrine and phenylpropanolamine are potentiated because they release large amounts of intraneuronal noradrenalin which cannot be metabolized because of the MAO insufficiency. Reserpine and L-dopa are also potentiated by MAOIs. Again, cessation of MAOI therapy 2–3 weeks prior to elective surgery is wise. If not possible, indirectly acting amines should be avoided.

The interaction of MAOIs with pethidine can cause agitation, hypertension, headache, rigidity, hyperpyrexia, and fits; this is possibly due to elevated 5-HT levels in the brain. A wide range of opioids, including pethidine, can interact to cause coma and respiratory depression. The mechanism in this case is inhibition by the MAOI of enzymes other than monamine oxidase resulting in impaired metabolism of the opioid and effectively, an overdose. Naloxone is indicated. If a patient on an MAOI requires an opioid analgesic, very cautious dosage, say a fifth of usual, is advisable initially, with careful observation of the patient thereafter. Pethidine, however, is best totally avoided.

MAOIs also potentiate barbiturates, and phenelzine (but not other MAOIs) lowers plasma cholinesterase levels thereby potentiating suxamethonium.

Lithium salts

Lithium also potentiates suxamethonium (but not D-tubocurarine) prolonging neuromuscular blockade. Stopping lithium treatment a week before elective surgery is a wise precaution.

Antipsychotic drugs

Like the TCAs antipsychotic drugs can alter the actions of sympathomimetic drugs. In this case, drugs such as chlorpromazine and thioridazine block the alpha effects producing vasodilatation and hypotension. Anticholinergic effects are also potentiated, especially in the elderly. Inhalation anaesthetics may be potentiated with an increased incidence of hypotension. The hypotensive effects of spinal or epidural block are also potentiated.

Narcotic analgesics are generally potentiated by antipsychotic medication although the mechanism is not clear. Cautious analgesic dosage is required to avoid respiratory depression and marked hypotension. Barbiturates and other sedative/hypnotics are also potentiated.

Sedative/hypnotic/tranquillizers

As a general rule, anaesthetic agents are potentiated by these drugs. In practice, however, tolerance may be quite marked, especially in the long-term user so that intravenous induction agents such as thiopentone sodium may need to be given in higher than usual dose. Alcoholics also show tolerance to intravenous induction agents.

References

Al-Kaisi, A.H., and McGuire, R.G. (1974). The effect of sulthiame on disturbed behaviour in mentally subnormal patients. *British Journal of Psychiatry* **124,** 45–49.

Azrin, N.H., Sisson, R.W., Meyers, R., and Godley, M. (1982). Alcoholism treatment by disulfiram and community reinforcement therapy. *Journal of Behaviour Therapy and Experimental Psychiatry* **13,** 105–12.

Blumer, D., Heilbronn, M., and Himmelhoch, J. (1988). Indications for carbamazepine in mental illness: atypical psychiatric disorder or temporal lobe syndrome? *Comprehensive Psychiatry* **29,** 108–22.

Borg, V. (1983). Bromocriptine in the prevention of alcohol abuse. *Acta Psychiatrica Scandinavica* **68,** 100–10.

Borg, V., and Weinholdt, T. (1982). Bromocriptine in the treatment of the alcohol-withdrawal syndrome. *Acta Psychiatrica Scandinavica* **65,** 101–11.

Brodie, M.J. (1989). Management of status epilepticus in adults. *Prescribers' Journal* **29,** 48–56.

Brown, L.M., Rowe, A.E., Ryle, P.R., Majumdar, S.K., Jones, D., Thomson, A.D., and Shaw, G.K. (1983). Efficacy of vitamin supplementation in chronic alcoholics undergoing detoxification. *Alcohol and Alcoholism* **18,** 157–66.

Bungay, G.T., Vessey, M.P., and McPherson, C.K. (1980). Study of symptoms in middle life with special reference to the menopause. *British Medical Journal* **281,** 181–3.

Chadwick, D., and Reynolds, E.H. (1985). When do epileptic patients need treatment? Starting and stopping medication. *British Medical Journal* **290,** 1885–88.

Charney, D.S., Riordan, C.E., Kleber, H.D., Murberg, M., Braverman, P.,

Sternberg, D.E., Heninger, G.R., and Redmond, D.E. (1982). Clonidine and naltrexone. A safe, effective, and rapid treatment of abrupt withdrawal from methadone therapy. *Archives of General Psychiatry* **39,** 1327–32.

Charney, D.S., Redmond, D.E., Galloway, M.P., Kleber, H.D., Heninger, G.R., Murberg, M., and Roth, R.H. (1984). Naltrexone-precipitated opiate withdrawal in methadone addicted human subjects: evidence for noradrenergic hyperactivity. *Life Sciences* **35,** 1263–72.

Ciraulo, D.A., Sands, B.F., and Shader, R.I. (1988). Critical review of liability for benzodiazepine abuse among alcoholics. *American Journal of Psychiatry* **145,** 1501–6.

Clare, A.W. (1983). Psychiatric and social aspects of premenstrual complaint. *Psychological Medicine (Monograph Supplement)* **4,** 1–58.

Collaborative Group for Epidemiology of Epilepsy (1986). Adverse reactions to anti-epileptic drugs: a multicentre survey of clinical practice. *Epilepsia* **27,** 323–330.

Committee on Safety of Medicines (1987). Fatal interaction between heminevrin (chlormethiazole) and alcohol. *Current Problems* **20,** 2.

Coope, J., Thomson, J.M., and Poller, L. (1975). Effects of 'natural oestrogen' replacement therapy on menopausal symptoms and blood clotting. *British Medical Journal* **4,** 139–43.

Duncan, J.S., Shorvon, S.D., and Trimble, M.R. (1988). Withdrawal symptoms from phenytoin, carbamazepine and sodium valproate. *Journal of Neurology, Neurosurgery and Psychiatry* **51,** 924–928.

Edwards, G., and Grant, M. (eds.) (1980). *Alcoholism treatment in transition.* Croom Helm, London.

Feely, M., and Gibson, J. (1985). Intermittent clobazam for catamenial epilepsy: avoid tolerance. *Journal of Neurology Neurosurgery and Psychiatry* **47,** 1279–82.

Fuller, R.K., Branchey, L., and Brightwell, D.R. (1986). Disulfiram treatment of alcoholism: a Veterans Administration cooperative study. *Journal of the American Medical Association* **256,** 1449–55.

Fuller, R.K., and Neiderhiser, D.H. (1981). Evaluation and application of a urinary diethylamine method to measure compliance with disulfiram therapy. *Journal of Studies in Alcohol* **42,** 202–6.

Fuller, R.K., and Roth, H.P. (1979). Disulfiram for the treatment of alcoholism: an evaluation in 128 men. *Annals of Internal Medicine* **90,** 901–4.

Garfinkel, P.E., and Garner, D.M. (eds.) (1987). *The role of drug treatments for eating disorders.* Brunner/Mazel, New York.

Gath, D., and Iles, S. (1988). Treating the premenstrual syndrome. *British Medical Journal* **297,** 237–38.

Gawin, F.H. *et al.* (1989). Desipramine facilitation of initial cocaine abstinence. *Archives of General Psychiatry* **46,** 117–21.

Gonzalez, J.P., and Brogden, R.N. (1988). Naltrexone. A review of its pharmacodynamic and pharmacokinetic properties and therapeutic efficacy in the management of opioid dependence. *Drugs* **35,** 192–213.

Goodridge, D.M.G., and Shorvon, S.D. (1983). Epileptic seizures in a population of 6000. *British Medical Journal* **287,** 641–647.

Greenblatt, R.B., Nezhat, C. Roesal, R.A., and Natrajan, P.K. (1979). Update on the male and female climacteric. *Journal of the American Geriatrics Society* **27,** 481–90.

Griffiths, R.A., Touyz, S.W., Mitchell, P.B., and Bacon, W. (1987). The treatment of bulimia nervosa. *Australia and New Zealand Journal of Psychiatry* **21,** 5–15.

Heather, N., and Robertson, I. (1985). *Problem drinking: The new approach.* Penguin Books, London.

Henderson, G., and McFadzean, I. (1985). Opioids—a review of recent developments. *Chemistry in Britain* Dec., 1094–7.

Hollister, L.E. (1986). Health aspects of cannabis. *Pharmacological Reviews* **38,** 1–21.

Hunt, K. (1988). Perceived value of treatment among a group of long-term users of hormone replacement therapy. *Journal of the Royal College of General Practitioners* **38,** 398–401.

Huon, G.F., and Brown, L.B. (1984). Bulimia: the emergence of a syndrome. *Australia and New Zealand Journal of Psychiatry* **18,** 113–26.

Janowsky, E.C., Risch, C., and Janowsky, D.S. (1981). Effects of anaesthesia on patients taking psychotropic drugs. *Journal of Clinical Psychopharmacology* **1,** 14–20.

Johnson, C., Stuckey, M., and Mitchell, J. (1983). Psychopharmacological treatment of anorexia nervosa and bulimia. Review and synthesis. *Journal of Nervous and Mental Disease* **171,** 524–34.

Kallen, B., and Tandberg, A. (1983). Lithium and pregnancy—a cohort study on manic-depressive women. *Acta Psychiatrica Scandinavica* **68,** 134–9.

Kleber, H.D. (1988). Cocaine abuse. *Journal of Clinical Psychiatry*, **49,** Suppl. 1–40.

Kramp, P., and Rafaelsen, O.J. (1978). Delirium tremens: a double-blind comparison of diazepam and barbital treatment. *Acta Psychiatrica Scandinavica* **58,** 174–90.

Lam, W., Sze, P.C., Sacks, H.S., and Chalmers, T.C. (1987). Meta-analysis of randomised controlled trials of nicotine chewing-gum. *Lancet* **2,** 27–30.

Loudon, J.B. (1987). Prescribing in pregnancy. Psychotropic drugs. *British Medical Journal* **294,** 167–9.

McInnes, G.T. (1987). Chlormethiazole and alcohol: a lethal cocktail. *British Medical Journal* **294,** 592.

Martin, W.R. (1984). Pharmacology of opioids. *Pharmacological Reviews* **35,** 283–304.

Mattes, J.A. (1986). Psychopharmacology of temper outbursts. A review. *Journal of Nervous and Mental Disease* **174,** 464–470.

Miller, W.C., and McCurdy, L. (1984). A double-blind comparison of the efficacy and safety of lorazepam and diazepam in the treatment of the acute alcohol withdrawal syndrome. *Clinical Therapeutics* **6,** 364–71.

Murray, J.B. (1986). An overview of cocaine use and abuse. *Psychological Reports* **59,** 243–64.

Norton, R., and Colliver, J. (1988). Prevalence and patterns of combined alcohol and marijuana use. *Journal of Studies on Alcohol* **49,** 378–80.

O'Brien, C.P., Childress, A.R., Arndt, I.O., McLellan, A.T., Woods, G.E., and Maany, I. (1988). Pharmacological and behavioural treatments of cocaine dependence: controlled studies. *Journal of Clinical Psychiatry* **42,** (Suppl), 17–22.

O'Brien, P.M.S. (1987). *Premenstrual syndrome.* Blackwell, Oxford.

O'Brien, P.M.S. (1985). The premenstrual syndrome. A review. *Journal of Reproductive Medicine* **30,** 113–26.

Peachey, J.E., and Naranjo, C.A. (1984). The role of drugs in the treatment of alcoholism. *Drugs* **27,** 171–82.

Peachey, J.E., O'Brien, J.F., Roach, C.A., and Loomis, C.W. (1981). A comparative review of the pharmacological and toxicological properties of disulfiram and calcium carbimide. *Journal of Clinical Pharmacology* **1,** 21–6.

Penick, E.C., Powell, B.J., Liskow, B.I., Jackson, J.O., and Nickel, E.J. (1988). The stability of co-existing psychiatric syndromes in alcoholic men after one year. *Quarterly Journal of Studies on Alcohol* **49,** 395–405.

Pollack, M.H., Brotman, A.W., and Rosenbaum, J.F. (1989). Cocaine abuse and treatment. *Comprehensive Psychiatry* **30,** 31–44.

Raw, M. (1985). Does nicotine chewing gum work? *British Medical Journal* **290,** 1231–2.

Reid, A.H., Naylor, G.J., and Kay, D.S.G. (1981). A double-blind, placebo controlled crossover trial of carbamazepine in overactive, severely mentally handicapped patients. *Psychological Medicine* **11,** 109–113.

Reid, R.L. (1985). *Premenstrual syndrome.* Year Book Medical Publishers, Chicago.

Reid, R.L. (1987). Premenstrual syndrome. *American Association for Clinical Chemistry* **5,** 1–12.

Reynolds, E.H. (1975). Chronic antiepileptic toxicity: a review. *Epilepsia* **16,** 319–52.

Reynolds, E.H. (1982). The pharmacological management of epilepsy associated with psychological disorders. *British Journal of Psychiatry* **141,** 549–57.

Ritson, B., and Chick, J. (1986). Comparison of two benzodiazepines in the treatment of alcohol withdrawal: effects on symptoms and cognitive recovery. *Drug and Alcohol Dependence* **18,** 329–34.

Robinson, G.E., Stewart, D.E., and Flak, E. (1986). The rational use of psychotropic drugs in pregnancy and postpartum. *Canadian Journal of Psychiatry* **31,** 183–90.

Rubinow, D.R., and Roy-Byrne, P. (1984). Premenstrual syndromes: overview from a methodological perspective. *American Journal of Psychiatry* **141,** 163–172.

Shorvon, S.D., and Reynolds, E.H. (1982). Early prognosis of epilepsy. *British Medical Journal* **285,** 1699–701.

Silverstone, T. (1983). The clinical pharmacology of appetite—its relevance to psychiatry. *Psychological Medicine* **13,** 251–3.

Simopoulos, A.M., Pinto, A., Uhlenhuth, E.A., McGee, J.J., and De Rosa, E.R. (1974). Diphenylhydantoin effectiveness in the treatment of chronic schizophrenics. *Archives of General Psychiatry* **30,** 106–11.

Slade, P. (1984). Premenstrual emotional changes in normal women: fact or fiction? *Journal of Psychosomatic Research* **8,** 1–7.

Smail, P., Stockwell, T., Canter, S., and Hodgson, R. (1984). Alcohol dependence and phobic anxiety states: a prevalence study. *British Journal of Psychiatry* **144,** 53–7.

Stephens, J.H., and Schaffer, J.W. (1970). A controlled study of the effects of diphenylhydantoin on anxiety, irritability and anger in neurotic outpatients. *Psychopharmacologia* **17,** 169–181.

Strassman, R.J. (1984). Adverse reactions to psychedelic drugs. A review of the literature. *Journal of Nervous and Mental Disease* **172,** 577–95.

Stromgren, L.S., and Boller, S. (1985). Carbamazepine in treatment and prophylaxis of manic-depressive disorder. *Psychiatric Developments* **4,** 349–367.

Thiels, C. (1987). Pharmacotherapy of psychiatric disorder in pregnancy and during breastfeeding: a review. *Pharmacopsychiatry* **20,** 133–46.

Wagman, A.M.I., and Allen, R.P. (1977). Effects of alcohol ingestion and abstinence on slow wave sleep of alcoholics. *Advances in Experimental Biology and Medicine* **59,** 453–66.

Weinstein, M.R. (1980). Lithium treatment of women during pregnancy and in the post delivery period. In: *Handbook of lithium therapy* (ed. F.N. Johnson) pp. 421–9. MTP Press, Lancaster.

Wilson, A., Blanchard, R., Davidson, W., McRae, L., and Maini, K. (1984). Disulfiram implantation: a dose response trial. *Journal of Clinical Psychiatry* **45,** 242–7.

Young, R.L., and Goldzieher, J.W. (1987). Current status of postmenopausal oestrogen therapy. *Drugs* **33,** 95–106.

19. Epilogue: changing perspectives

The modern era of psychopharmacology dates back to about 1950, the extant physical treatments such as ECT a decade further still. The intervening period has seen some increases in our understanding of the actions of these physical therapies and drugs although the crucial questions concerning them have not been answered. We still do not know how they effect clinical improvement. For example, how does inhibition of monoamine oxidase result in alleviation of panic attacks?

Much of this progress depends on the enormous strides which we have made in understanding brain function especially at the neuronal and even molecular level. But again, it has proved difficult to translate such insights into understanding the major psychiatric illnesses or their empirically developed treatments. We must remember with humility the extreme complexity of the human brain in terms of both structure and function. We must bear in mind that quite subtle changes in those structures or functions might result in profound abnormalities in emotional or cognitive behaviours. Our techniques, especially those applicable to man, still fall far short of the precision which is probably needed to uncover the abnormalities underlying most psychiatric disorders. Even in the severe dementias, the biochemical lesions appear quite complex, a possible exception being Huntington's chorea.

Innovation in psychopharmacology

It has been repeatedly emphasized in this book that practically all the physical therapies were discovered by chance. Even now, possible major developments generally come from unexpected quarters. For example, 5-HT_3 receptor antagonists were developed for their antiemetic potential. Studies in laboratory animals suggest that these compounds may have some antianxiety and antipsychotic potential (Editorial 1987). If this promise is fulfilled in man, yet another advance will owe a lot to serendipity.

Despite the complexities of the problems in developing new therapies, a mood of optimism pervades the world-wide pharmaceutical industry (Stahl 1987). Many large companies are continuing to devote substantial resources to developing new chemical entities for use in psychiatric disorders. Although some of this effort is uninspired (yet another benzodiazepine!) most companies are aware of the shortcomings of current therapies and concentrate their energies on novel approaches.

However, from time to time, an old drug is found to have a new use. An example is carbamazepine in the treatment of manic-depressive disorders. Another is the use of clonidine in the management of alcohol and opioid withdrawal. It is worth remembering that many drugs used to treat non-CNS conditions nevertheless have central effects. These effects are generally an unwanted nuisance but occasionally can be exploited therapeutically.

Although the greatest successes in discovering effective physical therapies have arisen by chance, research into developing new compounds tends to follow one of three paths. First, an existing compound can be taken as a starting point and its risk/benefit ratio improved. This is not the same as developing a 'me-too' compound, providing new chemical entities which possess only marginal advantages are discarded. Because of the haphazard way in which many drugs were discovered, they possess a range of unwanted effects due to accidental properties such as binding to cholinoceptors. For example, lofepramine is a derivative of imipramine in which the side chain has been extended so that affinity to cholinoceptors is low. The consequence is a worthwhile reduction in anticholinergic side effects in depressed patients treated with lofepramine rather than imipramine.

Second, a known biochemical or physiological function can be altered and the consequences studied for possible therapeutic uses. The classic example is the development of the beta-adrenoceptor antagonists. It was not clear which disorders such a drug might help, and the first of the series, propranolol, was found to have therapeutic indications such as the treatment of hypertension whose mechanism of action is still ill-understood. A variety of selective compounds are being developed which bind to specific receptors in the CNS and act as agonists or antagonists. Their therapeutic properties then have to be established empirically.

The third method is the most rational one. Research is carried out to identify the biochemical lesion associated with a psychiatric disorder and drugs are subsequently developed to rectify that abnormality. This approach has not yielded any successes in psychiatry although the use of L-dopa in the treatment of parkinsonism shows that this approach can be productive.

The empirical second approach, therefore, is the one most likely to have the greatest research effort focused upon it. Data accumulated over the past decade or so show a plethora of putative neurotransmitters, receptor types and enzymes in the CNS. A host of compounds could theoretically be developed to potentiate or antagonize these natural functions with varying degrees of selectivity. The effects, therapeutic and unwanted, are then sought in a range of psychiatric disorders.

Stahl (1987) has set out his 'wish list' of desired major advances needed into the next century. More efficacious and more rapidly acting antidepressants are required and perhaps the biochemical approach here is to find compounds which can down-regulate receptors more rapidly and more selectively than existing tricyclic and related antidepressants.

The antipsychotic drugs remain limited in their effectiveness and troublesome in their side effects. Although symptoms of overactivity ('positive symptoms') are usually effectively combatted, the decline in social functioning, cognitive performance and motivation ('negative features') is less susceptible to therapeutic intervention. The former symptoms may be associated with dopaminergic overactivity; the mechanism for negative symptoms remains unclear, but may reflect structural brain damage. A therapeutic breakthrough is urgently needed and focus away from the dopaminergic systems might facilitate such an advance.

With the sedative/hypnotic/tranquillizer drugs, dependence and abuse remain a drawback. It may be, however, that newer compounds acting on 5-HT pathways such as buspirone will prove to have low or even negligible dependence potential.

Totally new classes of drug are being proposed such as the 'serenics' to combat aggression (Olivier *et al.* 1986). Whether all of human experience is or should be susceptible to pharmacological manipulation remains a philosophical question.

But the greatest need remains to find treatments for the cognitive disorders such as Alzheimer's disease and senile dementia. Childhood autism and some forms of mental handicap may also be susceptible to drug intervention. As the population ages, the dementias loom larger and larger in terms of human suffering and the need to provide extensive resources for the care of these patients. This together with AIDS dementia affecting primarily younger people could strain to the limit the resources of even affluent countries.

Better use of existing drugs

This book has attempted to provide guidelines for the sensible and perhaps rational use of a wide variety of physical therapies, mainly drugs. Perspectives are changing with respect to our use of the currently available drugs. A few examples must suffice.

It is becoming increasingly usual for new drugs to be monitored after their release on the market. This monitoring can take several forms of which post-marketing surveillance seems most popular (Rawlins 1984). Various ways of identifying patients taking a particular drug are available, the starting point being the prescribing doctor, the dispensing chemist or the dispensed prescription. Several thousand patients are needed to establish the incidence of even quite common untoward effects. In view of the wide variety of such effects seen with psychotropic drugs, and the withdrawal of a few over the years, such monitoring is appropriate to many of these compounds, especially to new classes being introduced.

Drug treatments in psychiatry are often unnecessarily complex. With a difficult patient, another drug may be added without a previous one being discontinued. Eventually so many drugs are being given that it is impossible to ascribe any therapeutic benefit to any one drug. Although there may be some rationale for two-drug combinations (Rapp and Kaplan 1981), too often several drugs of the same type are given without a convincing reason. Surveys of prescribing practice have not been reassuring. In one for example, one-fifth of patients receiving long-acting depot neuroleptic injections also had oral preparations (Michel and Kolakowska 1981; Edwards and Kumar 1984) but the symptoms of the patients must also be taken into account (Morgan and Gopalaswamy 1984). Such audits should be followed by discussion of the more extreme examples of polypharmacy, with the hospital pharmacist or pharmacologist advising on ways of rationalizing the prescriptions.

Without such self-monitoring, prescribing policies may be imposed either locally or nationally. Drug formularies have been introduced in many general hospitals in attempts to cut costs (Petrie and Scott 1987) but such lists can also help to rationalize prescribing. National restrictions are also increasing in scope and number with limited lists of drugs being drawn up (Smith 1985). Although, again, the primary objective is cost-cutting, more rational prescribing can result as a by-product.

Thought must also be given to the wider consequences of drug treatments, both for medical practice and in a more general ecological sense. The widespread use of psychotropic drugs increases the work-load in acute medical services: for example parasuicide has been a major cause of acute medical admission for two decades. On the other hand, non-psychotropic drugs used against physical disease can cause behavioural disturbance. In a study of hospitals in three countries, of 26 000 intensely monitored patients 0.6 per cent were shown to have hallucinations, psychosis, and depression due directly to the drugs used during hospitalization (Danielson *et al.* 1981). Wider consequences are difficult to foresee and, to judge from the experiences of industry and agriculture, there is likely to be a delay before serious consequences are detected (consider the history of tardive dyskinesia and of benzodiazepine dependence). An instructive and well-studied example is provided by the contraceptive pill (Gunn 1987) associated as it is with physical and emotional morbidity in the user, with considerable impact on population changes, on the lives of women, ethical debate and social mores, not forgetting the occupational opportunities for lawyers, the cost of litigation now inhibiting research into a safer contraceptive pill! Drugs, including psychotropics, are now important agents in human society and are likely to remain so.

Conclusion

Physical treatments have maintained their popularity despite reservations over their efficacy, concern over their unwanted effects, and qualms over administering them to patients in whom informed consent may be incomplete. Most of these treatments have been rigorously evaluated, especially drugs introduced in the last 20 years. Although some have been used in a cavalier fashion at some times in some places by some doctors, most have been administered to patients with exemplary caution. However, indications often remain unclear and with many therapies it is difficult to predict the responders.

As a second issue, physical treatments provide an empirical basis upon which to attempt to build hypotheses concerning the pathogenesis of the conditions treated (Johnstone 1987). We should not, however, allow such hypotheses to dictate our treatments or perhaps even to influence unduly the directions which our future research efforts will take.

References

Danielson, D.A., Porter, J.B., Lawson, D.H., Soubrie, C., and Jick, H. (1981). Drug-associated psychiatric disturbances in medical inpatients. *Psychopharmacology* **74,** 105–8.

Editorial (1987). 5-HT_3 receptor antagonists: a new class of antiemetics. *Lancet* **1,** 1470–1.

Edwards, S., and Kumar, V. (1984). A survey of prescribing of psychotropic drugs in a Birmingham psychiatric hospital. *British Journal of Psychiatry* **145,** 502–7.

Gunn, A.D.G. (ed.) (1987). *Oral contraception in perspective. Thirty years of clinical experience with the pill.* Parthenon, Carnforth.

Johnstone, E.C. (1987). Physical treatments. *British Medical Bulletin* **43,** 689–703.

Michel, K., and Kolakowska, T. (1981). A survey of prescribing psychotropic drugs in two psychiatric hospitals. *British Journal of Psychiatry* **138,** 217–21.

Morgan, R., and Gopalaswamy, A.K. (1984). Psychotropic drugs: another survey of prescribing patterns. *British Journal of Psychiatry* **144,** 298–302.

Olivier, B., van Dalen, D., and Hartog, J. (1986). A new class of psychotropic drugs: Serenics. *Drugs of the future* **11,** 473–94.

Petrie, J.C., and Scott, A.K. (1987). Drug formularies in hospitals. *British Medical Journal* **294,** 919.

Rapp, M.S., and Kaplan, A. (1981). Polypsychopharmacy revisited. *Canadian Journal of Psychiatry* **26,** 569–73.

Rawlins, M.D. (1984). Postmarketing surveillance of adverse reactions to drugs. *British Medical Journal* **288,** 879–80.

Smith, T. (1985). Limited lists of drugs: lessons from abroad. *British Medical Journal* **290,** 532–4.

Stahl, S.M. (1987). Needs and opportunities for innovation in psychopharmacology. *Journal of the Royal Society of Medicine* **80,** 413–7.

Index